Headache

A Clinician's Guide to Diagnosis, Pathophysiology and Treatment Strategies

Edited by
Alan M. Rapoport, M.D.
and
Fred D. Sheftell, M.D.
New England Center for Headache
Stamford, Connecticut

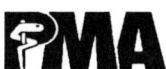

PMA Publishing Corp.
Costa Mesa, California

Copyright © 1993 by PMA Publishing Corp.
Distributed by SafetyLine/PMA
    4332 Cerritos Ave   Ste 100
    Los Alamitos, CA 90720
    (714) 220-6400

All rights reserved. This book is protected by copyright. No part of it may be reproduced, stored in a retrieval system or transmitted in any form or by any manner or means: electronic. electrostatic, magnetic tape, mechanical, photocopying, recording or otherwise, without written permission from the publisher.

NOTICE: The editors, contributors, and publisher of this work have made every effort to ensure that the drug dosage schedules and/or procedures are accurate and in accord with the standards accepted at the time of publication . Readers are cautioned, however, to check the product information sheet included in the package of each drug they plan to administer. This is particularly important in regard to new or infrequently used drugs. The publisher is not responsible for any errors of fact or omissions in this book.

Library of Congress Cataloging in Publication Data

Headache: a clinicians guide to diagnosis, pathophysiology, and treatment
   strategies / edited by Alan M. Rapoport and Fred D. Sheftell.
     p. cm.
   Includes bibliographical references and index.
   ISBN 1-56262-009-6
   1. Headache. I. Rapoport, Alan M., 1942-   . II. Sheftell, Fred D. , 1941-
    [DNLM: 1. Headache — diagnosis. 2. Headache — physiopathology.
   3. Headache — therapy.   WL 342 H43157 1993]
   RB128.H433   1993
   616.8'491 — dc20
   DNLM/DLC
   for Library of Congress   93-17688
                                                                                  CIP

Dedication

To Arja, TJ, Mark, and Sabrina:

Who have sacrificed some time with me so I could produce a quality work, thanks for your support and your love.

Alan

To Karen, Jason, and Lauren:

Thanks for your support, encouragement, and most of all …your love.

Fred

Contributors

Frances Arrowsmith, R.N., The New England Center for Headache, Stamford, CT

Steven M. Baskin, Ph.D., The New England Institute for Behavioral Medicine, Stamford, CT

Barry S. Baumel, M.D., Miami Beach, FL

Seymore Diamond, M.D., Director, Diamond Headache Clinic, Chicago, IL

Arthur H. Elkind, M.D., Director, Elkind Headache Center, Mt. Vernon, NY

Marek J. Gawel, M.D., Department of Neurology, Sunnybrook Medical Center, Toronto, Ontario, Canada

Amos D. Korczyn, M.D., Chairman, Department of Neurology, Ichilov Hospital, Tel Aviv, Israel

Lee Kudrow, M.D., Director, California Medical Clinic for Headache, Encino, CA

Ninan T. Mathew, M.D., Director, Houston Headache Clinic, Houston, TX

Stephen J. Peroutka, M.D., Ph.D., Associate Director, Clinical Reasearch Genentech, Inc., South San Francisco, CA

Alan M. Rapoport, M.D., Director, New England Center for Headache, Stamford, CT

Joel Saper, M.D., Director, Michigan Headache and Neurological Institute, Ann Arbor, MI

Fred D. Sheftell, M.D., Director, New England Center for Headache, Stamford, CT

Seymour Solomon, M.D., Director, Headache Unit, Montefiore Medical Center, Bronx, NY

Egilius L.H. Spierings, M.D., Director, Headache Section Division of Neurology, Brigham and Women's Hospital, Boston, MA

L. Jay Turkewitz, M.D., Midwest Center for Headpain Management, Piqua, OH

Randall E. Weeks, Ph.D., Clinical Psychology, The New England Institute for Behjavioral Medicine, Stamford, CT

Marcia Wilkinson, M.D., City of London Migraine Clinic, London, England

Contents

	Contributors	v
	Preface	ix
	Acknowledgements	x
1	The Pathophysiology of Head Pain *Alan M. Rapoport*	1
2	The Biochemistry of Migraine *Marek J. Gawel*	9
3	Serotonin Receptor Pharmacology in Migraine *Stephen J. Peroutka*	19
4	The Headache History *Steven M. Baskin*	25
5	The Neurological Examination *Larry S. Eisner & Barry Baumel*	35
6	Diagnostic Testing in Headache *Ninan T. Mathew*	43
7	Headache Physiology and the Pharmacology of Anti-Headache Medications *Egilius L.H. Spierings*	63
8	Migraine: Diagnosis, Pathogenesis, and Treatment *Egilius L.H. Spierings*	83
9	Tension-Type Headache *Seymour Diamond and Glen D. Solomon*	101
10	Cluster Headache: Diagnosis, Pathogenesis, and Treatment *Lee Kudrow*	111

11	Headache Due to Pain Sensitive Structures Within the Head *Seymour Solomon*	129
12	Miscellaneous Headache: More Unusual Types *Arthur H. Elkind and Mitchell S. Elkind*	139
13	Analgesic Rebound Headache *Alan M. Rapoport and Randall E. Weeks*	157
14	Ergotamine Dependency as a Cause for Refractory Recurring Migraine *Joel R. Saper*	167
15	Treatment of Chronic Daily Headache *Joel R. Saper*	175
16	Headaches in Children *Marcia Wilkinson*	185
17	Post-Traumatic Cephalalgia *Morris Levin and L. Jay Turkewitz*	197
18	Drug-Induced Headache *Amos D. Korczyn*	207
19	Behavioral Medicine Approach to Headache *Randall E. Weeks*	215
20	Psychological Considerations in Evaluation and Treatment of Headache Disorders *Fred D. Sheftell*	223
21	Ongoing Treatment Considerations in the Management of Headache Patients *Frances M. Arrowsmith*	235
22	A Comprehensive Approach to Headache Treatment *Alan M. Rapoport and Fred D. Sheftell*	243
23	The Inpatient Headache Treatment Unit *Alan M. Rapoport and Randall E. Weeks*	257
	Index	263

Preface

Several books have been written for physicians on the subject of headache, but none has been written by multiple international experts as a readable and practical book with appropriate references for the non-specialist. This book is designed especially for the physician, psychologist, nurse, or student who is treating or interested in learning about headache patients, but is not a headache specialist. This includes medical students and house officers in the fields of medicine, neurology, and psychiatry, as well as private practitioners and academicians.

We have attempted to discuss the major controversies in a straightforward and simplified form. The very question of where migraine originates, i.e., is it a cerebral dysfunction, or due to a change in blood vessels, or related to afferent nerve fibers and neurogenic inflammation, has been carefully discussed. The anatomy and physiology of migraine and other types of head pain have been reviewed. The latest information on serotonin receptors and the trigeminovascular system is presented. How to diagnose and treat standard and more difficult headache problems is detailed. Difficult treatment issues are discussed in the chapters on analgesic rebound headache, psychological considerations in headache, ongoing treatment considerations, behavioral medicine and headache, and post-traumatic cephalgia.

Acknowledgements

We thank the contributors, our publisher, and the hard work and tireless efforts of Pat Bushie, Grey Walklin, Elissa Migliaccio, and Karen Krane, without whom there would be no manuscript.

1

The Pathophysiology of "Vascular" Head Pain

Alan M. Rapoport

The pathophysiology of "vascular" head pain is as controversial today as it was when the pioneers of this century, such as Harold Wolff and Wilder Penfield, studied it over 40 years ago. For many years, throbbing headaches were presumed to arise from a disturbance in cephalic blood vessels. This was deduced from the observations that strokes, aneurysms, and arteriovenous malformations all produced headaches similar to migraine and clinical research indicated that blood vessels were the only structures within the cranium that, when stimulated, could cause pain resembling vascular head pain. In the first half of this century, investigators concentrated on mapping the pain-sensitive structures within the human cranium. The mechanical and electrical stimulation studies by Penfield in 1932 and Ray and Wolff in 1940 established the importance of the cerebral coverings, the dura and pia mater, as possible causes of headache [1]. The trigeminal nerve was identified as the major afferent pathway transmitting pain messages from the dura mater to the brain stem.

In 1938, Graham and Wolff demonstrated that the pulse amplitude of the superficial temporal artery increased during the headache phase of migraine, and that these increases could be abolished by ergotamine. Their conclusion was that the pain was caused by a stretching of the nerves in the walls of the distended arteries, and that the ergotamine was working as a vasoconstrictor. It was felt that the extracranial cephalic vessels were the most likely source of the pain. Although there has been limited supporting evidence over the years, this explanation of the cause of head pain and the rationale for the use of ergotamine has been widely accepted. Many studies on cerebral blood flow, including recent studies using xenon flow and single photon emission tomography, have not shown any direct correlation between vasodilation and head pain. Other scientific developments that have shaped migraine pain research include techniques to measure blood vessel contractility in vitro, the ability to measure levels of circulating hormones and biogenic amines, and the ability to assess platelet function.

In 1979, Moskowitz published a hypothesis that provided direction for his research in the last thirteen years and followed the leads provided by neuroscientists in the first half of this century [2]. He pointed out that the circumscribed unilateral headaches and pain referral to the cutaneous receptive field of the first trigeminal division suggested an important role for the trigeminal nerve in pain transmission and possibly in blood flow. He also suggested that the circle of Willis and its tributaries might be the primary source of pain because migraine headaches follow a disturbance in brain metabolism and flow (the aura), and may be reminiscent of the headaches observed with cerebrovascular occlusions, ruptured arteriovenous malformations, or aneurysms. He suggested that pial fibers were of trigeminal origin, and he postulated that perivascular fibers contained vasoactive neuropeptides such as substance P. The release of this chemical into the vessel wall could increase blood flow and vascular permeability causing pain, not by vasodilation, but by excitation of afferent nerve fibers.

This neural system, which is a final common pain pathway interrelating the brain stem with the cerebral blood vessels, has been termed the trigeminovascular system (see Fig. 1.1). Several mechanisms that are potential modulators of this system include biochemical (bradykinin, serotonin, histamine, progesterone, estrogen), mechanical (severe stretch), immunological (allergies), ionic (potassium), and neural (sympathetics and opiate-containing fibers). Although the exact cause of the vascular pain is still not clear, it seems to be mediated by a neural pathway that can be stimulated by multiple triggers, each of which activate (depolarize) perivascular sensory axons that are peripheral terminations of fifth nerve sensory afferents.

Most anatomical and biochemical studies have been performed on animals, not man. Axonal tracing studies of Mayberg revealed that most trigeminal fibers arise from ganglion cells within the first division of the semilunar (5th nerve) ganglion. These cells send widely ramifying axonal processes to innervate one or more ipsilateral large vessels of the circle of Willis. Trigeminal fibers are distributed to the anterior, middle, and posterior cerebral arteries, the anterior and posterior communicating arteries, and the rostral basilar and superior cerebellar arteries, all on the same side. Fibers also cross to innervate the contralateral anterior cerebral artery. Such an organization may explain the

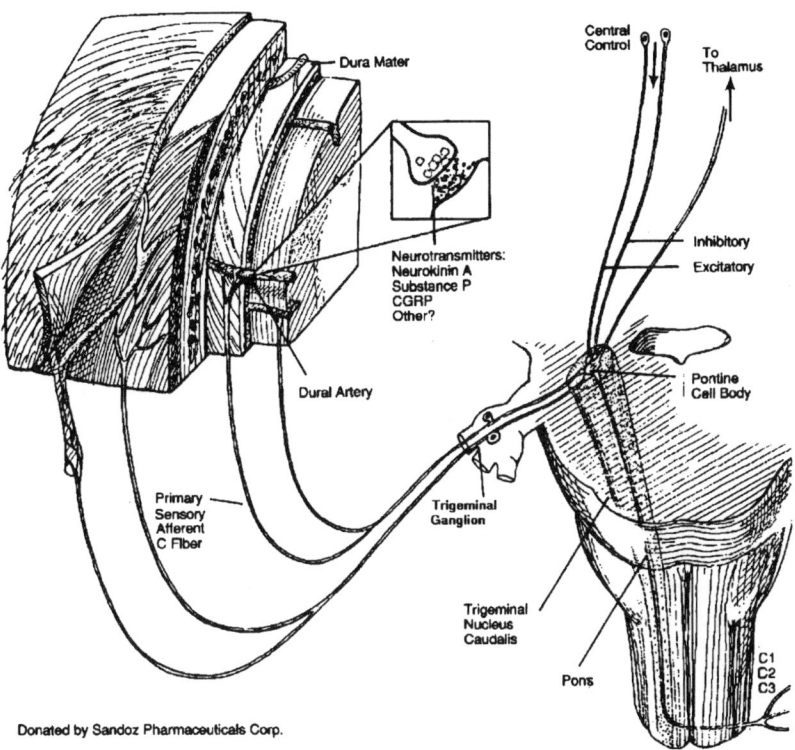

Figure 1.1 Diagram of the trigeminovascular system.

strictly unilateral distribution of many vascular headaches, the diffuse quality of the pain, and the difficulties in distinguishing between the pain patterns produced by each of the vessels. Some ganglion cells project divergent axon collaterals to innervate both the middle meningeal and middle cerebral arteries, according to O'Connor and van der Kooy. This explains the difficulties distinguishing between pain of pial and dural origin.

Dural vessels also receive rich trigeminal and upper cervical projections. Mayberg found that the middle meningeal artery is innervated by the ipsilateral trigeminal ganglia, primarily from cells within the first division [3]. He also found that the superior sagittal sinus receives a bilateral innervation, a finding that agrees with other reports in humans. The anterior cerebral artery also may receive a bilateral innervation. The first and second trigeminal divisions innervate the dura within the anterior fossa, the second and third divisions project to the middle cranial fossa, whereas upper cervical nerves (human and cat) as well as vagus and trigeminal nerves (cat) innervate dural structures within the posterior fossa.

Clinical Anatomical Correlations

The origin and distribution of perivascular afferent fibers suggest several of the following unique explanations for vascular headache patterns experienced by man:

- The predominantly ipsilateral distribution of trigeminal fibers explains the strictly unilateral distribution of many vascular headaches.
- The bilateral innervation of certain vessels (anterior cerebral artery and superior sagittal sinus) suggest the possibility that disturbances within the cranium produce bilateral headaches. Previous interpretations emphasize blood or some circulating nociceptor. The discovery of the dual innervation provides at least one alternative to this possibility. Theoretically, a vessel that is bilaterally innervated could also cause a contralateral headache, perhaps an explanation for the rare wrong-sided headache of migraine with aura.
- The trigeminal innervation of the superior cerebellar artery provides an explanation for the frontal headache experienced by patients with cerebellar tumors.
- The dual innervation of the superior cerebellar as well as the rostral basilar arteries (i.e., from upper cervical dorsal roots and trigeminal fibers) provides an anatomical explanation for the coexistence of occipital and frontal headaches, a second alternative to the convergence of descending trigeminal impulses with inputs from upper cervical cord segments.
- The observation that some dural and pial arteries receive divergent axon collaterals from single trigeminal neurons may account for the difficulty in distinguishing the source of pain in vascular headaches. The same sensory ganglia cell would discharge with appropriate stimulation in both circulations.

Only one study has traced the brain stem terminations of trigeminovascular fibers innervating cephalic blood vessels. Arbab showed that trigeminal ganglion cells projecting to the middle cerebral artery terminate within the trigeminal nuclear complex, the nucleus tractus solitarius, dorsal motor nucleus of the vagus, and C_2 dorsal horn. Cells projecting to the basilar artery terminate within the C_2 dorsal horn, nucleus tractus solitarius and dorsal motor nucleus of the vagus. Those cells projecting to the trigeminal nuclear complex are likely to mediate pain. Fibers terminating within the nucleus tractus solitarius may mediate arterial blood pressure responses induced by trigeminal activation and perhaps, autonomic disturbances during headache.

Careful anatomical dissections of the cavernous sinus in monkeys by Ruskell and Simons provide new anatomical data that may be relevant to migraine and cluster headache [4]. Within the sinus, ophthalmic branches join a plexus (cavernous plexus) composed of sympathetic and parasympathetic fibers. From this plexus, fibers from all three sources distribute to the internal carotid artery and the rostral basilar artery and caudal circle of Willis. In addition, this plexus receives a few recurrent axons that arise from the orbitociliary nerve (a branch of the maxillary nerve) within the sphenopalatine fossa. These recurrent axons join the cavernous plexus after reentering the cranium via the infraorbital foramen. Hence, the cavernous sinus provides an interesting confluence of venous blood, sympathetic, parasympathetic as well as sensory fibers, and the carotid artery. The afferents are derived from sensory nerves, some of which innervate the forehead and cheek. The sympathetics innervate the forehead, pupil and eyelid, and the parasympathetic fibers arise from the sphenopalatine ganglia that control lacrimation and nasal discharge. Thus, the typical constellation of symptoms and signs of cluster headache may be explained by a small pathophysiological focus located in the superior pericarotid cavernous sinus plexus. In this plexus can be found fibers from: the ophthalmic trigeminal division, the maxillary trigeminal division (a small branch of the orbitociliary nerve), the superior cervical ganglion controlling pupil and lid function, and the sphenopalatine ganglion. The typical signs of cluster headache are conjunctival injection, lacrimation, nasal congestion, rhinorrhea, forehead and facial sweating, miosis, ptosis, and eyelid edema. Pain is often referred to the first, and sometimes the second, trigeminal division, and forehead sweating is preserved.

Neuropeptides and the Trigeminal Vascular System

To date, five putative neurotransmitters have been identified within the nerve fibers comprising the trigeminovascular system. The tachykinin substance P was shown first by immunohistochemistry following trigeminal sectioning. The others include cholecystokinin-8, calcitonin gene-related peptide, galanin, and neurokinin A.

Substance P is composed of eleven amino acids and was first identified in 1931 by von Euler, and later proposed as a neurotransmitter in primary sensory neurons by Lembeck. It was isolated, sequenced and chemically synthesized in the 1970s. It is present in 10% to 15% of primary sensory neurons, including trigeminal ganglion cells. After synthesis in cell bodies, substance P is transported in both retrograde and anterograde directions to peripheral and central axons, respectively. Seventy-five percent of the newly synthesized transmitter is found in afferent processes. In the periphery, substance P is contained within unmyelinated C fibers or poorly myelinated A delta fibers. In spinal cord, substance P-containing fibers are concentrated in the dorsal horn. Release from within the spinal cord has been demonstrated with potassium-induced depolarization in a calcium-dependent manner or by electrical stimulation. Morphine and related opioid analgesics inhibit potassium-induced release of substance P from the trigeminal nucleus and from dorsal root ganglia cells grown in culture. This may be the mechanism by which opiates exert their therapeutic effectiveness at the spinal level.

Jansco found that injection of capsaicin, the pungent ingredient in Hungarian and chili peppers, causes activation of unmyelinated fibers, especially those that respond to chemical irritants, and induces substance P release. Tissue levels of substance P decrease and remain low for days to weeks or permanently in the case of neonates after exposure to capsaicin. Somatostatin, like the opiates, inhibits the release of substance P from afferent fibers.

Substance P is a mediator of vasodilation and plasma protein extravasation when injected intravenously or when released from perivascular axons following electrical or chemical stimulation of sensory fibers [5]. It also has potent effects on circulating cells involved in the inflammatory response. It degranulates mast cells, thereby promoting histamine release, and it stimulates phagocytosis by human polymorphonuclear leukocytes. Both dilation and extravasation are prevented by desensitization with capsaicin or by the administration of substance P antagonists such as somatostatin or enkephalin analogs.

Possible Relationships between Findings in the Trigeminovascular System in Animals and Vascular Headaches in Humans

The established relationship between the large cerebral arteries and the trigeminal nerve in the cat could explain some poorly understood clinical aspects of migraine headaches in humans. Specifically:
- It could provide an anatomical basis for the unilateral distribution of vascular headaches.
- It might explain why pain is referred to trigeminal receptive fields when pain is preceded by a visual aura or symptoms of posterior circulation dysfunction (because the posterior cerebral, superior cerebellar, and upper basilar arteries are innervated by the first trigeminal division).
- It would diminish the potential significance of blood flow in headache pathogenesis and emphasize the perivascular sensory innervation.
- It might suggest that the trigeminal nerve or the central nervous system, via the trigeminal nerve, can provoke unilateral vascular headaches.
- It would challenge the concept that the pain of vascular headache is due to dilating blood vessels. Dilation, which can be painful and sometimes accompanies headache, is probably not the cause of pain, but the result of depolarization-induced release of vasodilating substances such as substance P from sensory fibers.
- It could emphasize the importance of nociceptive afferents in vascular inflammation, and suggests their importance in other inflammatory conditions affecting cerebral arteries.
- It could suggest at least one rational approach to the prophylaxis and treatment of vascular headaches and certain inflammatory conditions (e.g., the development of substance P-receptor blocking drugs).

The concept of a neurogenically induced substance that is released from sensory nerve endings during the headache phase of migraine is not new. In 1960, Chapman found a polypeptide in fluid aspirated from tender regions of the head during the headache phase of migraine. The compound exhibited features similar to those of substance P and bradykinin and was termed neurokinin. These experiments have not been repeated using recent techniques.

The Effects of Antimigraine Drugs

Recently, the ability of ergot alkaloids to block neurogenic plasma extravasation in the rat dura mater was reported by Markowitz [6]. A single injection of ergotamine or dihydroergotamine, or chronic administration of methysergide blocked neurogenic inflammation (local vasodilation and plasma extravasation) in dura mater induced either by trigeminal electrical stimulation or by capsaicin. The conclusion from these findings was that ergots decrease neurogenic plasma extravasation by a C fiber-dependent mechanism, perhaps by blocking tachykinin release from perivascular fibers. Hence, an action of the ergots on sensory transmission has been suggested.

Nonsteroidal anti-inflammatory drugs block neurogenic inflammation in the dura mater as well. Drugs such as aspirin, indomethacin, and corticosteroids are useful in treating migraine, and indomethacin and corticosteroids have been helpful in cluster headache. The ability of ergots and the anti-inflammatory drugs to block this response in the coverings of the brain suggest that neurogenic inflammation is relevant to headache pathophysiology.

The experimental drug sumatriptan, which should be marketed in the U.S. as Imitrex in 1992, is a 5-HT_{1D} agonist and appears to work quickly, effectively and with few side effects to stop an acute migraine attack. Drs. Buzzi and Moskowitz showed that its effect may be attributed to its neurogenic mechanisms and its reaction with the trigeminovascular system [7]. When injected I.V. into rats, it inhibited the extravasation of labeled albumin from blood vessels. A similar effect was shown with guinea pigs when administered fifteen minutes before electrical stimulation of the trigeminal nerve and ten minutes before diffuse capsaicin stimulation. It did not block plasma extravasation in extracranial tissues or following the administration of serotonin, substance P or neurokinin A. So, it seems to be specific for neurogenic inflammation.

In the spring of 1991, Moskowitz presented a paper suggesting that sumatriptan and ergot alkaloids treat migraine by working on prejunctional 5-HT_{1D} receptors on unmyelinated C fibers, not by their vasoconstrictive effects [8]. He found that dihydro-ergotamine mesylate (D.H.E. 45) and sumatriptan (Imitrex) prevented the release of substance P (SP), calcitonin gene related peptide (CGRP), and neurokinin A from unmyelinated C fibers after electrical stimulation. Increased levels of CGRP were found in the sagittal sinus during electrical stimulation. D.H.E. 45 attenuated those levels. He also found that these drugs block platelet accumulation, endothelial vesicle and edema formation within postcapillary venules, and mast cell degranulation.

Another important and related action of these drugs is to block neural transmission within trigeminovascular neurons [9]. Following noxious stimulation of the meninges caused by injecting blood into the subarachnoid space, these drugs blocked expression of cellular activation within neurons of the trigeminal nucleus caudalis. Because blood in the subarachnoid space can cause severe headache and is associated with intense vasoconstriction, the data suggests that constriction of dilated vessels is not the relevant prerequisite for 5-HT_1-induced analgesia in vascular headaches.

Buzzi et al recently suggested that the 5-HT$_1$ receptor subtype mediating contraction of vascular smooth muscle may not be identical to the receptor which blocks neural transmission within trigeminovascular neurons [10].

Therefore, according to Moskowitz, it may be possible in the future to dissociate the two effects and to develop drugs which possess only the analgesic effects [9].

In summary, vascular headaches are among the most prevalent, yet poorly understood problems in clinical neurology. Cephalic blood vessels (pial and dural) are implicated as the most important source for all headaches and are innervated by sensory fibers that arise from ganglia also innervating the forehead, scalp, and neck. Trigeminal sensory fibers contain vasoactive neuropeptides that are released from peripheral (perivascular) and central terminations to mediate vasodilation and pain, respectively. The presence of vascular headache implies activation of this final common pain pathway that has been termed the trigeminovascular system (see Fig. 1.1). The existence of such a system clarifies certain pain patterns that develop following stimulation of cephalic blood vessels, suggests a mechanism to explain the referral of pain to the forehead, provides a mechanism to explain the action of certain antimigraine drugs, and suggests a local mechanism that enhances blood flow under certain pathological conditions.

References

1. Ray BS, Wolff HG. Experimental studies on headache: Pain sensitive structures of the head and their significance in headache. *Arch Surg 41*: 813-856, 1940.
2. Moskowitz MA, Reinhard JF Jr, Romero J, et al. Neurotransmitters and the fifth cranial nerve: Is there a relationship to the headache phase of migraine? *Lancet 2*: 883-885, 1979.
3. Mayberg MR, Langer RS, Zervas NT, et al. Perivascular meningeal projections from cat trigeminal ganglia: Possible pathway for vascular headache in man. *Science 213*: 228-230, 1981.
4. Ruskell GL, Simons T. Trigeminal nerve pathways to the cerebral arteries in monkeys. *J Anat 155*: 23-37, 1987.
5. Norregaard TV, Moskowitz MA. Substance P and the sensory innervation of intracranial and extracranial feline cephalic arteries: Implications for vascular pain mechanisms in pain. *Brain 108*: 517-533, 1985.
6. Saito K, Markowitz S, Moskowitz MA. Ergot alkaloids block neurogenic extravasation in dura mater: Proposed action in vascular headaches. *Ann Neurol 24*: 732-737, 1988.
7. Buzzi MG, Moskowitz MA. The antimigraine drug, sumatriptan (GR43175), selectively blocks neurogenic plasma extravasation from blood vessels in dura mater. *Br J Pharmacol 99*: 202-206, 1990.
8. Moskowitz MA, Buzzi MG, Theoharides TC, et al. Evidence that serotonin receptors on trigeminovascular axons mediate the anti-migraine effects of ergot alkaloids and sumatriptan. *Neurology 41 suppl 1*: 164, 1991.
9. Moskowitz MA. Interpreting changes in vessel diameter in vascular headaches. *Cephalalgia 12*: 5-7, 1992.
10. Buzzi MG, Moskowitz MA, Peroutka SJ, et al. Further characterization of the putative 5-HT receptor which mediates blockade of neurogenic plasma extravasatoin in rat dura mater. *Br. J. Pharmacol. 103*: 1421-1428, 1991.

2

The Biochemistry of Migraine

M.J. Gawel

Migraine is a complex disorder comprised of various symptoms and physical changes. It is also a paroxysmal disorder, and most patients are apparently symptom free during the interictal period. The thresholds for developing a migraine attack are likewise variable. On some days some patients may be able to consume wine and cheese with impunity while on other days the slightest indiscretion will spark off a headache.

Approaches to studying the biochemistry of migraine have largely revolved around finding an abnormality or deviation in the activity or level of serum factors during or between attacks and comparing these to non-migrainous controls. More recently, attention has focused on the state and activity of receptors in vivo and in vitro.

Historical Perspectives

It has been known since the time of Wolff that there are changes in the cephalic circulation during the migraine attack [1]. Intracranial vasoconstriction caused the "ischemic" aura, and extracranial vasodilation caused the pain. Heyck's concept of shunts in the cutaneous circulation conveniently explained the pallor that patients often exhibit [2]. A decreased pain threshold in migraineurs helped explain why the dilated arteries were painful, while arteries dilated by heat were not. Chapman's experiments with subcutaneous perfusates of tender and aching regions of the head demonstrated a "neurotensin" that caused painful reactions when injected subcutaneously [3]. They could not characterize this substance but were able to distinguish it from acetylcholine, histamine, bradykinin, etc.

The aura has always been a source of controversy. There have been proponents for an ischemic etiology and those for a dysrhythmic or neuronal etiology. The march of the "classical migraine" visual aura with its positive phenomena suggests some form of electrical disturbance. Demonstrated low cerebral blood flow and biochemical changes in the cerebrospinal fluid (CSF) compatible with ischemia following a migraine attack suggest a vasospastic origin that results in cerebral ischemia. Controversy still rages despite Olesen's demonstration of a wave of occipitally generated spreading oligemia in classical migraine suggestive of a neuronal etiology [4].

Are migraineurs more sensitive? There is evidence to suggest that they react differently to dopaminergic stimulation. Both dopamine agonists piribedil and bromocriptine mesylate (Parlodel) cause marked reductions in blood pressure in migraineurs but not in controls [5-7]. Many clinicians will testify that migraineurs will develop terrible side effects from minute doses of prophylactic medication while ingesting enough opiates to kill the clinician. This latter observation is reflected in the school of thought that strives to explain migraine on the basis of an opiate withdrawal model. The patients have low central opiate levels and develop a headache and nausea (withdrawal) [8]. This chapter will be devoted to examining salient evidence presented for these hypotheses or suppositions.

The Interictal State

There have been many efforts to demonstrate a biochemical defect or difference in migraine subjects and controls. These studies center about both peripheral and central systems. Platelet monoaminoxidase b (MAOb) is lower in migraine subjects than in controls [9]. Plasma phenylsulphatransferase is lower in some migraine subjects [10]. Beta endorphin has been found to be lower in patients with classical migraine, but not in those with common migraine [11]. Plasma dopamine -hydroxylase activity is elevated in migraine subjects [12]. Enkephalinase is lower in migraine patients during migraine-free periods [13]. None of these differences have been of clinical significance, but taken as a whole they may point to a slight difference in biochemical responsiveness in migraine patients compared to non-migraineurs. It is difficult to interpret many of these studies appropriately because classification of the patients varies so much and there is often little record of other medications that the patients may be taking. Many of these changes, for instance the finding of low MAOb in patients with migraine, or the finding of increased cortisol production in these patients, are also found in certain patients with depression and other psychiatric disorders.

The response of the patients to various stimuli is taken as a means of assessing central processes. For instance, the pupil of a migraineur responds differently to pharmacological manipulation, suggesting sympathetic denervation. Dopamine agonists such as piribedil and bromocriptine mesylate (Parlodel) exert a profound hypotensive effect in migraine patients differentiating them from controls and so called "tension headache" [5]. Patients with migraine have been found to be more sensitive to the pressor effect of tyramine [14]. Peripheral veins of migraineurs showed greater reactivity to catecholamines and serotonin [15]. Patients with migraine are more sensitive to the hallucinogenic actions of LSD [16]. All these findings fit into an overall suggestion of central diminution in 5 hydroxytryptamine (5-HT) and opiates resulting in a hyperresponsiveness of the sensory system [17]. This view is supported by the electrophysiological findings of increased amplitude in the visual and auditory evoked potentials and increased negativity of the contingent negative variation (CNV) in migraine patients [18,19]. Do people with migraine really go about in a state of sensory nudity? Clinically, there seems to be some support for such a concept.

Does this occur all the time? There is certainly some evidence that there are fluctuations in the tendency to have migraine. It is possible that these minor biochemical variations are also cyclical.

The Migraine Attack

Prior to the attack, various changes begin to unfold. It is difficult to produce a synthesis of these and probably many are nonspecific, arising as a result of stress rather than as part of the migraine attack. The precipitants of migraine are extremely varied yet probably act finally through the sympathetic nervous system. Historically, the release of 5-HT from platelets is said to be the first event. This is then excreted rapidly as homovanillic acid (HVA). The role of this 5-HT is unclear and the relevance of its release uncertain. Is it released from platelets mirroring a neuronal release or is it the release reaction to platelet activation, and is this merely a normal sequel to sympathetic stimulation? Hsu and colleagues have demonstrated a nocturnal rise in catecholamines on those nights in which the patients wake with a headache [20]. Anthony has described an increase in free fatty acid concentration prior to an attack [21]. Sympathetic stimulation produces an increase in free fatty acids and many of the changes found in the migraine attack. Similar changes have been observed following an infusion of norepinephrine.

Recent work by Moskowitz has highlighted the importance of the trigeminal vascular innervation of the intracranial blood vessels [22]. Fibers of the noradrenergic locus ceruleus project to all the blood vessels. It is possible that the control of the vascular changes during the attack is mediated by activation of the locus ceruleus, as postulated by Lance [23]. The pain is appreciated via the fibers of the first division of the fifth cranial nerve. The spinal nucleus of the fifth nerve has inputs from the second and third cervical sensory roots. Thus, pain may arise in the neck and be referred to behind the eye and vice versa. Local factors released into the areas of pain and associated with swelling may be prostaglandins and kinins, as originally postulated by Wolff.

Platelets are involved in the attack. It appears, taking all the experiments and methodologies together, that they are more active between attacks, they aggregate at the beginning of the attack, and become refractory to aggregation later into the attack and after the attack. Whether these changes are secondary to sympathetic stimulation or represent a primary platelet disorder is still controversial. The observation that migraine in patients with thrombocytopenia can be helped by splenectomy lends some strong circumstantial support to the latter hypothesis.

Serotonin appears to be released by a factor in the plasma that is involved in the platelet release reaction.

Platelet MAOb is further decreased during the attack, a decrease not explained by changes in platelet population. Angiotensin converting enzyme activity becomes elevated at this stage. In some studies there is, at this stage, an increase in endorphin levels.

Sicuteri and colleagues suggest that the migraine attack has parallels with opiate withdrawal [25]. He discusses the similarities in symptoms between the two. In actual fact, there are great differences. Nevertheless, the idea does have some attraction since it proposes a synthesis and a centralized hypothesis. In migraine, there is a reduction in serotonergic and endorphinergic tone resulting in a failure of modulation of sensory input. This results in an overactive sympathetic activity that occurs in the background of a peripheral denervation hypersensitivity. The presence of this hypersensitivity is evidenced by work on the pupil by Fanciullacci and by Sicuteri's experiments using venous response to a variety of catecholamines [15,26].

The nausea and vomiting that occur during the attack may be mediated by the action of serotonin or dopamine on the area postrema in the floor of the 4th ventricle in the medulla, a vomiting center in many animals.

The prodrome, or the aura, and the neurological manifestations that may occur are more difficult to explain or correlate with biochemistry. If one accepts the vascular ischemic hypothesis of these changes, then the action on the blood vessel innervation by the platelets' release products could cause local hypoxia and neuronal malfunction. It is more difficult to explain how the changes in biochemistry previously described involving the sympathetic system and the central 5-HT and endorphin systems could lead to a wave of neuronal disturbances demonstrated by Olesen [4]. The analogy of opiate withdrawal and hallucinatory states is perhaps of some relevance. Sicuteri described production of a migraine aura with pentazocine (Talwin) and its cessation with naloxone HCl (Narcan) [27]. It is possible that there is an opiate-mediated cortical shutdown mechanism that comes into play. Hosobuchi, in his early reports, indicated that naloxone could dramatically reduce the neurological signs produced by ischemia in some patients, although this has not been supported by later experiments.

The Mechanism of Pain

The peripheral role of the peptidergic system is being rapidly unraveled. There appear to be peptidergic neurons containing substance Y impinging on the cerebral arterioles interacting with the noradrenergic inputs from the locus ceruleus.

It is now known that there are fibers from the trigeminal nucleus innervating the extracranial vessels of the pia and dura. Stimulation of these nerves produces a release of peptides from the nerve terminals [32,33,34]. These peptides can be identified in dural vascular preparations after *in vitro* stimulation. Goadsby et al [35] have demonstrated an increased release of neuropeptide Y, vasoactive intestinal peptide, substance P, calcitonin and gene related peptide in the jugular but not in the cubital vein of humans during attacks of both common and classical migraine, now termed migraine without and with aura.

These peptides probably act on the mast cells in close apposition to the vessels and cause the release of vasoactive algogenic substances. There is a 5-HT$_{1D}$ receptor on the presynaptic portion of the trigeminal nerve abutting the extradural blood vessels. Stimulation of these receptors blocks release of peptides from the nerves following electrical stimulation of the fifth nerve sensory fibers. Both dihydroerotamine (D.H.E.-45) and a new experimental drug, sumatriptan, have the ability to stimulate these receptors and, hence, block release of peptides in the above model [36]. Sumatriptan has been shown to be effective in the treatment of both migraine and cluster headache[36A].

Goadsby and Gundlach have recently demonstrated a high specific binding site for D.H.E.-45 in the area of the brain associated with pain control (the dorsal and median raphé nuclei of the midbrain)[37]. Other binding sites were in the dorsal horn of the cervical spinal cord, in the medulla, associated with the tractus solitarius, the area postrema and the descending spinal trigeminal nucleus, in the mesencephalon and the cerebral cortex.

This binding suggests that D.H.E.-45 probably has a central role, as well as the peripheral one previously described. With more knowledge of the receptor affinities of a variety of hitherto pragmatically used drugs it is to be hoped that a new knowledge of the fundamental biochemistry of migraine will emerge.

Enkephalinase activity has been measured in the plasma and CSF of patients during and between migraine attacks. Plasma enkephalin is lowered in migraine patients during the free period and rises during attacks, reaching the same levels as those of controls. An increased level of plasma enkephalin has been observed during migraine attacks. Enkephalins and catecholamines are both liberated from the medulla in stress. Plasma changes in enkephalinase can be attributed to the discomfort of the stress. Enkephalin in the central nervous system (CNS) does not increase after stress. Sicuteri infers that enkephalinase, angiotensin converting enzyme, and cholinesterase, which are not altered either, are not involved in the central changes [13]. On the other hand, he felt that the reduced concentration of beta endorphin in plasma and CSF suggests that these opiates play a more important role in the mechanism.

Gastrin levels are slightly lower in migraine subjects, especially in those that have nausea and vomiting during the headache. The pain of the attack may therefore be related to altered central opiate tone, however there are many factors pointing to more local mechanisms. The presence of local tenderness in the arteries of migraineurs, Wolff's bradykinin released locally, and local release of histamine from mast cells all point to secondary local mechanisms. It was thought that prostaglandin may be involved at this level. Certainly the success of nonsteroidal anti-inflammatory agents in symptomatic treatment and prophylaxis would suggest this. However, attempts at demonstrating a primary involvement of prostaglandin in pain genesis have not been very successful. For instance, infusion of large doses of prostacyclin into migraineurs and non-migraine volunteers failed to induce a headache, despite marked vascular changes [29].

The Post Attack Phase

What happens at the end of the attack? This is less frequently studied but certainly some elements of a refractory period pertain. This is evidenced by changes in the responsiveness of platelets to aggregating stimuli. The work of Couch, Hassanein, and Kalendashi support this as does that of Carroll [30,31]. It seems that this refractory period may last up to several weeks. Some patients feel better when they go to sleep. Others find that the action of vomiting will abort the attack. Although the biochemical and psychological basis of migraine is still poorly understood, the pieces are gradually falling into place.

Suggested Reading

SEROTONIN

Anthony M. Role of individual free fatty acids in migraine. *Res Clin Study Headache 6*: 110-116, 1978.

Anthony M. Plasma free fatty acids and prostaglandin E1 in migraine and stress. *Headache 16*: 58-63, 1976.

Anthony M, Hinterberger H, Lance JW. Plasma serotonin in migraine and stress. *Arch Neurol 16*: 544-522, 1967.

Anthony M, Lance JW. The role of serotonin. In: Pearce J, (ed). *Modern Topics in Migraine*, pp 107-123. London, W Heinermann Medical Books, 1975.

Curran DA, Hinterberger J, Lance JW. Total plasma serotonin, 5-hydroxyindoleacetic acid and p-hydroxy-m-methoxymandelic acid excretion in normal and migrainous subjects. *Brain 88*: 997-1010, 1965.

Hyyppa MT, Kangasniemi P. Variation of plasma free tryptophan and CSF 5-HIAA during migraine. *Headache 17*: 25-27, 1977.

Sicuteri F, Testi A, Anselmi B, et al. An enzyme (MAO) defect on the platelets in migraine. *Int Arch Allergy 15*: 300-307, 1959.

VASCULAR CHANGES

Blau JN, Davis E. Small blood vessels in migraine. *Lancet 2*: 740-742, 1870.

Elkind AH, Friedman AP, Grossman J. Cutaneous blood flow in vascular headache of the migraine type. *Neurology 14*: 24-30, 1964.

Hachinski VC, Norris JW, Edmeads J, et al. Ergotamine and cerebral blood flow. *Stroke 9*: 594-596, 1978.

Hachinski VC, Olesen J, Norris JW, et al. Cerebral hemodynamics in migraine. *Can J Neurol Sci 4*: 245-249, 1977.

Matthew NT, Hrastnik F, Meyers JS. Regional cerebral blood flow in the diagnosis of vascular headache. *Headache 15*: 252-260, 1976.

Norris JW, Hachinski VC, Cooper PW. Changes in cerebral blood flow during a migraine attack. *Br Med J 3*: 676-684, 1975.

O'Brien MD. Cerebral blood changes in migraine. *Headache 10*: 139-143, 1971.

Olesen J. Vascular aspects of migraine pathophysiology. In: Clifford Rose F, (ed). *Migraine. Proc 5th Int Migraine Symp, London, 1984*, pp 130-137. Basel, Karger, 1985.

Tunis MM, Wolff HG. Studies on headache: Long term observation of the reactivity of the cranial arteries in subjects with vascular headache of the migraine type. *Arch Neurol Psychiat 70*: 551-557, 1953.

NEURONAL CHANGES

Gowers WR. Prodromes of migraine. *Br Med J 2*: 1400-1403, 1909.

Grafstein B. Mechanism of spreading cortical depression. *J Neurophysiol 19*: 154-171, 1965.

Hare EH. Personal observations on the spectral march of migraine. *J Neurol Sci 3*: 259-264, 1966.

Lashley KS. Patterns of cerebral integration indicated by the scotomas of migraine. *Arch Neurol Psychiat 46*: 331-339, 1941.

Leao AAP. Spreading depression of activity in the cerebral cortex. *J Neurophysiol 7*: 359-390, 1944.

Leao AAP. Further observations on the spreading depression of activity in the cerebral cortex. *J Neurophysiol 10*: 409-419, 1947.

PLATELETS

Burnstein Y, Berns L, Heldenberg D, et al. Increase in platelet aggregation following a rise in plasma free fatty acids. *Am J Hematol 4*: 17-22, 1978.

Couch JR, Hassanein RS. Platelet aggregability in migraine. *Neurology 27*: 843-848, 1977.

Deshmukh SV, Meyer JS. Cyclic changes in platelet dynamics and the pathogenesis and prophylaxis of migraine. *Headache 17*: 101-108, 1977.

Gawel M, Burkitt M, Clifford Rose F. The platelet release reaction during migraine attack. *Headache 19*: 323-327, 1979.

Hilton BP, Cummings JN. 5-Hydroxytryptamine levels and platelet aggregation responses in subjects with acute migraine headache. *J Neurol Neurosurg Psychiat 35*: 505-509, 1972.

OPIATES

Jansen I, Uddman R, Hocherman M, et al. Localization and effects of neuropeptide Y, vasoactive intestinal polypeptide, substance P, and calcitonin gene-related peptide in human temporal arteries. *Ann Neurol 20*: 496-501, 1986.

Kangasniemi P, Riekkinen P, Rinne UK. Kallikrein-like esterase and peptidase activities in CSF during migraine attacks and free intervals. *Headache 12*: 66-68, 1972.

Nappi G, Facchinetti F, Martignoni E, et al. Failure of central opioid tonus in migraine: Modulation of steroid milieu. In: Clifford Rose F, (ed). *Migraine. Proc 5th Int Migraine Symp, London, 1984*, pp 72-78. Basel, Karger, 1985.

Sicuteri F, Spillantini MG, Fanciullacci M. "Enkephalinase" in migraine and opiate addiction. In: Clifford Rose F, (ed). *Migraine. Proc 5th Int Migraine Symp, London, 1984*, pp 86-94. Basel, Karger, 1985.

References

1. Tunis MM, Wolff HG. Studies on headache: Long term observations of the reactivity of the cranial arteries in subjects with vascular headache of the migraine type. *Arch Neurol Psychiat 70*: 551-557, 1953.
2. Heyck H. Pathogenesis of migraine. *Res Clin Stud Headache 2*: 1-28, 1969.
3. Chapman LF, Wolff HG. Studies of proteolytic enzymes in cerebrospinal fluid. *Arch Int Med 103*: 86-94, 1959.
4. Olesen J, Larsen B, Lauritzen M. Focal hyperemia followed by spreading oligemia and impaired activation of rCBF in classic migraine. *Ann Neurol 9*: 344-352, 1981.
5. Bes A, Guell A, Victor G, et al. Effects of dopaminergic agonist (Piribedil) on CBF in migraine patients. *J Cere Blood Flow Metab 1 suppl 1*: 549-550, .
6. Sicuteri F, Boccuni M, Fanciullacci M, et al. A new nonvascular interpretation of syncopal migraine. *Adv Neurol 33*: 199-208, 1982.
7. Hockaday JM, Peet KMS, Hockaday TDR. Bromocriptine in migraine. *Headache 16*: 109-114, 1976.
8. Nappi G, Facchinetti F, Martignoni E, et al. Failure of central opioid tonus in migraine: Modulation of steroid milieu. In: Clifford Rose F, (ed). *Migraine. Proc 5th Int Migraine Symp, London, 1984*, pp 72-78. Basel, Karger, 1985.
9. Sandler M, Youdim MBH, Hanington E. A phenylethylamine oxidizing defect in migraine. *Nature 250*: 335-337, 1974.
10. Littlewood J, Glover V, Sandler M, et al. Platelet phenolsulphotransferase deficiency in dietary migraine. *Lancet 1*: 983-986, 1982.
11. Gawel M, Fettes I, Kuzniak S, Edmeads J. Endorphin levels in headache syndromes. In: Clifford Rose F, (ed). *Migraine. Proc 5th Int Migraine Symp, London, 1984*, pp 66-71. Basel, Karger, 1985.
12. Anthony M, Earl JW, Hinterberger H. Dopamine-B-hydroxylase (DBH), cyclic adenosine monophosphate (cAMP) and plasma free fatty acids in migraine (abst). *The Migraine Trust 2nd International Symposium*, London, 1978.
13. Sicuteri F, Spillantini MG, Fanciullacci M. "Enkephalinase" in migraine and opiate addiction. In: Clifford Rose F, (ed). *Migraine. Proc 5th Int Migraine Symp, London, 1984*, pp 86-94. Basel, Karger, 1985.
14. Sicuteri F, Anselmi B, Bianco PL. 5-Hydroxytryptamine supersensitivity as new theory of headache and central pain: A clinical pharmacological approach with p-chlorophenylalanine. *Psychopharmacologia 29*: 347-356, 1973.
15. Sicuteri F, Fanciullacci M, Michelacci S. Decentralization supersensitivity in headache and central panalgesia. *Res Clin Stud Headache 6*: 19-33, Basel, Karger, 1978.
16. Sicuteri F. Migraine: A central biochemical dysnociception. *Headache 16*: 145-159, 1976.
17. Sicuteri F. Endorphins, opiate receptors and migraine headache. *Headache 17*: 253-256, 1978.
18. Kennard C, Gawel M, Rudolph N de M, Clifford Rose F. Visual evoked potentials in migraine subjects. In Friedman, Granger, Critchley, (eds). *Res Clin Stud Headache 6*: 73-80, Basel, Karger, 1978.

19. Schoenen J, Maertens A, Timsit-Bertier M, Timsit M. Contingent negative variation (CNV) as a diagnostic and physiopathologic tool in headache patients. In: Clifford Rose F, (ed). *Migraine. Proc 5th Int Migraine Symp, London, 1984*, pp 17-25. Basel, Karger, 1985.
20. Hsu LKG, Crisp AH, Kalucy RS, et al. Early morning migraine. Nocturnal plasma levels of catecholamines, tryptophan, glucose and free fatty acids and sleep encephalography. *Lancet 1:* 447-450, 1977.
21. Anthony M. Role of individual free fatty acids in migraine. *Res Clin Stud Headache 6:* 11-116, 1978.
22. Norregaard TV, Moskowitz MA. Substance P and the sensory innervation of the intracranial and extracranial feline cephalic arteries. *Brain 108:* 517-533, 1985.
23. Lance JW, Lambert GA, Goadsby PJ, et al. Brainstem influences in the cephalic circulation: Experimental data from cats and monkeys of relevance to the mechanism of migraine. *Headache 23:* 258-265, 1983.
24. Wolff HG, Tunis MM, Goodell H. Studies on headache: Evidence of tissue damage and changes in pain sensitivity in subjects with vascular headaches of the migraine type. *Arch Int Med 92:* 478-484, 1953.
25. Sicuteri F. Headache as the most common disease of the antinociceptive system, analogies with morphine abstinence. In: Bonica, Liebeskind, Albe Fessard, (eds). *Advances in Pain Research and Therapy*, Vol 3, pp 359-565. New York, Raven Press, 1979.
26. Fanciullacci M. Iris adrenergic impairment in idiopathic headache. *Headache 1979 19:* 8-13, 1979.
27. Sicuteri F, Boccuni M, Fanciullacci M, et al. Naloxone effectiveness on spontaneous and induced perceptive disorders in migraine. *Headache 23:* 179-183, 1983.
28. Holaday J, Faden A. Naloxone acts at central opiate receptors to reverse hypotension, hypothermia and hypoventilation in spinal shock. *Brain Res 189:* 295-299, 1980.
29. Pestfield R, Gawel M, Clifford Rose F. The effect of infused prostacyclin in migraine and cluster headache. *Headache 21:* 190-195, 1981.
30. Couch JR, Hassanein RS. Platelet aggregability in migraine. *Neurology 27:* 843-848, 1977.
31. Carroll JD, Coppen A, Swade CC, et al. Blood platelet 5-hydroxytryptamine accumulation and migraine. *Upsala J Med Sci suppl 31:* 10-12, 1980.
32. Jansen L, et al. Localization and effects of neuropeptide Y, vasoactive intestinal polypeptide, and calcitonin gene-related peptide in human temporal arteries. *Ann Neur 20:* 296-501, 1986.
33. Lembeck F, Holtzer P. Substance P as neurogenic mediator of antidromic vasodilation and neurogenic plasma extravasation. *Naunym-Schmiedebergs Arch Pharmacol 310:* 175-183, 1979.
34. Markowitz S, Saito K, Moskowitz MA. Neurogenically leakage of plasma protein occurs from blood vessels from dura mater but not brain. *J Neurosci 7:* 4129-4136, 1987.
35. Goadsby PJ, Edvinsson L, Ekman R. Vasoactive peptide release in the extracerebral circulation of humans during migraine headache. *Ann Neur 28(2):* 183-187, 1990.
36. Buzzi MG, Moskowitz MA. The antimigraine drug, sumatriptan (GR43175), selectively blocks neurogenic plasma extravasation from blood vessels in dura mater. *Br J Pharmacol 99:* 202-206, 1990.
36A. The Subcutaneous Sumatriptan International Study Group. Treatment of migraine attacks and sumatriptan. *New Eng J Med 325:*376-321, 1991.
37. Goadsby PJ, Gundlach AL. Localization of ^{3}H-dihydroergotamine-binding sites in the cat central nervous system: relevance to migraine. *Ann Neur 29:* 91-94, 1991.

3

Serotonin Receptor Pharmacology in Migraine

Stephen J. Peroutka

Alterations in serotonin (5-hydroxytryptamine [5-HT]) neurotransmission have been implicated in several human disorders including migraine, depression, and anxiety, as well as in normal human functions such as sleeping, sexual activity, and eating. Unfortunately, the scientific linkage between serotonin and these disorders has been largely speculative rather than definitive. Nonetheless, migraine and other headache disorders are one of the strongest links between abnormalities of serotonin neurotransmission and a human disease state.

A variety of molecular, biochemical, and physiological observations suggest that multiple serotonin receptors exist in the central nervous system [1,2]. 5-Hydroxytryptamine receptors can be generally divided into three main families: $5\text{-}HT_1$, $5\text{-}HT_2$, and $5\text{-}HT_3$ receptors. Within each of the three families, receptor subtypes have been described. The diversity of the 5-HT receptor subtypes offers a unique opportunity to clinical neuropharmacologists. Theoretically, each receptor subtype provides a target site in the central nervous system that can be pharmacologically manipulated. The goal of the basic scientific research is to identify the potential functional significance of each serotonin receptor subtype. The evolving hypothesis is that the clinical efficacy of antimigraine agents derives from their ability to stimulate a specific serotonin receptor subtype (i.e., the $5\text{-}HT_1$ receptor family), while prophylactic antimigraine agents share an ability to block $5\text{-}HT_2$ receptors.

5-HT₁ Receptors

The 5-HT_{1D} receptor is a 5-HT_1 receptor subtype that was initially characterized in 1987 and has been shown to be widespread in the human brain [3-6]. In fact, the 5-HT_{1D} receptors are the most common type of serotonin receptor subtype observed in the human brain [6]. The 5-HT_{1D} receptor also functions as the autoreceptor that controls release of serotonin and other neurotransmitters [7].

At the same time, vascular studies have identified a 5-HT_1-like receptor in the cranial vasculature that may be identical to the 5-HT_{1D} receptor [8-11]. Multiple vascular studies have implicated this 5-HT_1-like receptor in the constriction of cerebral blood vessels. In particular, a novel experimental serotonergic agent, sumatriptan (formerly called GR 43175), appears to be an extremely selective agonist of these vascular serotonin receptors [9]. Moreover, recent studies have indicated that sumatriptan is a potent and selective 5-HT_{1D} receptor agent [12,13]. Therefore, the 5-HT_1-like receptor in certain cerebral vessels may, in fact, be the 5-HT_{1D} receptor.

This observation is important since sumatriptan has recently been reported to be extremely effective on an experimental basis in the acute treatment of migraine. Doenicke and colleagues reported that 2 mg IV sumatriptan completely abolished migraine symptoms in the majority of patients [14]. Two theories have been proposed to explain the efficacy of 5-HT_{1D} receptor agonists in migraine. First, the receptor(s) stimulated by both ergots and sumatriptan has been implicated in the constriction of arteriovenous anastomoses [15]. Under the migraine model proposed by Heyck, as yet unknown events lead to the opening of carotid arteriovenous anastomoses in the head [16]. Blood is diverted from the capillary beds, and ischemia and hypoxia result. Based on this hypothesis of migraine, an effective antimigraine agent would close the shunts and restore blood flow. Indeed, Feniuk and colleagues have shown that sumatriptan is a selective vasoconstrictor of the carotid circulation in the dog [9]. As noted above, these receptors display marked pharmacological similarities to 5-HT_{1D} receptors defined in radioligand binding studies.

Alternatively, the 5-HT_{1D} receptor appears to be an auto-receptor that modulates neurotransmitter release [7]. Conceivably, the 5-HT_{1D} agonists like dihydroergotamine mesylate (D.H.E. 45) and sumatriptan may act by blocking the release, at the nerve terminal, of transmitters such as serotonin, norepinephrine, and/or acetylcholine. Indeed, Saito and colleagues have demonstrated that ergotamine and dihydroergotamine are able to block the development of neurogenic plasma extravasation in dura mater that follows depolarization of perivascular axons following capsaicin injection or unilateral electrical stimulation of the trigeminal nerve. The ability of potent 5-HT_{1D} agonists to antagonize endogenous transmitter release may, theoretically, account for both this effect as well as for their efficacy in the acute treatment of migraine [17,18].

Table 3.1. Hypothetical Role of 5-HT Receptor Families in Migraine Therapy

5-HT$_1$ Receptors	Acute migraine relief may result from agonist activity at 5-HT$_1$ receptor sybtypes (i.e., the 5-HT$_1$D receptor)
5-HT$_2$ Receptors	Prophylactic migraine relief may result from antagonist activity at 5-HT$_2$ receptor subtypes (i.e., 5-HT$_2$ and/or 5-HT$_1$C receptors)

5-HT$_2$ Receptors

The 5-HT$_2$ receptor family has been extensively characterized in vitro, and a number of potent 5-HT$_2$ antagonists have been marketed as prophylactic antimigraine agents. Methysergide maleate (Sansert), cyproheptadine HCl (Periactin), pizotifen (not available in the U.S.), and amitriptyline HCl (Elavil, Endep) are potent agents at the 5-HT$_2$ receptor in human brain, whereas verapamil HCl (Calan, Isoptin) and nifedipine (Adalat, Procardia) display slightly lower affinities for these sites. These data demonstrate that a number of antimigraine drugs display high or moderate affinity for the 5-HT$_2$ receptor subtype in the human brain.

Hypotheses have been proposed that may explain the efficacy of 5-HT$_2$ antagonists in the prophylactic treatment of migraine. First, the 5-HT$_2$ receptor has been shown to mediate contraction of smooth muscle in many vascular beds [19]. Second, Coughlin, Moskowitz, and colleagues have demonstrated that 5-HT can stimulate production of prostacyclin and other products of arachidonic acid metabolism in smooth muscle cells in vitro [20,21]. This action of 5-HT appears to be mediated by 5-HT$_2$ receptors, since methysergide, cyproheptadine, and pizotifen potently prevent this effect. The significance of this finding is that modulation of prostacyclin and arachidonic acid metabolism may have important effects on vascular tone and/or local inflammation [20,22]. In essence, 5-HT (via 5-HT$_2$ receptors) could stimulate arachidonic acid metabolism at the onset of a migraine attack, which would be expected to lead to a sterile inflammatory reaction in the brain vasculature. Theoretically, 5-HT$_2$ antagonists are able to inhibit 5-HT from inducing the inflammatory state. However, once the inflammatory reaction is initiated (i.e., and the migraine begins), 5-HT$_2$ antagonists would be of little benefit.

Most recently, it has been suggested that 5-HT$_1$C receptor antagonists, as opposed to the 5-HT$_2$ receptor antagonists, may play an important role in the pathophysiology of migraine [23]. This suggestion derives from the fact that 5-HT$_1$C receptors share similar pharmacological characteristics to 5-HT$_2$ receptors, since both sites are subtypes of the 5-HT$_2$ family of receptors. Unfortunately, currently available prophylactic antimigraine agents do not differentiate between 5-HT$_1$C and 5-HT$_2$ receptors. Therefore, selective 5-HT$_1$C antagonists must be identified and developed before this interesting hypothesis can be tested in clinical trials.

Conclusions

Since a satisfactory animal model for migraine does not exist, attempts to determine a common mechanism of action for effective antimigraine agents may be of benefit in elucidating the pathogenesis of this neurological syndrome. As summarized in Table 3.1, antimigraine drugs share an ability to interact with specific serotonin receptor subtypes. These observations offer a novel approach to the analysis of antimigraine agents. Drugs could be selected for use in clinical migraine studies based on their selectivity for a specific 5-HT receptor subtype. For example, an agent that displays both a high affinity and selectivity for 5-HT$_{1D}$ receptors could be clinically evaluated. Its effectiveness, or lack thereof, could indicate the importance of this specific serotonin receptor site in the pathogenesis of migraine. Future attempts to determine a common mechanism of action for effective antimigraine agents should elucidate the pathogenesis of this neurological syndrome.

References

1. Peroutka SJ. 5-Hydroxytryptamine receptor subtypes. *Ann Rev Neurosci 11*: 45-60, 1988.
2. Schmidt AW, Peroutka SJ. 5-Hydroxytryptamine receptor families. *FASEB J 3*: 2242-2249, 1989.
3. Heuring RE, Peroutka SJ. Characterization of a novel ^{3}H-5-hydroxytryptamine binding site subtype in bovine brain membranes. *J Neurosci 7*: 894-903, 1987.
4. Waeber C, Schoeffter P, Palacios JMH, et al. Molecular pharmacology of 5-HT$_{1D}$ recognition sites: Radioligand binding studies in human, pig and calf brain membranes. *Naunyn Schmiedebergs Arch Pharmacol 337*: 595-601, 1988.
5. Waeber C, Dietl MM, Hoyer D, et al. Visualization of a novel serotonin recognition site (5-HT$_{1D}$) in the human brain by autoradiography. *Neurosci Lett 88*: 11-16, 1988.
6. Peroutka SJ, Switzer JA, Hamik A. Identification of 5-hydroxytryptamine$_{1D}$ binding sites in human brain membranes. *Synapse 3*: 61-66, 1989.
7. Hoyer D, Middlemiss DN. Species differences in the pharmacology of terminal 5-HT autoreceptors in mammalian brain. *Trends in Pharmacological Science (TIPS) 10*: 130-132, 1989.
8. Humphrey PPA, Feniuk W, Perren MJ, et al. GR43175, a selective agonist for the 5-HT$_1$-like receptor in dog isolated saphenous vein. *Br J Pharmacol 94*: 1123-1132, 1988.
9. Feniuk W, Humphrey PPA, Perren MJ. The selective carotid arterial vasoconstrictor action of GR43175 in anaesthetized dogs. *Br J Pharmacol 96*: 83-90, 1989.
10. Parsons AA, Whalley ET, Feniuk W, et al. 5-HT$_1$-like receptors mediate 5-hydroxytryptamine-induced contraction of human isolated basilar artery. *Br J Pharmacol 96*: 434-449, 1989.
11. Connor HE, Feniuk W, Humphrey PPA. Characterization of 5-HT receptors mediating contraction of canine and primate and basilar artery by use of GR43175, a selective 5-HT$_1$-like receptor agonist. *Br J Pharmacol 96*: 3790387, 1989.
12. Peroutka SJ, McCarthy BG. Sumatriptan (GR43175) interacts selectively with 5-HT$_{1B}$ and 5-HT$_{1D}$ binding sites. *Eur J Pharmacol 163*: 133-136, 1989.
13. McCarthy BG, Peroutka SJ. Comparative neuropharmacology of dihydroergotamine and sumatriptan (GR43175). *Headache 29*: 420-422, 1989.
14. Doenicke A, Brand J, Perrin VL. Possible benefit of GR43175, a novel 5-HT$_1$-like receptor agonist, for the acute treatment of severe migraine. *Lancet 1*: 1309-1311, 1988.

15. Saxena PR, Ferrari MD. 5-HT$_1$-like receptor agonists and the pathophysiology of migraine. *TIPS 10*: 200-204, 1989.
16. Heyck H. Pathogenesis of migraine. *Res Clin Stud Headache 2*: 1-28, 1969.
17. Saito K, Markowitz S, Moskowitz MA. ERgot alkaloids block neurogenic extravasation in dura mater: Proposed action in vascular headaches. *Ann Neurol 24*: 732-737, 1988.
18. Moskowitz MA. The neurobiology of vascular head pain. *Ann Neurol 16*: 157-168, 1984.
19. Peroutka SJ. Vascular serotonin receptors: Correlation with 5-HT$_1$ and 5-HT$_2$ binding sites. *Biochem Pharmacol 33*: 2349-2353, 1984.
20. Coughlin SR, Moskowitz MA, Antoniades HN, et al. Serotonin receptor-mediated stimulation of bovine smooth muscle cell prostacyclin synthesis and its modulation by platelet-derived growth factor. *Proc Nat Acad Sci USA 78*: 7134-7138, 1981.
21. Coughlin SR, Moskowitz MA, Levine L. Identification of a serotonin type 2 receptor linked to prostacyclin synthesis in vascular smooth muscle cells. *Biochem Pharmacol 33*: 692-695, 1984.
22. Peatfield RC, Fozard JR, Rose FC. Drug treatment of migraine. In: Rose FC, (ed). *Handbook of Clinical Neurology*, vol 4, pp 173-216. New York, Raven Press, 1986.
23. Fozard JR. The development and early clinical evaluation of selective 5-HT$_3$-receptor antagonists. In: *The Peripheral Actions of 5-Hydroxytryptamine*. Oxford, Oxford University Press, 1989.

4

The Headache History

Steven M. Baskin

Proper headache diagnosis is essential to providing safe and effective treatment. A detailed headache history is the clinician's most valuable diagnostic tool, and subtle but thorough questioning is necessary.

Many patients often have a fear of significant brain pathology and/or worry that the clinician thinks their problem is psychogenic. These patients may distort the history in relation to their own naive conceptualization of headache and may omit or alter certain key points. Some patients have consulted with many other professionals and nonprofessionals (family, friends, etc.) and have many misconceptions about the nature of head pain as well as the various therapeutic alternatives. Some are taking many medications, either self-prescribed or prescribed by a physician, which may paradoxically increase their headache frequency, intensity, and duration, and may reduce the effectiveness of other interventions. To encourage honest and open doctor-patient communication, certain points must be included in all interviews to ensure a reliable history. The following chapter will outline and discuss the essential parts of a good headache history. A detailed diagnostic interview will help ensure that you do not become another stop along some patient's long and fruitless search for an underlying medical condition.

Table 4.1. The Headache Diagnostic Interview

1. Types of Headache
2. Onset
3. Characteristics of Pain
   a. Frequency and intensity
   b. Location and laterality
   c. Character
   d. Time of onset and duration
   e. Prodromal symptoms
   f. Associated symptoms
   g. Behavior during the attack
4. Precipitating Factors
5. Medication History
6. Medical History
7. Habit History
8. Family History
9. Behavioral Assessment
   a. Assessment of sleep
   b. Assessment of depression
   c. General coping style factors

The Headache Diagnostic Interview (see Table 4.1)

TYPES OF HEADACHE

Since many patients suffer from more than one type of headache, it is essential that the clinician help the patient identify all types of headaches that may coexist. Patients with chronic headache often refer to the problem as "my headache" without accurately differentiating two different headache types. These patients, typically, have had episodic common migraine (migraine without aura) attacks over the years that have become complicated by a daily constant headache between attacks as well as by chronic, often excessive, analgesic usage. Many patients with chronic daily headache believe that if they do not take frequent analgesics, all of their headaches will be incapacitating. This is usually more fear than fact. Other patients may have distinct, easy-to-separate attacks of migraine and tension-type headache. During the interview it is often helpful for the clinician to differentiate these headache types along an intensity dimension. It is very helpful to question the patient along a four point intensity scale. For example, the following questions are often helpful:

- What is the frequency of headache that will either incapacitate you or dramatically decrease your ability to function?
- How often do you have a headache that is moderate to severe in intensity but does not significantly affect your functional capacity?
- How often do you have a dull headache?
- How often are you clear-headed, with no trace of head discomfort?

ONSET

It is important to establish the age and circumstances of onset for each headache type. Headaches that begin in childhood or in young adulthood are often of a migrainous type. A female may note that her headaches began at the time of menarche and were absent during the last two trimesters of pregnancy. Certainly, a recent onset of pain that began suddenly with other neurological symptoms should alert the physician to a possible acute neurological problem. It is important for the clinician to determine the duration of symptoms for each headache type.. It is also important to note a qualitative change in symptoms in a chronic headache sufferer. A common problem is an increased frequency of migraine, from a stable pattern, and the onset of daily head pain soon after the migraine frequency increase.

Often, the circumstances in a patient's life can trigger the headache. If a 20-year old college sophomore, with a history of infrequent migraine reports that her daily headaches began in the fall of her senior year in high school, when she was applying to colleges and feeling very anxious, then a psychological trigger may be entertained.

Trauma, either physical or emotional and occurring near the time of the onset of headache, may be an important factor in determining headache type. Headache may coexist with a severe medical illness as well as major depression., When headache presents for the first time in geriatric patients, one must consider organic disease such as temporal arteritis or cervical spine problems.

CHARACTERISTICS OF PAIN FOR EACH HEADACHE TYPE

Frequency and Intensity

It is important to delineate the specific frequencies of each type of headache along an intensity dimension. It is helpful to look at the frequency of attacks both in the past and present and note when they increased in frequency.

The most notable aspect of migraine is its paroxysmal or episodic nature. The frequency of migraine is rarely more than once or twice a week, and many patients report one to two attacks a month. Women often have attacks right before or at the start of their menses.

Cluster headaches typically present in clusters of one to three attacks per day for a four-to-eight week period, followed by long periods of remission. The attacks often begin at the same time each year. About 10% of people with cluster headache develop the chronic form, defined by the absence of a remission period.

Chronic tension-type headache is often daily and constant. If the frequency or intensity of headache increases after a stable pattern, one must be alert to any new organic or emotional development, or to the abuse of analgesics.

Location and Laterality

Migraine presents unilaterally in approximately 50-70% of the cases, although many migraine patients report bilateral pain. It is often located temporally, retro-orbitally, or generalized throughout the cranium. Cluster headache is always unilateral and often periorbital in location. Pain may radiate over one side of the head or into the cheek or mastoid area. The pain is most often localized to the eye alone. A bilateral fronto-occipital band-like distribution of head pain is typical of tension-type headache. Often there is concomitant neck tightness. It can occasionally be unilateral but that should raise a red flag and prompt a thorough investigation for organic causes of headache.

Character of Pain

Migraine is often reported as a severe throbbing, pulsating, and deep pain. Cluster headache is described as excruciating in severity and boring, sharp, and non-throbbing in character as though a hot poker is being thrust through the eye. The pain of chronic tension-type headache is typically non-throbbing at dull-to-moderate intensity and is often described as a squeezing ache or steady pressure. Tic douloureux consists of short, severe, and sharp burning and lancinating pains that can last up to four minutes and recurs several times per hour. It usually increases in intensity to a peak and then decreases only to occur again in wavelike fashion over several minutes.

Time of Onset and Duration

Migraine may occur at any time of the day, but patients often awaken with it. A migraine usually lasts anywhere from six hours to three days; although there are rare cases lasting up to two weeks or longer. It averages 12-24 hours.

Cluster attacks often begin at the same time each year and often at the same time each day. Attack duration ranges from 30 to 90 minutes and attacks tend to occur most often during sleep. They awaken the patient most commonly 90 minutes after falling asleep, which is coincident with the onset of the first period of rapid eye movement (REM) sleep. Often cluster patients will have attacks upon awakening from a nap in the afternoon. Cluster headaches may present a pattern of multiple attacks within a 24-hour period.

Tension-type headache may present as either episodic or chronic. Most people experience episodic tension-type headaches during the day under conditions of acute emotional, physical, or mental stress. They last from a few minutes to up to 12 hours. Chronic tension-type headaches, on the other hand, usually occur on a daily basis, constantly or waxing and waning, for periods lasting months or even years. The patient may awaken with a headache or develop it as the day progresses.

Tic douloureux pain usually occurs during the day, more so in the morning after being triggered by touching the face, speaking, swallowing, etc. The pain lasts from seconds to four minutes.

Aura Symptoms

These warning symptoms are typical of classical migraine (migraine with aura) and usually last 20 to 30 minutes, quickly followed by a headache. The symptoms are largely limited to visual phenomena such a scintillating scotomata made up of flashing colored lights that move across the visual field from the center to the periphery. Some headaches are preceded by bright, colored zigzag lines that are called fortification spectra. The headache begins as the aura fades. Neurological symptoms such as paresthesia, vertigo, ataxia, oculomotor paralysis, and hemiparesis may be part of the aura symptoms but more commonly develop during the headache. In common migraine (migraine without aura) there is no visual aura and if a prodrome exists, it is usually vague and may precede the attack by several hours or days. Prodromal symptoms may include psychological changes, fatigue, nausea, yawning, palpitations, and fluid retention. However, many patients experience the headache without any prodromal symptoms. Cluster pain is almost always sudden, without warning, and no prodromal symptoms are noted in tension-type headache or tic douloureux.

Associated Symptoms

Most migraineurs typically have some gastrointestinal symptoms, most notably nausea and/or vomiting, as an essential feature of the disorder. Other associated features include anorexia, diarrhea, polyuria, pallor, dizziness, sensitivity to sound, sensitivity to light, cold extremities, and fatigue.

The associated symptoms in cluster headache are unilateral and consist of ipsilateral reddening and tearing of the eye, ptosis, miosis, and stuffiness and/or rhinorrhea of the ipsilateral nostril. Cluster headache predominates in men who have certain specific physical characteristics. These men typically have a ruddy complexion, deep skin furrows, a leonine (lion) appearance, orange peel thick skin, and acromegaloid look with large nose or jaw. Approximately 38% of cluster patients have hazel eye color, which is significantly greater than the general population. Patients with tension-type headache more often have associated anxiety, depression, and sleep disorder.

Behavior During the Attack

Migraine patients tend to hibernate during a headache, getting into bed in a dark room and avoiding sounds, lights, and movements. A major criterion used in the diagnosis of cluster headache is the constant movement of the patient during the attack. The patient is typically unable to lie still and usually paces, rocks, or bangs his head on a hard object. There is no other primary headache disorder in which this type of behavior occurs.

PRECIPITATING FACTORS

Patients with migraine often recognize various factors that may trigger a headache attack. These include weather changes, altitude, alcohol ingestion, red wine, fasting or delaying food intake, lack of or excess sleep, weekends and vacation, and certain foodstuffs. Food containing tyramine, MSG, or sodium nitrate can be triggering factors. Psychological events may also play a role in headache induction. Careful questioning involving the amount and type of recent life changes may explain an increase in headache frequency. Many migraine sufferers notice that their headaches may occur during the let-down period after a prolonged period of stress, rather than during it. An episode of anxiety or depressive disorder may increase or change the headache pattern.

Frequently, migraine first appears during menarche. In children, the male to female ratio for migraineurs is 60:40, but the disorder becomes progressively more frequent in females after puberty, reaching 25:75 male to female in adults. There is an increased incidence of migraine perimenstrually. After the first trimester of pregnancy, many women report being free of migraine attacks. These data suggest a hormonal relationship to the disorder. Many women begin having migraine headaches only after starting birth control pills, and some notice an increased frequency on cyclical estrogen replacement therapy.

Physical exertion and sexual activity may also precipitate a headache. Certain medications may be vasoactive and increase migraine frequency or induce an attack such as vasodilators in cardiac patients. Many analgesic agents are significant maintenance factors in chronic headache.

MEDICATION HISTORY

It is important to take a careful history of medication usage, both abortive and preventative. Note the exact dosages of these medications as well as the length of treatment in order to assess whether the patient received an adequate trial. One must carefully assess whether the patient has ever had an adequate ergotamine trial.

The physician should document the current use of abortive agents for headaches such as the off the shelf and/or prescription analgesics as well as the ergotamine preparations. Many patients are habitual analgesic users, and these drugs will often paradoxically perpetuate and worsen their head pain. This paradoxical effect of analgesics has been termed analgesic rebound headache. Chronic use of these agents often interferes with standard, usually effective preventative pharmacological therapy. Recent investigations suggest that ergotamine rebound pain may begin in some patients chronically taking as little as 4 mg of ergotamine tartrate per week, if used more than one to two days per week. These ergotamine habituation headaches usually resemble the original migraine headache. Patients will use ergotamine effectively for these headaches, maintaining the rebound effect.

It is also important to look at medications that might in themselves cause headache. Migraine and cluster patients are particularly susceptible to vasodilator medications such as nitrates and histamine-containing agents. Vasoconstrictor drugs such as caffeine and ergotamine can cause a withdrawal headache. Reserpine, used in hypertensive therapy, may precipitate or increase the frequency of the headache. Oral contraceptives have been repeatedly observed to trigger or increase the frequency of migraine. Progesterone and the cyclical administration of estrogen replacement therapy may also increase the frequency of migraine. The use of sympathomimetics, such as amphetamines, cocaine, and over use of certain oral or nasal decongestants may increase migraine frequency. The xanthines may also adversely affect headache frequency.

MEDICAL HISTORY

The physician should know if a patient has had prior trauma to the head or loss of consciousness. Questions about a history of seizure disorder or other neurological problems are indicated. Episodic vomiting and motion sickness as a child are often precursors of migraine. The clinician should note if the patient is hypertensive or has any cardiovascular disease. Any previous or coexisting psychiatric problems should be noted. Sinus, dental, temporomandibular joint, or cervical spine problems should be detailed.

The patient's previous medical history can influence the treatment of the headache problem. If a patient has a history of respiratory problems such as asthma, non-selective beta blockers are contraindicated. Also, many patients with a history of daily headache and gastrointestinal problems, such as ulcer disease or irritable bowel syndrome, often do well on the antihistaminic tricyclic antidepressants. Patients should be questioned about the results of any previous diagnostic tests done for their headache problem. Previous surgery for a tumor may suggest metastatic disease as a possible cause of headache.

Habit History

It is important to assess alcohol and recreational drug usage. Patients in a cluster period are very sensitive to alcohol, which will often induce a cluster attack immediately after ingestion. The amount of caffeine ingested in coffee and soft drinks should be noted. Many patients are aware that caffeine in abortive migraine medications will have an antimigraine effect. It must be explained to them, however, that caffeine taken on a daily basis will increase the frequency of headache, due to caffeine withdrawal. It is also helpful to ask the patient about cigarette smoking, which can increase headache.

Family History

Patients with migraine will often present a family history of headaches. Most experts believe that over 70-90% of migraineurs have a close relative with migraine. It may be helpful to ask the patient if any member of his family has had a sick headache. It is also helpful to get a family history of psychiatric disorders, most notably depression, as well as neurologic disease, general medical problems, alcohol/drug abuse, and cardiovascular problems.

Behavioral Assessment

Assessment of Sleep

Sleep problems, such as difficulty falling asleep, frequent awakening during the night, and early awakening in the morning, are associated with depression. Often changes in sleep pattern such as hypersomnia or lack of sleep are significant headache triggers. A normal sleep/wake cycle is very important in cluster headache. It should be determined if the patient's insomnia is related to a depressive or anxiety disorder.

Assessment of Depression

The clinician must evaluate the symptoms of major depression. These include depressed mood, decreased interest or pleasure in most activities, significant weight loss or weight gain, chronic insomnia or hypersomnia, psychomotor agitation or retardation, fatigue or loss of energy, excessive guilt or feelings of worthlessness, decreased concentration, and recurrent suicidal ideation.

General Coping Style Factors

It is helpful to determine the psychological background of the headache sufferer. Careful questioning of family and marital relationships, occupational history, social/environmental stresses, and recent life changes, both positive and negative, should be undertaken. It is important to ascertain why the person is currently seeking help and his/her motivation for treatment. Disability and litigation issues should be noted. Careful observation of appearance, mannerisms, cognitive functioning, abstraction ability, rhythm and rate of speech, insight, judgment, and affective style is useful. It is often helpful to notice how the patient describes pain, e.g., killing me, searing, etc. Confrontation is of limited usefulness during the initial headache interview. It is always more helpful to ask about psychological symptoms that may be secondary to chronic headache rather than as a primary cause.

5

The Neurological Examination

Larry S. Eisner and Barry Baumel

The key to proper diagnosis, in headache patients as in all of medicine, lies in careful history taking coupled with a thorough physical examination. Together, the history and physical provide the basic information for evaluating the headache patient and formulating a plan for care. Although the time required for history taking is quite variable, an adequate general examination and neurological survey can be performed within 10 to 15 minutes.

The carefully obtained *headache history* is invaluable in directing diagnostic skills. Symptoms must be analyzed in terms of their characteristics, the time and mode of onset, the duration and variability, the factors that exacerbate and ameliorate. The presence of factors that occur episodically and are not associated with major neurological impairment are suggestive of the benign primary headache disorders. Conversely, progressively more severe symptoms of insidious onset and progressive neurological deficits are of ominous significance. A careful review of systems is also helpful in searching for clues that might reveal the presence of an underlying systemic or neurological systems disorder that contributes to the development of headache as a secondary phenomenon. The detailed methods of analyzing the headache history are reviewed in Chapter 4.

General Examination

The general examination should include recording vital signs, with particular attention to blood pressure evaluated in each arm both supine and sitting or erect. Examination of the neck should include inspection of position, motility, and configuration. Abnormalities should be recorded. Palpation of the neck for muscle tonus, tenderness, meningismus, and for the presence of abnormal masses is imperative. Auscultation of the anterior neck for carotid bruits and of the head in frontal, temporal, and occipital zones and over the orbit for intracranial bruits is recommended. The cranium should be inspected for deformity and for the presence of externally visible lesions. General examination of the heart, lungs, abdomen, breasts, and limbs are no different in headache patients than in those presenting with other complaints. Back and spine are examined for deformity, lesions, mobility deficits, or muscular spasm.

Neurological Examination

The neurological examination is divided into seven components. These include assessment of mental status, cranial nerve function, motor systems, coordination, station and gate, sensory systems, and reflexes.

MENTAL STATUS

Beginning with a mental status examination, the physician determines the level and assesses the content of consciousness. Level of consciousness can be categorized as awake and alert, awake but not fully alert, lethargic, delirious, stuporous, obtunded, or comatose. Categorization is based on awareness and response to external stimuli rather than specific content.

Content of consciousness should include an assessment of orientation in the spheres of person, place, and time. Intellect is assessed on the basis of an individual's ability to process information. Tests employed are numerous and variable. Efficient methods of evaluating intellect include quick assessments of calculation, patient's description of similarities and differences in classes of objects, interpretations of current events, and vocabulary.

Attention is graded on the basis of an individual's ability to maintain relevant conversation and to perform serial calculations such as subtracting 7s serially from 100. Judgment is often assessed through the interpretation of proverbs. Favorite proverbs among neurologists include, "A stitch in time saves nine" and "People who live in glass houses should not throw stones." Also, questions such as, "What would you do if you were in a movie theater and smelled smoke?" or "What would you do if you found a stamped addressed envelope on the street?" are useful. Affect is graded on the basis of an evaluation of the patient's mood (euphoric, normal, or depressed); the examiner uses his or her own judgment in assessing the appropriateness of the patient's responses to situations which, in the normal individual, would lead to either happy or sad responses. Language function is assessed for prosody, the ability to produce syllables within a fixed period of time. A normal individual should produce a minimum of 60 syllables within a 60-second interval. Also, diction or choice of words is assessed for appropriateness as is the presence or absence of paraphasia. Pronunciation is assessed for the presence of dysarthria. The ability to repeat simple and complex sentences or phrases such as, "No ifs, ands, or buts," plus naming, spelling, and following simple commands, completes the brief language assessment.

Memory should be tested for short- and long-term recall. Short-term immediate recall is easily tested through the dictation of progressively longer series of numbers. A normal individual should be able to inscribe into and immediately recall from memory a series of seven numbers. Intermediate memory is assessed by asking the patient to repeat three objects such as ball, flag, tree; and to repeat them after one minute. Retest again after three minutes, during which time other cognitive testing is performed. Long-term memory is easily assessed by evaluating the patient's past medical history and social history for cohesiveness.

Abnormalities in mental status testing seldom localize a headache complaint to a lesion in a specific area of the brain, but the presence of abnormalities on the mental status portion of neurological assessment demands further investigation. Evidence of aphasia may help to localize the lesion.

Cranial Nerve Function

The cranial nerve examination assesses function of each of the 12 pairs of nerves emanating from the base of the brain. The first or olfactory nerve is tested by requesting a patient to identify substances based on their odor. Each nostril is tested separately with the other nostril occluded by the examiner's or the patient's finger placed firmly on the side of the nose, compressing the ala nasae against the septum. The patient should be able to identify most common aromas either by specific name or by general description.

The second cranial, or optic, nerve is evaluated by confrontation perimetry, assessment of central visual acuity, and direct examination of the fundus by ophthalmoscope.

Cranial nerves III, IV, and VI are usually tested as a group by evaluating ocular motility. The third cranial nerve also controls pupillary constriction and the position of the eyelid as mediated by the levator palpebra muscle. The palpebral fissures are compared side to side for equality. Pupils are observed in a darkened room and size estimated and equality assessed. A bright light is cast upon each pupil directly to assess responsivity. The light source is quickly removed to the opposite pupil so that both the direct and the consensual light response can be recorded. Ocular motility should be full with the limbus of the iris being buried in the respective inner or outer canthus of the eye for the adducting or abducting eye, respectively. There should be no nystagmus at rest, nor any sustained nystagmus on extremes of gaze. Rotatory, vertical, and traction nystagmus are invariably abnormal. The fourth, or trochlear, nerve is difficult to assess as it controls only one muscle: the superior oblique. Its function is to turn the eye down and in (clockwise on the right and counterclockwise on the left). However, its function cannot be seen while the oculomotor nerve is intact, as that nerve controls the medial and inferior rectus muscles; these muscles, when activated together, effect the same directional movement of the eye. The sixth, or abducens, nerve abducts the eye. Thus, the entire oculomotor-trochlear-abducens system is tested by asking the patient to bring his eyes into full right, left, up, and down gaze.

The fifth cranial nerve, the trigeminal, has both motor and sensory function. It controls those muscles that clench the jaw and move it from side to side. It is also, through its three major sensory divisions (ophthalmic, maxillary, and mandibular), the major sensory nerve for the anterior scalp and forehead, the mid face, and the lower face and jaw area. It is tested by assessment of strength of jaw closure and side-to-side movements, controlled by the masseter and temporalis muscles, and the pterygoid muscles, respectively. Its sensory function is tested by tactile, vibratory, pain and temperature sensation in the skin over the three divisions.

The seventh, or facial, nerve is tested by observation of symmetry of the static and mimetic expression of the face. Upper and lower portions of the face are evaluated independently. The facial nerve also controls glandular secretion, the sensation of taste over the anterior two-thirds of the tongue, dampening of loud noise through contraction of the stapedius muscle, and variable sensory function in and about the external auditory meatus. Though helpful in a detailed neurological examination, these functions of the nerve are often overlooked in the screening neurological examination.

The eighth, or acoustic, nerve controls hearing and contributes to the controls of balance and equilibrium. Hearing is easily tested with a 256 cycles per second (CPS) tuning fork held first on the mastoid process behind each ear until the sound is no longer appreciated, and then directly next to the external auditory meatus, to compare bone conduction and air conduction. In normal individuals, air conduction should be better than bone conduction (Rinne test).

The ninth, or glossopharyngeal, and tenth, or vagus, nerves are usually tested as a unit. They function together and are responsible for the deglutition mechanism elicited in the gag reflex. Modulation of voice tone for varying pitch depends upon the recurrent laryngeal branch of the vagus nerve.

The eleventh, or spinal accessory, nerve controls the trapezius and sternocleidomastoid muscles. They are tested by the confrontation method, evaluating resistance of the shoulder shrug maneuver and the movement of the head from side to side as the chin is brought in approximation with the shoulder. In the normal individual, each of these muscles is quite strong.

The twelfth, hypoglossal, nerve is easily tested by asking the patient to protrude the tongue directly forward. The tongue should protrude in the midline and wag on request symmetrically. No fasciculations should be noted in the resting state, with the tongue resting on the floor of the mouth.

MOTOR SYSTEMS

The evaluation of the motor system is important in the headache patient since lesions and diseases of the central nervous system that cause headache may have either subtle or gross effects on motor function. Attention is directed to pyramidal and extrapyramidal systems, lower motor neurons in brain stem and spinal cord, and cerebellar function as well.

Motor system evaluation begins with an assessment of muscle tone. Tonus can be evaluated by observation of the patient under voluntary movement conditions and by passively moving the major joints such as shoulder, elbow, wrist, knee, and ankle.

Spastic tonus involves opposing muscle groups to different degrees such that one muscle group has increased tonus while the other is easily passively overcome. In conditions of rigidity, both flexors and extensors have simultaneously increased resistance to passive movement. Hypotonicity is a condition in which there is loss of normal muscle tone. Motor strength is most easily assessed by confrontation measurement of power. The examiner requests the patient's maximal effort in the flexion and extension of major joints while the examiner applies equal but opposite effort to the joint. The patient's strength can thus be compared to the force of gravity or to the examiner's counterforce and graded on a numerical scale from zero (no muscular strength) through five (normal strength for body habitus). Intermediate grades of one (muscular activity without joint movement), two (joint movement with gravity eliminated), three (strength sufficient to resist the force of gravity), and four (strength in excess of gravity but less than normal) complete the scale. An additional quick assessment of subtle deficits in motor strength include the arm roll test and assessments of rapid alternating movements. The capacity to perform alternating movements (diadochokinesis) should be symmetrical.

COORDINATION TESTING

Coordination testing is most easily performed by observing the patient in the performance of stereotyped movements. Commonly used tests of the finger-to-nose test in which the patient touches the tip of his index finger alternately to the tip of his own nose and to the tip of the examiner's finger. This is performed with the eyes open. Another finger-to-nose test is performed with eyes closed, asking the patient to touch his index finger to the tip of his nose at varying rates from different positions in space. The pronation-supination test is performed with the patient in the sitting position tapping the knee alternately with the palm and dorsum of the hand at varying rates of speed. In the heel-to-knee test, the patient lies in a supine position, lifts the tested leg high in the air, and gently taps the opposite knee with the heel of the test foot. Varying the speed of testing helps to assess for subtle asymmetry. Rapid alternating movements are used to test for dysdiadochokinesia. Finger wiggle, tongue wiggle, and foot-tap tests may be helpful. The patient should be observed for involuntary movements. Tremors are rhythmic spontaneous, rapid, irregular, and purposeless movement of small joints. Ballistic movements have similar characteristics to those described as choreiform but are more proximal, of greater amplitude, and considerably more violent. Athetoid movements are slow, sustained, writhing movements affecting primarily distal portions of extremities. Dystonic movements involve spasms of more proximal and axial muscles.

STATION AND GAIT

Station and gait are assessed by observation of the patient's posture, stance, and motility. The carriage of the head and limbs at rest, sitting, standing, and walking are noted. The size, meter, and stability of steps are significant.

SENSORY SYSTEMS

In the sensory examination, the primary modalities routinely tested include pain, position, vibratory sensation, soft touch, and temperature. Assessment for right-left symmetry and lack of distal loss are made for each modality. Pain sensation is tested more easily through the use of a clean, sharp pin or sharpened wooden stick. The patient is asked to compare the acuteness of the pin prick between homologous areas of the body, looking for asymmetry, subjective, or objective sensory loss. The Wartenburg wheel is a handy accessory device that provides repetitive, relatively constant degrees of stimulation over large areas of the body.

Vibratory sensation is tested with a tuning fork of 128 CPS frequency. The base of the instrument is placed on major bony prominences. Position sensation is tested by small amplitude movements of the distal interphalangeal joints of the hands and feet. If there is impairment, more proximal joints should be tested as well. Soft touch is assessed using a wisp of cotton or, more objectively, a series of graded diameter filaments known as Von Frey Hairs. In this manner, soft-touch deficits can be quantitatively reported. Temperature sensation is quickly assessed, using metallic objects that have been warmed or cooled in warm water of ice water, by comparing the subjective response over different body parts. Comparison is made between report of proximal and of distal sensation in trunk and limbs. Lateralizing sensory asymmetries suggest disease of the central nervous system, while peripheral sensory loss usually indicates peripheral neuropathy.

Secondary sensory modalities include the ability to localize a point of touch, the discrimination of two distinct pin pricks at variable linear separations, the capacity to report double simultaneous stimulation over widely spaced body parts, and stereognosis, the ability to identify an object by handling it.

REFLEXES

Reflex examination is performed by using the deep tendon tap technique. The muscle stretch reflexes most often tested include jaw jerk, biceps, brachioradialis, triceps, quadriceps femoris (knee jerk), gastrocnemius-soleus (ankle jerk), hamstrings, and Hoffman (finger flexor). Reflexes are graded 1 through 4. Grade 1 reflexes are hypoactive; grade 2 are normal; grade 3, hyperactive; and grade 4, hyperactive to the point of clonus. Superficial reflexes may be included in the routine examination. These include the corneal reflexes, superficial abdominal reflexes, and anal wink reflex. Pathological reflexes should be sought, including the Babinski. The plantar surface of the foot is stroked with the fingernail, a key, or a relatively sharp instrument along the lateral border and across the ball of the foot toward the base of the great toe. Variations on the Babinski reflex include the Chaddock (stimulation along the lateral aspect of the foot), the Oppenheim (stimulation with firm pressure of knuckles over the shin from the knee down to the ankle), and the Stransky reflex (in which the little toe is slowly abducted to extreme, then quickly released). In each of these reflexes, a flaring of the toes and upward movement of the great toe constitute an abnormal or positive response. A positive snout reflex is the puckering of the lips following a tap above the upper lip.

Through the performance of the above maneuvers, the examiner may discover abnormal function in the central and peripheral nervous system. An inventory of such abnormalities suggests the locus of pathology within the nervous system. Through further application of the history and general physical examination, etiological alternatives and differential diagnoses are suggested. In this manner, the neurological examination, coupled with a careful patient history, is the key to unlocking the proper diagnosis in the headache patient.

References

De Gowin, De Gowin. *Bedside Diagnostic Examination*. London, The Macmillan Company, 1969.
DeJong. *The Neurologic Examination*, 4th Ed. Hagerstown, MD, Harper & Row Publishers, 1979.

6

Diagnostic Testing in Headache

Ninan T. Mathew

The diagnosis of headache is based on a thorough history of headache, general medical history, and a detailed physical and neurological examination. Some primary headache syndromes such as migraine and cluster headache are usually easily recognizable and laboratory tests may play only a minor role. In other headaches that do not fit specific patterns, appropriate diagnostic tests should be performed. In addition to ruling out structural or organic conditions that cause headache, these tests serve as a reassurance to an anxious patient who is worried about an impending serious illness as the cause of headache. Fear of a brain tumor, aneurysm, or other structural abnormality is common among the headache population. Patients go to a physician not only for relief of pain but for an explanation of their pain [1]. Therefore, reassurance is important in the successful management of patients with chronic recurrent headache, once organic causes have been ruled out.

Indications for Diagnostic Work-Up in Migraine

There are special situations in a migraine patient, even when the history is typical of migraine with and without aura, that would warrant diagnostic testing. Recent changes in the clinical features of the attacks or findings of an abnormal neurological sign are indications for further selected investigations. In cases of complicated migraine, where there are associated visual, labyrinthine, and cerebral symptoms, further investigation to exclude a structural lesion and to reassure both the patient and the physician is important. Diagnostic work-up is particularly important in patients with transient visual symptoms without headache, sometimes termed acephalalgic migraine, and in patients with recurrent and prolonged monocular or binocular visual defects, persistent visual defects, and recurring ocular palsies associated with headaches.

A young person's first attack of hemiparetic migraine, even with a typical clinical history and a possible family history of hemiplegic migraine, demands exclusion of occlusive or hemorrhagic cerebral vascular events. Therefore, full investigations are necessary.

The characteristics of basilar artery migraine, which consist of rapid development of visual symptoms, vertigo, incoordination of gait, and culminate in rapid impairment of consciousness, usually in a young person, are of great concern and require an immediate work-up. Appropriate tests include an electroencephalogram (EEG), computerized tomography (CT scan), or magnetic resonance imaging (MRI scan). The return of any abnormal finding to normality, after the recovery of symptoms, permits a confident diagnosis of basilar artery migraine. Many patients develop rotational vertigo and illusions of movement during an attack and, in some, these symptoms may occur without associated headache. They require a neuro-otological work-up that may reveal certain abnormalities. In most cases, the patient's attack profile and family history indicate that the vertigo is part of the migraine syndrome [2]. A diagnostic work-up including a neuropsychological evaluation is indicated in patients with confusion, inattention, impairment of intellectual functioning during attacks of severe migrainous headache, and in patients with uncommon variants of complicated migraine manifesting as severe and prolonged disorientation, amnesia, phobias, agitation, and hallucinations. In some cases with prolonged mental symptoms and focal neurological signs, a cerebrospinal fluid (CSF) examination is indicated to exclude viral meningitis [3,4].

Timing and Selection of Diagnostic Tests

The timing and selection of appropriate tests are usually determined by the clinical profile. Clinical presentation of headache can be divided into three categories: acute severe headache, occurring for the first time; a short history of headache that gradually becomes progressively severe; and a long history of recurrent or persistent headache.

FIRST OCCURRENCE OF HEADACHE OF SUDDEN ONSET

Pain of instantaneous onset resulting in a very severe headache, which may become excruciating, occurs in conditions such as acute subarachnoid hemorrhage due to a ruptured intracranial aneurysm or arteriovenous malformation (AVM) and acute intracerebral hemorrhage. It may also happen in benign situations such as coital headache or orgasmic cephalgia. A careful history and neurological examination will differentiate subarachnoid hemorrhage from orgasmic cephalgia. In any doubtful case, if the patient is seen during or shortly after the headache, it is of vital importance to detect an intracranial hemorrhage. A CT scan should be performed immediately, followed by spinal tap. The blood-stained CSF is spun down in a centrifuge to detect xanthochromia, which will develop within several hours of a subarachnoid hemorrhage and will persist for a week or more, depending on the volume of blood spilled into the subarachnoid spinal fluid. A CT scan will usually fail to detect a very small warning leak. Fluid from the spinal tap performed within an hour or two of the small subarachnoid hemorrhage may be clear because the blood may not have reached the subarachnoid space in the lumbar sac. A high degree of suspicion of subarachnoid hemorrhage should lead to further studies including contrast enhanced CT scan and cerebral arteriogram to detect an aneurysm or AVM. If blood is seen in the non-contrast scan, it is not necessary to perform a spinal tap since diagnosis of intracranial hemorrhage is clear.

Warning headache may occur in aneurysmal subarachnoid hemorrhage. Thirty consecutive patients with aneurysmal subarachnoid hemorrhage (SAH), 20 with ischemic stroke and 100 control patients, were interviewed about previous episodes of sudden headache [5]. Thirteen patients with SAH (43%) had a history of a forewarning headache, compared with only one of the patients with ischemic stroke and none of the controls. The interval between the warning headache and the admission rupture was one to two months in all but one patient with SAH. Only half of the 13 patients with a warning headache consulted their physician. Verweij and colleagues concluded that warning headaches may occur in patients with SAH, and they recommended measures to increase the recognition of certain headaches as a warning sign of aneurysmal subarachnoid hemorrhage [5].

In patients with coital headache or orgasmic cephalgia, a good history and detailed neurological examination is all that is necessary to make a diagnosis and reassure the patient. However, in doubtful cases, even with the slightest suspicion of subarachnoid hemorrhage, investigations are in order.

Less sudden onset of headache is not likely to be due to intracranial hemorrhage. However, conditions such as meningitis and encephalitis must be kept in mind, though these are usually accompanied by fever and neck stiffness. A spinal tap is indicated in such a situation after a non-contrast CT scan is obtained. In most situations, a non-contrast CT scan is sufficient for emergency purposes, as it will enable one to rule out a space-occupying lesion producing mass effect or ventricular enlargement. In the emergency room when a patient presents with a severe headache for the first time, it is safe to perform a spinal tap if the non-contrast CT scan is normal. Even if a parenchymal or extracerebral lesion is present, the risk of herniation is slight under these circumstances, since it is not deforming the ventricular system. An enhanced scan can be obtained later, if necessary. Many radiologists are reluctant to perform contrast-enhanced scans outside of regular hours, since an allergic reaction to a contrast medium can be better managed during regular hours when all ancillary and supportive help is available.

In a young patient, if the rapid-onset, first-time headache is hemicranial, with associated nausea and vomiting, migraine is the most likely diagnosis. The patients should undergo observation and further diagnostic testing including CT scan and EEG, especially if the headache does not subside with appropriate pharmacological therapy, such as ergotamine.

Most patients are seen after the acute headache has subsided. A neurological examination at that time is usually normal; if the history suggests a serious underlying cause for the headache of sudden onset, a complete investigation including brain imaging is in order. A CT scan of the brain is very useful in detecting acute sinusitis in various paranasal sinuses. Blood count, chemistry profile, and endocrine studies may be performed, depending on the type of history obtained.

SHORT HISTORY OF PROGRESSIVE, RECURRENT, OR PERSISTENT HEADACHE

Headache occurring as a new symptom, especially if it becomes progressively severe, is likely to be highly significant; in such instances, neuroimaging techniques, either MRI or CT scan with and without contrast, is indicated [5]. If the neuroimaging tests are normal, then infectious, toxic, metabolic, and systemic conditions must be ruled out.

CHRONIC RECURRENT HEADACHE

The longer a headache has been recurring, the less likely it is due to a demonstrable lesion. However, patients with a long history of recurrent or persistent headache should have a CT or MRI scan of the brain. The scan should be repeated if the nature of the headache changes. The knowledge that the scan is normal can be very reassuring to many patients. Other tests, such as cervical spine x-rays and tomograms of the temporomandibular joint, may be ordered to detect factors responsible for triggering a tension-type headache.

Neuroimaging in Headache

Neuroimaging using MRI or CT is the single most useful test in the evaluation of headache and most other neurological symptoms. The indications for neuroimaging in patients with headaches are: acute headache of sudden onset occurring for the first time and without a previous history of headache; headache of recent onset that is progressively worsening; and, in patients with recurring headache such as migraine, when the clinical picture raises suspicions about an alternate diagnosis such as cerebral tumor or infarction, symptomatic migraine in which an arteriovenous malformation may be considered, complicated migraine in which there are prolonged transient or permanent focal cerebral symptoms, and in patients who present to the emergency room with impaired consciousness.

CT Scan of the Brain

A normal scan does not rule out meningeal conditions such as meningitis and carcinomatous infiltration of the meninges. If these conditions are suspected, further testing including spinal tap must be performed. CT scan with and without contrast will help to rule out space-occupying lesions such as primary or secondary parenchymal tumors, intracerebral hematomas, areas of cerebral infarction, abscess formation, hydrocephalus, tumors of the pineal and pituitary regions, and tumors of the cranial nerves. Acute epidural and subdural hematoma can also be detected easily. However, when it comes to a chronic subdural hematoma, the diagnosis can become difficult because of the isodense stage of the hematoma in which there is no difference between the density of the brain and the density of the hematoma [7]. This is especially problematic when the chronic isodense subdural is bilateral, in which situation there is usually no shift of the midline or distortion of the ventricular system. One clue may be that the scan looks supernormal for the patient's age, since hematomas tend to compress the sulci thereby reducing the usual appearance of cortical atrophy in older patients. High-resolution scanning with high-dose contrast medium may help.

Lesions close to the base of the skull and posterior fossa are sometimes difficult to detect by CT scan. In the posterior fossa, the very dense petrous bone produces artifacts that cross the brain stem transversely from petrous apex to petrous apex, making lesions of the clivus and the adjacent posterior fossa difficult to detect. Lesions around the foramen magnum also are difficult to see on tomographic scans because of bony artifacts. These problems can be circumvented by using high-resolution scanning with thin cuts and high doses of contrast media, or by MRI scans.

Only about 70% to 80% of cerebral infarcts are detected by computerized tomography techniques, even when contrast enhancement is used. It is important that serial scans are done to make the diagnosis of cerebral infarction, as the timing is very important. In a cerebral infarction, the CT scan may not show an infarct in the first 24 hours. The infarction and the cerebral edema become much more evident after the second and third day. A negative CT scan in a patient with headache and a history suggestive of stroke is of vital importance as it indicates that the lesion is not a hemorrhagic infarction or a primary hemorrhage. Small quantities of blood can be detected very reliably by CT scan. It is estimated that 10 to 15 cc of blood in the subarachnoid space can be detected by CT scan.

Normal CT scans are obtained from the majority of patients with migraine in the intervals between attacks, even from those with exceptionally severe headaches. If a CT scan can be obtained during the initial period of an attack of complicated migraine, it is likely to provide evidence of focal edema or ischemia. A follow-up CT scan during the next few weeks will show signs of recovery if initial diagnosis of complicated migraine was correct. There have been a number of reports in the literature of evidence of cerebral infarction and edema demonstrated on the CT scan of patients with complicated migraine [8-12]. Repeated cerebral ischemic insults as a result of migraine may result in focal cerebral atrophy [8,9].

Magnetic Resonance Imaging

Magnetic resonance imaging of the brain, craniovertebral junction, and upper cervical spine serves a useful purpose in the diagnosis of headache from many points of view. Conditions such as Arnold-Chiari malformation, which may present with recurrent headaches, especially cough headache or exertional headache, can easily be diagnosed by MRI scan. Sagittal sections through the skull can clearly demonstrate the foramen magnum region allowing easy identification of abnormalities in Arnold-Chiari malformation and other lesions such as meningioma. Type I Arnold-Chiari malformation may be encountered sometimes with the tonsils of the cerebellum slightly below the level of the foramen magnum.

The clinical significance of this finding may sometimes become difficult to evaluate. In true herniation of the cerebellar tonsils there is a pinched appearance of the tonsil rather than the normal rounded appearance.

Ventricular pathways, the third ventricle, the aqueduct of Sylvius, and the fourth ventricle are clearly seen on MRI scan. Conditions such as aqueductal stenosis with hydrocephalus that may present as a recurrent or chronic headache can be more accurately diagnosed using MRI scan. Third ventricular tumors and colloid cysts of the third ventricle and particularly lesions of the pituitary gland are much better delineated by MRI than by CT scans. Microadenomas of the pituitary gland, which may be prolactin-secreting tumors, are easily detected by MRI scan of the pituitary area. Subdural hematoma, when isodense and especially when bilateral, may be totally missed by a CT scan. However, MRI scans are very useful in detecting them. Thus, there is no doubt that MRI has revolutionized the diagnostic capability in chronic recurrent headache because of its ability to rule out conditions that might be missed by CT scan.

There are reports of unidentified bright objects (UBOs) in the white matter in patients with headache [13]. It is a rather nonspecific finding that is seen even in otherwise healthy patients. They may indicate small ischemic lesions in the white matter or possibly demyelination due to some underlying pathology. The significance of UBOs in the migraine patient is not adequately understood and should not cause great concern when evaluating MRI scans in migraine patients.

However, when such abnormalities are seen in headache patients, it is important to rule out collagen diseases such as systemic lupus erythematosus (SLE), manifesting as microinfarcts in the brain and headache [14]. Headache is a common presentation of SLE, with the reported frequency as high as 64% [15]. Recently, much attention has been given to a syndrome associated with the presence of antiphospholipid antibodies and a migraine-like headache [16,17]. Patients exhibiting this syndrome may show MRI abnormalities in the form of multiple small areas of increased signal density or even frank infarctions of larger areas of the brain.

Cranial X-Rays

Skull, sinus, mandibular, and spinal x-rays, though performed less frequently since the advent of CT and MRI, are useful in selected patients. Enlargement of the sella turcica, bone lesions of the calvarium, and congenital or developmental anomalies of the skull are well demonstrated on x-rays. Platybasia or basilar invagination may be associated with conditions such as Arnold-Chiari malformation, which can give rise to a certain type of occipital headache. Localized bone lesions as a result of dermoids, epidermoids, metastases, and myeloma may produce localized pain and may cause plain radiographic defects in the skull. Paranasal sinus abnormalities and nasopharyngeal soft tissues can be examined with plain x-rays. Basal views of the skull may show bony erosion from various malignant conditions, especially nasopharyngeal carcinoma that infiltrates into the base of the skull causing facial pain and cranial nerve paralysis. Paget's disease and hyperparathyroidism are other conditions that show radiographic abnormalities in the skull. In general, skull x-rays are adequate for preliminary evaluation and are more cost-effective than the imaging techniques.

Sinus x-ray series help in the diagnosis of infection in the paranasal sinuses, erosion of the bony walls, enlargement of the sinus cavity, and periosteal reactions that may indicate malignant infiltration. Intrasinus tumors can range from carcinoma of the lining to benign osteoma. CT examinations sometimes help to identify sinus lesions better than sinus x-rays, especially when one is dealing with sphenoid sinusitis. Kennedy suggests that CT scanning should be done with coronal reconstriction to visualize the area lateral to the middle turbinate of the nose to the greatest advantage [18]. One of the major reasons for obtaining sinus x-rays is to help convince patients that headaches are not due to sinus disease, a common myth or a misdiagnosis of migraine.

The role of the cervical spine in the production of headache is controversial. However, most would agree that constant or recurrent occipital and nuchal pain can result from degenerative and traumatic changes in the discs and facet joints of the upper cervical spine. Head pain without neck pain rarely has a cervical cause. Osteoarthritis of the atlanto-axial or atlanto-occipital articulations can cause occipital pain, occipital neuralgic symptoms, and can be readily visualized by appropriate cervical spine views. On the whole, cervical spine x-rays are useful in identifying degenerative diseases including rheumatoid disease resulting in osteoporosis of the odontoid process. MRI of the cervical spine may provide more detailed information of the region.

Plain x-rays and tomograms of the temporomandibular joint are sometimes used in the evaluation of headaches. Degeneration of the joint may lead to the temporomandibular joint syndrome, but the presence of radiologically demonstrable changes in the joint should not be taken as proof that this syndrome is the cause of the patient's headaches. Patients that suffer from various forms of migraine, mixed headache syndrome, and tension-type headaches are often diagnosed as having temporomandibular joint dysfunction, a diagnosis that is difficult to substantiate.

Radionuclide Scans

Radionuclide brain scans are not commonly performed because of the availability of CT and MRI scans. However, when such facilities are not available, radionuclide scans are still useful in the detection of subdural hematoma, primary or secondary brain tumors, and intracranial masses such as abscesses and meningiomas. Radionuclide bone scans are particularly useful in the detection of metastatic skull and cervical spine lesions. A gallium scan is useful in detecting osteomyelitis of the skull even though the majority of those lesions can be detected by plain skull x-rays.

Radionuclide Cisternography

Radionuclide cisternography is an occasionally useful procedure in the diagnosis of spontaneous cerebrospinal fluid leakage, even though in a number of cases it has been unsuccessful [19,20]. This is a rare condition that occurs as a result of a tear in the arachnoid membrane and the dura in the dorsal spinal regions, most commonly during violent sports or other physical activities such as lifting. It has also been known to follow a hard cough or sneeze. Spontaneous CSF rhinorrhea can occur as a result of defects in the dura of the cribriform plate of the ethmoid. This often follows trauma and can also occur in invasive malignant lesions. Patients with CSF leakage develop low CSF pressure resulting in headaches similar to those that occur following a spinal tap. The headaches occur while assuming an upright position and worsen the longer this posture is maintained. There is usually complete and rapid relief upon lying down. A radioisotope cisternogram is done by instilling radioactive ytterbium or indium through a lumbar puncture and scanning the entire neuraxis at four, eight, and 24 hours. Spontaneous leakage of cerebrospinal fluid through a tear in the spinal theca or the cribriform plate of the ethmoid bone can be detected.

Occasionally, leaking occurs through the mastoid bone passing down the eustachian tube into the nasopharynx.

Cerebral Angiography

Cerebral angiography has little place in the diagnosis of headache, except in very special situations. If an aneurysm is suspected, it should be confirmed or ruled out by angiography. Aneurysms of the cerebral arteries hardly ever cause periodic headaches with migrainous features, and angiography can not be considered a primary investigation in patients with migraine. Aneurysms may be suspected during the first attack of ophthalmoplegic migraine, and angiography may be required for exclusion.

The only other indication for angiography in headache is when CT or MRI already shows an abnormality, such as cerebral A-V malformation. Angiography may be necessary to define the depth and size and to demonstrate the feeding and the draining vessels of the vascular malformation so that an appropriate therapeutic approach by surgery or interventional radiology can be planned. An angiogram will almost never reveal a brain tumor in a patient who has had normal results on CT or MRI. Unilateral headache of rapid onset, felt retroorbitally, and associated with incomplete Horner's syndrome, may be due to internal carotid artery occlusion or dissection; carotid doppler may be helpful but angiography is needed for confirmation [21]. Segmental narrowing of intracerebral arteries during migraine attacks has been reported [22,23].

Is Cerebral Angiography Safe In Migraine?

Direct carotid puncture and use of more toxic contrast material in the early years resulted in a high morbidity rate following angiograms in patients with migraine [24]. Following Patterson's report, some reviewers commented on the risk of angiography in migraine [24-26]. Also, temporary deterioration of neurological symptoms and signs following arteriography have been documented in migraine patients [27-31]. Recently, new radiological techniques, safer contrast dyes, and increased awareness of complications have helped decrease the side effects of angiography for all patients [32,33]. To assess the risk of angiography in migraine patients, Shuaib and Hachinski have reviewed the charts of 148 patients with migraine who underwent arteriogram. Transient neurological events were seen in five patients: transient amnesia in one, hemisensory changes in one, hemiparesis in one, global confusion in one, and angina in one [34]. Focal cerebral events occurred in 2.6% of cases and this compared with a rate of complications of 2.8% caused by angiography in a prospective study of 1,002 patients from their own center. According to Shuaib and Hachinski, a history of migraine does not increase the risk of complications caused by angiography [34]. Angiography during acute episodes of headache would also appear to be a safe procedure. Transient focal neurological symptoms, however, are not infrequent, especially in cases of migraine with aura following angiography.

Electroencephalography

Electroencephalography may be of no major diagnostic value in the investigation of headaches since there is no definite diagnostic EEG pattern associated with any type of headache. An abnormal EEG may occasionally help in differentiating an organic disease from a functional problem and syncope from an epileptic process. It is doubtful that even the new technique of computerized EEG topography (EEG brain mapping) will prove to be useful in diagnosing headache types, as its usefulness in the diagnostic evaluation of individual patients with various neurological problems is questionable [35].

Various diffuse and focal EEG abnormalities are more commonly seen in migrainous than non-migrainous subjects [36]. Such abnormalities are more common in patients suffering from migraine with aura than in those suffering from migraine without aura. But there is no EEG pattern specific for a diagnosis of migraine. Abnormalities in migraine include focal slow and sharp wave activity that sometimes agrees with focal visual, motor, or sensory symptoms; nonspecific episodic slow frequencies; or recurrent bursts of sharp waves, slow and sharp wave complexes, and occasional spike activity. Excessive response to hyperventilation and photic stimulation has also been reported [37]. Occasional patients with sharp waves and paroxysmal EEGs have responded to anticonvulsant medication: some headache specialists use EEG results to help guide pharmacologic treatment of migraineurs. In some complicated migraine patients with focal neurological symptoms, transient or even permanent focal abnormalities have been noted. EEGs usually improve a few days after the complicated migraine attack has subsided. The relatively high frequency of abnormalities in the EEG in patients with migraine may indicate that the primary pathogenesis of migraine is neural. Further research is necessary to explore this concept.

Cerebrospinal Fluid Examination

Cerebrospinal fluid examination has no known value in the routine investigation of primary headache disorder. In fact, it may be better to avoid a spinal tap in patients with primary headache disorders such as migraine and tension-type headache since it may lead to more problems by causing post-spinal headache. However, there are definite indications for spinal tap in a patient who presents with headache. These include acute subarachnoid hemorrhage, acute meningitis, encephalitis, chronic meningitis of various types including carcinomatous and fungal meningitis, sarcoid, other suspected diseases such as neurosyphilis, benign intracranial hypertension, and low cerebrospinal fluid pressure headache due to spontaneous cerebrospinal fluid leak. Patients with acquired immune deficiency syndrome (AIDS), when presenting with increasing headache, should have a spinal tap after excluding space-occupying lesions. It is important to measure the pressure of the fluid with the patient in a horizontal, fully relaxed condition. Appropriate cytological, serological, and biochemical tests should be performed, depending on the clinical suspicion. Patients with headache after spinal tap should lay flat in bed for at least 24 hours and drink a lot of liquids. Post-spinal headaches can become a problem in the primary headache disorder population and can be prolonged for a number of days. Strict bed rest in a flat position is probably the most effective treatment. Epidural blood patch can be performed if the condition persists more than five to seven days. It works rapidly to relieve low-pressure headache and has a high rate of success [38-40].

There have been a few case reports in which a patient with a known history of migraine presents with sudden severe headache and neck rigidity; cerebrospinal fluid examination may show increased lymphocytes [41,42]. Rapid recovery from both headache and neck rigidity occur within two to three days and the pleocytosis disappears. The mechanism of production of this cerebrospinal fluid abnormality is not know.

Blood Tests

Sedimentation rate is an essential test when one suspects temporal or giant cell arteritis. Headache of recent onset and visual problems in the elderly female should raise the suspicion of temporal arteritis. Serial examinations are important in order to follow the clinical exacerbations and remissions of the headache. Sedimentation rate can also be used as a therapeutic guide for dose titration of corticosteroids in the treatment of temporal arteritis. A temporal artery biopsy may be necessary.

If a person with episodic headache has associated unusual behavior or impairment of consciousness, hypoglycemia due to insulinoma or diabetes should be suspected, and blood glucose and insulin levels should be measured. Headache patients who have irregular menstrual cycles or amenorrhea with or without associated galactorrhea should have measurements of prolactin and other hormone levels to rule out hypophyseal dysfunction. Serum protein electrophoresis and immunoelectrophoresis would help in the diagnosis of myeloma and other immune-related disorders that may have some bearing on the headache. Arterial blood gases may help in explaining headaches in chronic obstructive pulmonary disease. Carboxyhemoglobin levels may be an indication of exposure to carbon monoxide from the heating system accounting for early morning headaches during the cold weather [43]. This is especially relevant if several members of the family are similarly affected by headache.

Central nervous system syphilis and Lyme disease should be kept in mind as causes of chronic persistent headache; therefore, serological tests of both blood and cerebrospinal fluid may be in order. Other tests of importance in patients with chronic headaches, especially those who are habituated to various medications, are estimations of drug and alcohol levels in blood. Determinations of lead and vitamin A levels are also important as lead poisoning and vitamin A excess can lead to chronic headache [44-47]. Because a number of patients with chronic recurrent headache are also depressed, biological markers of endogenous depression such as a positive dexamethasone suppression test may be helpful in the overall assessment of depression associated with chronic headache [48].

Urine Tests

Estimations of urinary concentrations of vanillylmandelic acid, metanephrines, and other catecholamines are indicated when a pheochromocytoma is suspected. Additional tests are indicated when there is a high level of these compounds in the urine. Urinary estimations of drugs and heavy metals and metabolites of porphyrins are also important in the diagnosis of toxic and metabolic causes of headache.

Temporal Artery Biopsy

If the sedimentation rate is elevated in a headache patient, temporal artery biopsy may be indicated. The surgeon should take out at least 3 cm to 5 cm of the artery, as temporal arteritis tends to be segmental. If only a small piece is taken out, the diagnosis may be totally missed. If the microscopic examination fails to confirm the diagnosis and if the index of suspicion is very high, opposite arteries should be removed for examination.

The diagnosis of temporal arteritis should be determined with extreme care since it is a serious disease with potential permanent visual loss, and treatment involves long-term, high-dose corticosteroid therapy.

Evoked Potentials

Visual evoked potential (VEP) is an important diagnostic test for specific neurological disorders. VEP latencies measure conduction velocities in the optic nerve and the central optic pathways to the level of the visual cortex, while the amplitude of the VEP represents the number of receptors stimulated in the retina and the excitability of the visual cortex. Several studies have found increased VEP amplitudes in patients with migraine, which were interpreted as evidence for the increased excitability of the occipital cortex in migraine [49-53]. Other reports were not in agreement with the above observation [54,55].

Alterations have been found more frequently with flash VEP than with pattern-shift VEP [56-60]. Rudino did not find any statistically significant differences in mean P-wave latency or in mean P-wave amplitude in migraine patients using pattern-reversal stimuli [54]. However, he found changes in individual cases, especially when the visual evoked potentials were obtained close in time with the migraine attack. It has been pointed out that pattern-shift VEPs are more altered during migraine attacks or in patients with numerous and recent migraine attacks [58,59]. Nevertheless, Dean and colleagues did not find VEP alterations in dietary migraineurs during their migraine attacks [55].

Although previous reports have indicated statistical differences between groups of migraine patients and controls, VEP has not helped, on an individual basis, either in the diagnosis of migraine per se or in differentiating between migraine types [49-53]. Marsters and colleagues attempted to evaluate VEP as a diagnostic test for migraine, and used complex calculations integrating flash frequency, flash amplitude, pattern frequency, and pattern amplitude to arrive at fast-wave coefficient (FWC) [61]. They reported that they could distinguish classic migraine, common migraine, and the control group using FWC. Their results need to be reproduced before any reliable diagnostic value can be assigned to VEP in migraine patients [61].

From the literature review, it appears that the abnormalities reported in migraine patients have been found more easily with flash VEP than with pattern-shift VEP. The components of pattern-shift VEP are mediated by geniculostriate pathways, and they are generated in the occipital lobe [62,63]. Visual cortex is probably the processing area for the flash P1 component; however, the flash P2 component has different characteristics and may be processed by a different system, possibly a completely separate non-geniculate pathway [64]. The greater frequencies of alterations in flash VEP than in pattern-shift VEP probably reflect a greater alteration in non-geniculate pathways. The greater frequencies of alterations in VEPs recorded close to a migraine attack probably results from alterations in either ischemic changes and/or abnormalities in neurotransmitters.

Isolated reports of alterations in brain stem auditory evoked potential (BAEP) have appeared in the literature; there are reported transient alterations in one case of basilar migraine, and alterations in BAEP during attacks of migraine but not between attacks in a series of cases [65,66]. Ganji, on the other hand, reported posterior slowing in the EEG, but normal VEP, BAEP, and somatosensory evoked potentials (SSEP) in one case of basilar artery migraine. Alterations on BAEP, like that of VEP, are by no means diagnostic for migraine. BAEP may be abnormal in some patients with cluster headache.

Transcranial Doppler

Transcranial Doppler has been used recently for studying the intracranial hemodynamics in patients with cluster headache [68]. Interhemispheric asymmetry was found to be greater in the cluster headache group compared with controls. Within the patient groups, velocities in the middle cerebral artery and posterior cerebral artery were significantly faster on the headache side, and this increased velocity was thought to be due to narrowing of the vessel most probably due to spasm [68]. Swollen arterial wall is the other possible explanation for narrowing of the vessels. Narrowed carotid artery due to possible swollen and edematous arterial wall has been observed in the carotid siphon area by Ekbom and Greitz during cerebral arteriography in a cluster headache patient [70].

While there may be statistical differences in the intracranial flow velocities during headache, the flow changes are not diagnostic in individual cases; therefore the diagnostic value of transcranial Doppler is questionable. However, it appears to be a very useful research tool to study intracranial hemodynamics noninvasively, and it may be useful in determining and evaluating the effects of medications. Thomas and colleagues have recently shown that migraineurs during the headache-free interval demonstrated excessive cerebrovascular reactivity to CO_2, evidenced by an increase in middle cerebral artery blood flow velocity (MCAFV) by 47% ± 15% compared with 28% ± 14% in controls (P = 0.026) [71].

Psychological and Behavioral Tests

Kudrow and Sutkus demonstrated that severity of the Minnesota Multiple Personality Inventory (MMPI) changes rose in sequence through patients with the following diagnoses: migraine and cluster headaches, muscle contraction headache (tension-type headache), mixed migraine and muscle contraction headaches, post-traumatic headache, and conversion headaches [72]. This was seen as a consequence of chronic illness, pain, and suffering. Sternbach and colleagues found that vascular headache patients obtained lower MMPI scores than muscle contraction and mixed headache patients, possibly due to more frequent and longer pain-free intervals [73]. These findings were confirmed by Weeks and colleagues [74]. The most frequent combination of elevated scores are on scale I (hypochondriasis), scale II (depression), scale III (hysteria), and in some cases, scale VII (psychasthenia). Even though MMPI is used very frequently in the evaluation of chronic headache and pain, there are many inherent weaknesses to the MMPI [75-77]. Whether a neurotic personality is antecedent or a consequence of the experience of living with chronic pain has been a topic of great debate. Arena and colleagues, using a number of psychological test parameters, concluded that the characteristic personality traits often found in headache sufferers are not a result of pain experience, but in fact are present before the emergence of pain [78]. It is generally agreed by headache specialists that MMPI by itself has no diagnostic value, and that even though there are inherent weaknesses and difficulties in interpretation, it serves as a guideline in the overall assessment of the personality profile and helps in the behavioral and psychological management of patients with chronic headache.

Apart from MMPI, depression scales are helpful. The most commonly used depression scales are the Beck Depression Scale and the Zung Depression Scale [79,80]. In general, patients with chronic headaches have higher depression scale scores compared with patients with episodic headache such as migraine or cluster headache.

Type A behavioral pattern described by Friedman and Rosenman is seen in a considerable number of patients with chronic recurrent headaches [81]. An evaluation of the type A personality behavior may be of value in the overall management of headache.

Thermography in Headache

Medical electronic thermography is a noninvasive procedure for observing and photographing heat energy emission patterns. Radiating from the skin surface of the human body is an infrared energy proportional to the amount of vascular supply below the skin. A thermography device transforms this invisible infrared energy into electrical energy and amplifies it so that it may be converted into light and photographed. An infrared camera and Polaroid photographic techniques are used.

Various thermographic abnormalities are seen in the headache population. Lance and Anthony noted asymmetrical heat patterns in the forehead of migraine patients [82]. They observed reduced heat emission at the start of the migraine attack and increasing heat emission as the attack progresses. Mathew and Alverez showed that asymmetrical heat patterns in the forehead are seen in a larger percentage of migraineurs and other vascular headache patients compared with nonvascular headache patients [83]. Swerdlow and Dieter established a significant correlation between cold patches and vascular-related headaches, maintaining that they are a valid diagnostic marker for vascular headaches as they are a persistent constituent of the thermal geography of the face [84]. Cold patches persist during headache-free intervals and are best seen in the supraorbital area of the forehead. A cold patch is generally accepted as a facial hypothermic asymmetry that has a temperature 0.5° C cooler than the surrounding area. The mechanism producing a cold patch is not clear. Changes in the vascular dynamics, including arteriovenous shunting or arteriolar narrowing may account for the reduced circulation and subsequent reduced heat emission. Kudrow, using Doppler techniques, demonstrated vasoconstriction in the forehead area supplied by the branch of the external carotid artery in patients with cluster headache who had ipsilateral cold patches between attacks during the cluster period [85].

During an acute attack of migraine and cluster headache, increased heat emission is usually noted. Drummond and Lance examined 11 patients thermographically during spontaneous attacks of cluster headache and 22 during cluster headache induced by nitroglycerin or alcohol [86]. Increased heat emission was recorded from the affected orbital region, which, in some patients, spread above and below the eye. They noted that the thermographic changes usually followed the onset of pain, indicating that extracranial vascular changes are probably secondary phenomena. During migraine attacks, the majority of patients show increased heat emission even though not all patients exhibit this phenomenon [87].

In summary, the current state of knowledge regarding thermography establishes that there are measurable heat changes during attacks of migraine and cluster headache, the majority showing increased heat emission indicating extracranial vascular dilation. Between attacks, asymmetrical heat patterns with cold patches also seem to be a common finding. In the hands of experienced thermographic clinicians, this technique may have some diagnostic validity, as it enables one to record the part of the pathophysiological changes that occur during vascular headaches. The most valid information is obtained from changes that occur in the supraorbital, orbital, and temporal areas. Posterior cervical thermographic abnormalities have no correlation with chronic headache syndromes [88].

References

1. Packard RC. What does the headache patient want? *Headache 10*: 370-374, 1979.
2. Kuritzky A, Toglia UJ, Thomas D. Vestibular function in migraine. *Headache 21*: 110-112, 1981.
3. Bartleson JD, Swanson JW, Whisnant JP. A migrainous syndrome with cerebrospinal fluid pleocytosis. *Neurology 31*: 1257-1262, 1981.
4. Brattstrom L, Hindfelt B, Nilsson O. Transient neurological symptoms associated with mononuclear pleocytosis of the cerebrospinal fluid. *Acta Neurol Scand 70*: 104-110, 1984.
5. Verweij RD, Wijdicks EFM, Gijn JV. Warning headache in aneurysmal subarachnoid hemorrhage: A case control study. *Arch Neurol 45*: 1019-1020, 1988.
6. Sargent JD, Silbach P. Medical evaluation of migraineures: Review of the value of laboratory and radiologic tests. *Headache 23*: 62-65, 1983.
7. Amendola MA, Ostrium BJ. Diagnosis of isodense subdural hematoma by computed tomography. *AJR 129*: 693-697, 1977.
8. Mathew NT, Meyer JS, Welch KMA, et al. Abnormal CT scans in migraine. *Headache 16*: 272-279, 1977.
9. Hungerford GD, du Boulay GH, Zilkha KJ. Computerized axial tomography in patients with severe migraine: A preliminary report. *J Neurol Neurosurg Psychiat 39*: 990-944, 1976.
10. Cala LA, Mastaglia FL. Computerized axial tomography in the detection of brain damage; II: Epilepsy, migraine and general medical disorders. *Med J Aust 2*: 616-620, 1980.
11. Dorfman LJ, Marshall WH, Enzmann DR. Cerebral infarction and migraine: Clinical and radiology correlations. *Neurology 29*: 317-322, 1979.
12. Selby G, Fryer JA. Fatal migraine. *Clin Exp Neurol 20*: 85-92, 1984.
13. Goldstein J. Multiple bilateral tiny areas of increased white matter, signal intensity/UBO's (unidentified bright objects) found on MRI scan in a migraine patient. *Headache 26*: 311, 1986.
14. Adelman DC, Saltiel E, Klinenberg J. The neuropsychiatric manifestations of systemic lupus erythematosus: An overview. *Semin Arthritis Rheum 15*: 185-199, 1986.
15. Abel T, Gladman DD, Urowitz MB. Neuropsychiatric lupus. *J Rheumatol 7*: 325-333, 1980.

16. Levine SR, Welch KMA. The spectrum of neurological diseases associated with antiphospholipid antibodies. *Arch Neurol 44*: 876-883, 1987.
17. Shuaib A, Barklay L, Lee MA, et al. Migraine and antiphospholipid antibodies. *Headache 29*: 42-45, 1989.
18. Kennedy DW. Functional endoscopic sinus surgery. *Arch Otolaryngol III*: 643-649, 1985.
19. Labadie EL, Van Antwerp J, Bamford CR. Abnormal lumbar isotope cisternography in an unusual case of spontaneous hypoliquorrheic headache. *Neurology 26*: 135-139, 1976.
20. Baker CC. Headache due to spontaneous low spinal fluid pressure. *Minn Med 66*: 325-328, 1983.
21. Morki B. Sundt TM, Houser OW. Spontaneous internal carotid dissection, hemicrania and Horner's syndrome. *Arch Neurol 36*: 677-680, 1979.
22. Serdaru M, Chiras J, Lhermite F. Isolated benign cerebral vasculitis or migrainous vasospasm? *J Neurol Neurosurg Psychiat 47*: 73-76, 1984.
23. Schon F, Harrison MJH. Can migraine cause multiple segmental cerebral artery constructions. *J Neurol Neurosurg Psychiat 50*: 492-494, 1987.
24. Patterson RH Jr, Goodell H, Dunning HS. Complications of carotid arteriography. *Arch Neurol 10*: 513-520, 1964.
25. Kendall B. Neuro-radiological investigations. In: Warlow C, Morris PJ, (eds). *Transient Ischemic Attacks*, p 154. New York, Marcel Dekker Inc, 1982.
26. Diamond S, Dalessio DJ. *The Practicing Physician's Approach to Headache*, ed 3, p 39. Baltimore, Williams & Wilkins, 1982.
27. Dooling EC, Sweeney VP. Migrainous hemiplegia during breast feeding. *Am J Obstet Gynecol 118*: 568-570, 1974.
28. Ehyai A, Fenichel GM. Natural history of acute confusional migraine. *Arch Neurol 35*: 368-369, 1978.
29. Bartleson JD, Swanson JW, Whisnant JP. A migrainous syndrome with cerebrospinal fluid pleocytosis. *Neurology 31*: 1257-1262, 1981.
30. Lauritzen M, Olesen J. Regional cerebral blood flow during migraine attacks by Xenon-133 inhalation and emission tomography. *Brain 107*: 447-461, 1984.
31. Fitzsimons RB, Wolfeden WH. Migraine coma: Meningitic migraine with cerebral edema associated with a new form of autosomal dominant ataxia. *Brain 10*: 555-577, 1985.
32. Mani RL, Eisenberg RL, McDonald EJ Jr, et al. Complications of catheter cerebral angiography: Analysis of 500 procedures; I: Criteria and incidence. *AJR 131*: 861-865, 1978.
33. Huckman MS, Shenk GI, Neems PL, et al. Transfemoral cerebral angiography vs direct percutaneous carotid and brachial arteriography: A comparison of complications. *Radiology 132*: 93-97, 1979.
34. Shuaib A, Hachinski VC. Migraine and the risks from angiography. *Arch Neurol 45*: 911-912, 1988.
35. Report of American Academy of Neurology: Therapeutic and technology subcommittee. *Neurology 39*: 1100-1101, 1989.
36. Smyth VOG, Winter AL. The EEG in migraine. *Electroencephalogr Clin Neurophysiol 16*: 194-202, 1964.
37. Barolin GS. Bioelectric findings and migraines. In: Dalessio DJ, Dalsgaard-Nielsen T, Diamond S, (eds). *Proceeding of the International Headache Symposium*, pp 9-21, Basel, Sandoz, 1971.
38. Olsen KS. Epidural blood patch in the treatment of post lumbar puncture headache. *Pain 30*: 293-301, 1987.
39. Ostheimer GW. Headache in the postpartum period. In: Marx GF, (ed). *Clinical Management of Mother and Newborn*, pp 27-41. New York, Springer-Verlag, 1979.
40. Crawford JS. Experiences with epidural blood patch. *Anaesthesia 35*: 513-515, 1980.

41. Day TJ, Knezevic W. Cerebrospinal fluid abnormalities associated with migraine. *Med J Aust 141*: 459-461, 1984.
42. Raskin NH. *Headache*, ed 2, pp 81-91. New York, Churchill Livingston, 1988.
43. Beck HG, Schulze WH, Suter GM. Carbon monoxide: A domestic hazard. *JAMA 115*: 1, 1940.
44. Smith FR, Goodman DS. Vitamin A transport in human vitamin A toxicity. *N Engl J Med 294*: 805-808, 1976.
45. Whitfield CL, Ch'ien LT, Whitehead JD. Lead encephalopathy in adults. *Ann Intern Med 52*: 289, 1972.
46. Muenter MD, Perry JO, Ludwig J. Chronic vitamin A intoxication in adults: Hepatic, neurological and dermatologic complications. *Am J Med 50*: 129-136, 1971.
47. Stimson WH. Vitamin A intoxication in adults. *N Engl J Med 265*: 369-373.
48. France RD, Krishnan KRR. The dexamethasone suppression test as a biological marker of depression in chronic pain. *Pain 21*: 49-55, 1985.
49. Diener HC, Ndosi NK, Kiletzki E, et al. Visual evoked potentials in migraine. In: Pfaffenrath V, Lundberg PJ, Sjaastad O, (eds). *Updating in Headache*, pp 101-106. Berlin, Springer-Verlag, 1984.
50. Connolly JF, Gawel M. Rose FC. Migraine patients exhibit abnormalities in the visual evoked potential. *J Neurol Neurosurg Psychiat 45*: 464-467, 1982.
51. Kennard C, Gawel M, Rudolph N, et al. Visual evoked potentials in migraine subjects. *Res Clin Stud Headache 6*: 73-80, 1978.
52. Lehtonen JB. Visual evoked cortical potentials for single flashes and flickering light in migraine. *Headache 14*: 1-12, 1974.
53. Nyrke T, Kangasniemi P, Lang AH, et al. Steady state visual evoked potentials during migraine prophylaxis by propranolol and femoxetine. *Acta Neurol Scand 69*: 9-14, 1984.
54. Rudino F. Visual evoked potential in patients with migraine. *Headache 28*: 531-533, 1988.
55. Dean P, Chi-Wan L, Ziegler D, et al. Clinical and electrophysiological responses to dietary challenge in migraineurs. *Headache 27*: 287-288, 1987.
56. Richey ET, Kooi KA, Waggoner RW. Visually evoked responses in migraine. *Electroencephalogr Clin Neurophysiol 21*: 23-27, 1966.
57. Gawel M, Connolly JF, Rose FC. Migraine patients exhibit abnormalities in the visual evoked potential. *Headache 23*: 49-52, 1983.
58. Muller-Jensen A, Zschocka S. Pattern-induced visual evoked responses in patients with migraine accompagnee. *Electroencephalogr Clin Neurophysiol 50*: 37, 1980.
59. Wenzel D, Brandl U, Harms D. Visual evoked potentials in juvenile complicated migraine. *Electroencephalogr Clin Neurophysiol 53*: 59, 1982.
60. Polich J, Ehlers CL, Dalessio DJ. Pattern-shift visual evoked responses and EEG in migraine. *Headache 26*: 451-456, 1986.
61. Marsters JB, Good HND, Mortimer MJ. A diagnostic test for migraine using the visual evoked potential. *Headache 28*: 526-530, 1988.
62. Jeffreys DA, Axford JG. Source location of pattern specific components of human visual evoked potentials: Component of striate cortical origin. *Exp Brain Res 16*: 1-21, 1972.
63. Leserve N, Joseph JP. Modifications of the pattern evoked potentials (PEP) in relation to the stimulated part of the visual field (clues for the most probable origin of each component). *Electroencephalogr Clin Neurophysiol 47*:183-203, 1979.
64. Wright CE, Drasdo N, Harding GFA. Pathology of the optic nerve and visual association areas: Information given by the flash and pattern visual evoked potential and the temporal and spatial contrast sensitivity function. *Brain 110*: 107-120, 1987.
65. Yamada T, Dickins S. Arensdorf K, et al. Basilar migraine: Polarity-dependent alteration of brainstem auditory evoked potential. *Neurology 36*: 1256-1260, 1986.
66. Podoshin L, Ben-David J, Pratt H, et al. Auditory brainstem evoked potentials in patients with migraine. *Headache 27*: 27-29, 1987.

67. Ganji S. Basilar artery migraine: EEG and evoked potential patterns during acute stage. *Headache 26*: 220-223, 1986.
68. Gawel MJ, Krajewski A. Intracranial hemodynamics in cluster headache. *Headache 28*: 484-487, 1988.
69. Dahl A, Russell D. Transcranial Doppler examination of middle cerebral arteries during cluster headache attacks. *Cephalalgia 7* (suppl 6): 343-344, 1987.
70. Ekbom K, Greitz T. Carotid angiography in cluster headache. *Acta Radiol 10*: 177-186, 1970.
71. Thomas DT, Harpold GJ, Troost BT. Cerebrovascular reactivity in migraineurs as measured by transcranial Doppler (abstr). *Annual Meeting of American Neurological Association*, October 1987.
72. Kudrow L, Sutkus B. MMPI pattern specificity in primary headache disorders. *Headache 19*: 18-24, 1979.
73. Sternbach RA, Dalessio DJ, Kunzel M, et al. MMPI patterns in common headache disorders. *Headache 20*: 311-325, 1980.
74. Weeks R, Baskin S, Sheftell F, et al. A comparison of MMPI personality data and frontalis electromyographic readings in migraine and combination headache patients. *Headache 23*: 75-82, 1983.
75. Watson CPN, Evans RJ, Reed K, et al. Amitriptyline versus placebo in postherpetic neuralgia. *Neurology (NY) 32*: 671-673, 1982.
76. Naliboff BD, Cohen MJ, Yellen AN. Does the MMPI differentiate chronic illness from chronic pain? *Pain 13*: 333-341, 1982.
77. Merskey H, Brown A, Brown J, et al. Psychological normality and abnormality in persistent headache patients. *Pain 23*: 35-47, 1985.
78. Arena JG, Andrasik F, Blanchard EB. The role of personality in the etiology of chronic headache. *Headache 25*: 296-301, 1985.
79. Beck AT, Ward CH, Mendolshon M, et al. An inventory for measuring depression. *Arch Gen Psychiatry 5*: 561-571, 1961.
80. Zung WWK. A self rating depression scale. *Arch Gen Psychiatry 12*: 63-70, 1965.
81. Friedman M, Rosenman RH. Association of specific overt behavior patterns with blood and cardiovascular findings. *JAMA 169*: 1286-1296.
82. Lance JW. Anthony M. Thermography in vascular headache. *Med J Aust*: 240-243, 1971.
83. Mathew NT, Alverez L. The usefulness of thermography in headache. In: Rose FC, (ed). *Progress in Migraine Research*, pp 232-245. London, Pittman, 1984.
84. Swerdlow B, Dieter JN. The validity of the vascular "cold patch" in the diagnosis of chronic headache. *Headache 26*: 22-26, 1986.
85. Kudrow L. Thermography and Doppler flow asymmetry in cluster headache. *Headache 19*: 204-208, 1979.
86. Drummond PD, Lance JW. Thermographic changes in cluster headache. *Neurology 34*: 1292-1298, 1984.
87. Drummond PD, Lance JW. Extracranial vascular changes and source of pain in migraine headaches. *Ann Neurol 13*: 32-37, 1983.
88. Swerdlow B, Dieter JN. Posterior cervical thoracic thermograms pattern persistence and correlation with chronic headache syndrome. *Headache 27*: 10-15, 1987.

7

The Pathophysiology of Headache and the Pharmacology of Anti-Headache Medications

Egilius L.H. Spierings

Introduction

When headache is caused by a derangement in function rather than in structure of tissues of the head or neck, as in muscle contraction headache (now termed tension-type headache) or migraine headache, medications other than analgesics may be effective in relieving the pain. This chapter deals with the pharmacology, i.e., the mode of action, of these medications.

The medications which are effective in relieving headache can be divided into those that provide instant relief, like the vasoconstrictor agents, and those that prevent the occurrence of headaches when taken on a regular basis. The latter group represents the so-called preventive medications and includes agents of different signature, such as antiserotoninergics, beta-adrenoceptor blockers, tricyclic antidepressants, and calcium entry blockers.

Except for the vasoconstrictor agents, usually not all medications of a certain category are effective in relieving headache, which suggests a certain specificity. This specificity may help determine the relevant mode of action of the medications out of the array of pharmacological properties medications usually possess. This is especially important when the pathogenesis of the condition studied is not fully understood, as is the case with headache. Insight into the mode of action of effective medications may help unravel the pathogenetic mechanisms underlying the condition, as a certain specificity is implied.

This chapter focuses on an analysis of the mode of action of the medications effective in relieving headache. The evidence available to document the effectiveness of these medications will not be presented here. The discussion of the pharmacology of the medications will be historical.

Vasoconstrictors

The vasoconstrictor agents represent the oldest group of specific medications used in the treatment of headache. The ergot extract or extractum secalis cornuti aquosum, also known as ergotin, was already used for the treatment of migraine in the second half of the 19th century [1]. It was obtained from the compact mass of hardened mycelium, called sclerotium, which is formed by the fungus Claviceps purpurea in rye infected by it. The ergot extract was in use since the 16th century, especially by midwives, to quicken childbirth and to control postpartum hemorrhage.

The ergot extract was initially used only for the angioparalytic form of migraine, which was suggested by Moellendorf to be due to anenergia of the vasomotor nerves innervating the carotid artery, leading to relaxation of the artery and increased blood flow to the brain [2]. Eulenburg described this form of migraine as hemicrania vasomotoria and Berger called it hemicrania sympathicoparalytica, ascribing the vasodilation and increased blood flow to paralysis of the sympathetic innervation [3].

The angioparalytic form of migraine existed next to the migraine form described several years earlier by du Bois-Reymond as hemicrania sympathicotonica [4]. In this form of migraine the pain was considered to be due to spastic contraction of the blood vessels of the head, secondary to increased sympathetic activity, exerting pressure on adjacent sensory nerves.

What led to the use of the ergot extract in the treatment of the angioparalytic form of migraine was the understanding that the gangrenous form of ergotism, ergotismus gangraenosus, caused by the consumption of Claviceps purpurea-contaminated rye, is due to severe and persistent arterial vasoconstriction. This was revealed by Virchow and his student, von Recklinghausen, through histological studies in the early part of the second half of the 19th century.

In 1906, Dale demonstrated that preparations of the ergot extract caused not only vasoconstriction but also a specific paralysis of motor elements in sympathetically innervated structures [5]. It was also known at that time that responses similar to those obtained from sympathetic stimulation could be elicited by administration of adrenaline. Therefore, an antagonism between adrenaline and the ergot extract was suspected.

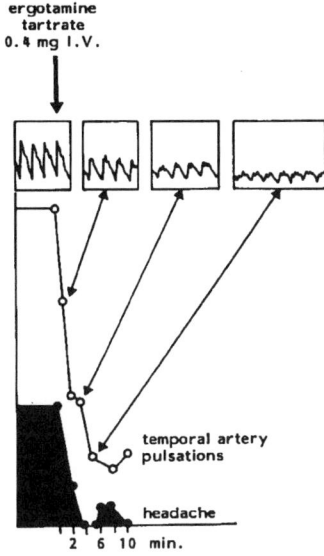

Figure 7.1. Effect of ergotamine tartrate, 0.4 mg intravenously, on the amplitude of pulsation of the superficial temporal artery on the one hand and the intensity of the migraine headache on the other. Note that the two effects of ergotamine are closely parallel to each other. Reproduced with permission from Graham and Wolff [9].

Ergotamine

In 1918, Stoll isolated from the ergot extract the substance ergotamine, which in animal experiments caused powerful contraction of the uterus and in toxic dosages also caused the gangrenous manifestations of ergotism. At that time the use of ergot extract for the treatment of migraine had been largely forgotten and consequently the medication was advocated for use in obstetrics only.

In 1925, Rothlin demonstrated that a pharmacological antagonism exists between ergotamine and adrenaline for sympathetically innervated structures, as had been supposed earlier for adrenaline and the ergot extract [6]. This observation led to the introduction of ergotamine in the treatment of migraine by Maier in 1926 on the basis of du Bois-Reymond's concept of the pathogenesis of the migraine headache [7]. The reasoning was that if the migraine headache is caused by increased sympathetic activity and ergotamine has a sympatholytic action, the medication should be beneficial in migraine. This beneficial effect was subsequently demonstrated in (open) clinical studies in Europe and in the United States [8].

One of the clinical studies performed in the United States was conducted by Lennox at the Boston City Hospital [8]. Subsequently, in 1938 Graham and Wolff established the mode of action of ergotamine in migraine, studying the effects of the medication on the pulsation amplitude of the extracranial arteries [9].

The involvement of the extracranial arteries in migraine was at that time concluded from the observation that the intensity of the migraine headache could be diminished by pressure exerted on the ipsilateral common carotid artery or on the artery at the site of the pain, and on the striking dilation of the temporal artery and vein, as was often seen during attacks of migraine.

In their study, Graham and Wolff showed that distention of the temporal artery by increasing the intramural pressure caused headache, and that manual pressure on the ipsilateral common carotid artery alleviated the pain and also reduced the pulsation amplitude of the ipsilateral temporal artery [9]. They demonstrated that ergotamine decreased the pulsation amplitude of the extracranial arteries but not that of the cranial cerebral arteries. The effect of ergotamine on the extracranial arteries in addition paralleled closely the decrease in headache intensity that followed the administration of the medication in the cases studied (Figure 7.1).

Similar observations were made with regard to adrenaline, and it was noted that dilation of the pupil on pinching the skin of the neck was as readily obtained after administration of ergotamine as it was before it, indicating total absence of a sympatholytic effect. So while it was the sympatholytic action of ergotamine that led to the introduction of the medication in the treatment of migraine, it was the vasoconstrictor effect that ultimately proved to be its relevant mode of action. This was also the mode of action of the ergot extract, the original source of ergotamine, that had been considered relevant more than half a century earlier when the extract was introduced in the treatment of migraine [1]. Today, ergotamine is thought to act by stimulating $5-HT_{1D}$ receptors.

Headache Pathogenesis

Graham and Wolff concluded, on the basis of their experiments, that the migraine headache is due to dilation of extracranial arteries [9]. Heyck objected to this view because of the clinical observation that patients look pale rather than flushed during migraine attacks. He hypothesized that the combination of dilated arteries and veins with relative paleness of the skin indicates specific opening of vascular structures known as arteriovenous anastomoses [10,11].

Arteriovenous anastomoses are vascular structures through which blood can pass directly from the arterial to the venous side of the circulation, bypassing the capillary bed. In man they are present in the skin of the forehead, nose, cheeks, lips, and ears, as well as in the dura mater [12,13]. The arteriovenous anastomoses have a diameter generally larger than 20 μm, which makes them wider than the capillaries that measure from 5 μm to 10 μm. Heyck hypothesized that these vascular structures open at the onset of the migraine attack and through a decrease in peripheral resistance lead to distention of the arteries and through a steal mechanism to decreased perfusion and ischemia of the surrounding tissues [10,11].

Heyck corroborated his hypothesis by measuring the arteriovenous oxygen content difference over the extracranial circulation, sampling blood from the external jugular vein. He showed that the arteriovenous oxygen content difference was significantly lower on the side of the headache than on the nonaffected side. Also, when administration of dihydroergotamine mesylate (D.H.E. 45), a hydrogenated derivative of ergotamine with basically the same mode of action, relieved the migraine headache, he found this beneficial effect to be associated with a significant increase in arteriovenous oxygen content difference [10,11].

Heyck's hypothesis was further experimentally investigated by Spierings and Saxena who studied the effects of both ergotamine and dihydroergotamine on the distribution of carotid blood flow in the cat using 15 μm microspheres [14,15]. These microspheres, when injected arterially, due to their size get trapped in the capillaries but pass through most arteriovenous anastomoses. It was revealed using this technique that both medications reduce the proportion of microspheres passing through the arteriovenous anastomoses, compatible with a constrictor effect on the arteriovenous anastomoses, as had been demonstrated for ergotamine through histological studies by Stolzenburg in 1937 [16].

While Spierings and Saxena's results indirectly supported Heyck's hypothesis, a question remained with regard to Heyck's original experiments. This question related to the significance of the arteriovenous oxygen content difference as an indication of arteriovenous anastomotic blood flow. To investigate this issue further, Spierings and Saxena analyzed the baseline data of their experiments for correlations with the arteriovenous oxygen content difference, measured over the extracranial circulation of the cat by drawing blood from the external jugular vein [15]. It was found that the arteriovenous oxygen content difference correlated significantly with the total amount of blood flow passing through the arteriovenous anastomoses, but this correlation was due to a correlation with the arterial blood flow rather than with the proportion of arterial blood flow shunted through the arteriovenous anastomoses. It was felt that these results had direct bearing on Heyck's observations and basically invalidated the conclusions that he had drawn, despite the fact that the pharmacological experiments with regard to the mode of action of ergotamine and dihydroergotamine were in favor of his hypothesis.

Receptor Pharmacology

Initially, attention was focused on the alpha-adrenoceptors because of the similarities in mode of action between ergotamine and noradrenaline, the alpha-receptor's endogenous substrate. In strips of canine femoral vein, it was found that both the contractions induced by ergotamine and noradrenaline could be blocked in a competitive way by the alpha-adrenoceptor blocker, phentolamine [17]. This suggested that these contractions were mediated through an interaction with alpha-adrenoceptors.

However, several years later when arterial strips were studied and the effects of ergotamine were compared not only with those of noradrenaline but also with those of serotonin, a different conclusion was reached [18]. In these experiments

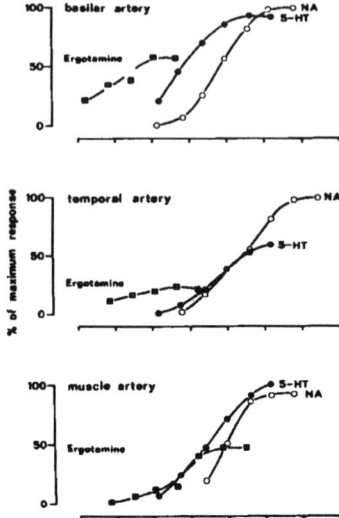

Figure 7.2. Dose-response curves for ergotamine, serotonin (5-HT), and noradrenaline (NA) on helical strips from different human arteries. Note that the maximum response to ergotamine is about half of that to serotonin in all preparations. Reproduced with permission from Mueller-Schweinitzer and Weidmann [18].

that involved bovine, canine, and human artery strips, it was found that ergotamine was the most potent agent in terms of effective concentrations causing contraction. Ergotamine stimulated the different arterial preparations in concentrations 100 times lower than serotonin and 600 times lower than noradrenaline, indicating a very high affinity of the medication for both serotoninergic and alpha-adrenergic receptors.

However, the maximum response elicited by ergotamine in any of the arterial preparations was considerably less than that with either serotonin or noradrenaline. This lower intrinsic activity was similar in the different arterial strips when expressed in terms of the maximum response to serotonin, but varied considerably when expressed in terms of the maximum response to noradrenaline (Figure 7.2). This suggested that ergotamine's vasoconstrictor effect is medicated through an interaction with serotoninergic rather than with alpha-adrenergic receptors as had been previously concluded [18].

Isometheptene Mucate

Another commonly used vasoconstrictor in the treatment of migraine is isometheptene mucate (Midrin), which is an indirectly acting sympathomimetic that releases noradrenaline from the postganglionic sympathetic nerve fibers. In experimental studies, the medication has been shown to decrease carotid blood flow without affecting cerebral blood flow, and similar to ergotamine, to divert blood from the arteriovenous anastomoses to the capillaries [19]. On a general cardiovascular level, isometheptene increases heart rate and blood pressure compatible with a sympathomimetic action of indirect nature involving stimulation of both alpha- and beta-adrenoceptors.

Antiserotoninergics

In an attempt to further elucidate the mechanism of the migraine headache, Wolff and colleagues demonstrated in 1953 that the deep pain threshold is decreased at the site of pain during attacks of migraine [20]. In 1957, Ostfeld and colleagues published evidence for involvement of a humoral factor in the lowering of the pain threshold as well as in the dilation of the blood vessels with adenosine triphosphate, serotonin, and bradykinin as possible candidates [21]. On the chance that serotonin was involved, Graham in 1958 and Ostfeld in 1959 investigated bromo-LSD as the first antiserotoninergic agent studied in the preventive treatment of migraine [22,23]. Graham found the medication to be ineffective but Ostfeld found it effective in a subpopulation of patients in whom intravenous administration of serotonin precipitated headache.

Methysergide maleate (Sansert) was the second antiserotoninergic agent studied in migraine prevention. It, like bromo-LSD, is a derivative of lysergic acid. Both medications come from the laboratories of Sandoz and were developed by Hofmann, who also discovered the hallucinogenic effects of LSD. LSD and bromo-LSD are potent antagonists of serotonin but are surpassed in this activity by methysergide, which is about four times more potent.

Methysergide was first studied in the treatment of migraine by Sicuteri in 1959 and found to be effective as a preventive medication [24]. Before that, Sicuteri had observed that when migraine attacks are precipitated by administration of a vasodilator, such as histamine or nitroglycerin, the onset of these attacks generally occurs many hours later, when the strong vasomotor response has already disappeared. He therefore suggested that, in addition to Wolff's hypothesis that the migraine headache is caused by dilation of extracranial arteries, local activation and/or release of humoral factors also plays a role. He supported this hypothesis by experiments in which he injected serotonin into the superficial temporal artery, causing intense flushing with slight edema in the temple associated with a very intense burning pain. This observation led him to test the potential beneficial effect of methysergide in the treatment of migraine.

Serotonin Agonists

A vasoconstricor medication recently introduced in the treatment of migraine is sumatriptan (Imitrex). It was first shown to be effective in the abortive treatment of migraine by Doenicke et al [24a]. It is a derivative of serotonin and selectively stimulates the type-1 serotonergic receptors which mediate contraction of the isolated canine saphenous vein [24b]. In experimental studies, sumatriptan has also been shown to decrease carotid blood flow [24c] and to divert blood from the arteriovenous anastomoses to the capillaries [24d]. In addition, it has been shown to decrease neurogenic inflammation in the dura mater, but not in the extracranial tissues [24e]. Ergotamine tartrate and dihydroergotamine mesylate (D.H.E. 45) are also 5-HT$_{1D}$ agonists.

Serotonin

In 1961, Sicuteri and colleagues reported that the urinary excretion of the serotonin metabolite, 5-hydroxyindoleacetic acid (5-HIAA), is increased during attacks of migraine [25]. This was confirmed in 1965 by Curran and colleagues, who also observed the platelet serotonin content to be significantly lower during attacks than in the headache-free interval [26]. The decrease in platelet serotonin content has been confirmed many times since and has become the best established biochemical change of the migraine attack [27]. It was also looked upon as the initial event of the migraine attack with the released serotonin causing cerebral vasoconstriction and the migraine aura, and the decrease in platelet (and plasma) serotonin content causing loss of extracranial vascular tone and the migraine headache [28].

The concept that the migraine aura is caused by cerebral vasoconstriction leading to hypoxia is based on the observation that inhalation of the cerebral vasodilator, amyl nitrite, is followed by transient regression of the symptoms [29,30]. This was also observed in experiments with inhalation of 10% carbon dioxide in air, since carbon dioxide also is a cerebral vasodilator [31].

The serotonin hypothesis of migraine was supported by the observation of Lance and colleagues in 1967 that intracarotid injection of serotonin, in man, reduces the pulsation amplitude of the ipsilateral superficial temporal artery [32]. A decrease in external carotid blood flow following intracarotid injection of serotonin was also observed in dogs and monkeys, but in baboons an increase was reported [33,34]. With regard to the internal carotid blood flow, intracarotid injection of serotonin was followed by a decrease in both baboons and monkeys [34-36].

When methysergide was studied on the craniovascular changes induced by serotonin, it was found that the medication attenuated the decrease in internal and external carotid blood flow in the monkey following intracarotid administration of serotonin [34]. In addition, it caused a transient reduction in blood flow in both arteries. A vasoconstrictor effect of methysergide on the external carotid artery was also demonstrated in dogs; in that study methysergide was also found to potentiate the vasoconstrictor effect of intracarotid injection of noradrenaline [33].

Methysergide's beneficial effect in migraine could therefore be due to an antagonism of serotonin-induced cerebral vasoconstriction, and an increase in extracranial vascular tone on the basis of a direct vasoconstrictor effect and a potentiation of the vasoconstrictor effect of noradrenaline. However, no such direct vasoconstrictor effect on the external carotid artery or potentiation of noradrenaline-induced vasoconstriction were observed for cyproheptadine (Periactin) and pizotifen (not available in the U.S.), the two antiserotoninergic agents introduced after methysergide for the prophylactic treatment of migraine [33,37]. Pizotifen, like methysergide, attenuates the decrease in internal carotid blood flow in monkeys following the intracarotid injection of serotonin [37].

The antagonism of cerebral vasoconstriction by the antiserotoninergic agents might have been the mechanism of their beneficial effect in migraine if it were not for the fact that when the cerebral blood flow was studied at a capillary level using the Xenon-clearance technique, it was found that intracarotid injection of serotonin in man does not affect cerebral blood flow [38]. In addition, the cerebral blood flow studies during the migraine aura failed to support the concept that the migraine aura is caused by vasoconstriction-induced cerebral hypoxia [39,40]. In contrast, these studies provided support for a primary neuronal mechanism, such as Leão's spreading depression, as the process underlying the migraine aura.

Central Involvement

In further exploring the role of serotonin in migraine, Sicuteri reported an interesting experiment involving the treatment of migraine with para-chlorophenylalanine, a selective depletor of central and peripheral serotonin [41]. He observed that in several of the patients treated, a pain syndrome developed consisting of deep and superficial hyperalgesia with spontaneous pains in the limbs, trunk, neck, and scalp. The development of such a pain syndrome had not been observed when the medication was administered to nonmigraine patients and therefore, a specific significance was attributed to it.

It had been shown that para-chlorophenylalanine reduced morphine-induced analgesia as had also been demonstrated for lesions of the midbrain raphe nuclei, the main locus of serotoninergic cell bodies in the central nervous system [42,43]. Sicuteri hypothesized that the observed sensitivity of migraine patients to the para-chlorophenylalanine with regard to its effect on pain threshold was due to a deficiency of serotonin in this system [41].

Serotonin has since been shown to exert an inhibitory effect on the transmission of pain signals from the primary sensory afferents to the spino- and trigeminothalamic tracts (Figure 7.3) [44]. This inhibition takes place in the dorsal horn and its rostral extension in the brain stem, the nucleus of the trigeminal tract. It is mediated through the activation of enkephalinergic interneurons, and while studies on the cerebrospinal fluid level of 5-hydroxyindoleacetic acid have been inconclusive [27], the level of enkephalin has been shown to be decreased during migraine attacks, suggesting a decreased activity of the enkephalinergic neurons [45]. Such decreased activity might be due to decreased serotoninergic activation of these neurons and may result in a

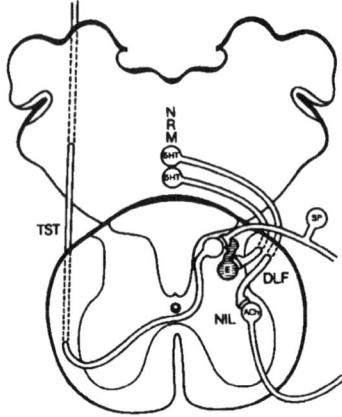

Figure 7.3. The transmission of pain signals from the primary sensory afferents to the spino- and trigeminothalamic tracts (TST) is inhibited by enkephalinergic (E) interneurons (shaded) through a mechanism of presynaptic inhibition. The enkephalinergic interneurons are innervated in turn by serotoninergic (5-HT) fibers originating from the nucleus raphe magnus (NRM) in the brain stem that also innervates the acetylcholinergic (ACh) preganglionic sympathetic fibers that originate from the nucleus intermediolateralis (NIL).

lowering of the pain threshold on a central level. This may be the mechanism involved in addition to the localized decrease in pain threshold at the site of the pain described above, to explain the painfulness of the dilation of the extracranial blood vessels causing the migraine headache.

The involvement of the central serotoninergic system suggests the possibility of another mode of action for the antiserotoninergic agents in migraine, as these medications, including methysergide, pizotifen, and cyproheptadine, at low concentrations potentiate the effects of serotonin, while they antagonize the amine in high concentrations [46]. The relative impermeability of the blood-brain barrier to the medications may determine their central nervous system levels to be significantly lower than their peripheral levels, explaining the difference in mode of action. It has been shown in rats that repeated administration of the above-mentioned antiserotoninergic medications increases brain serotonin levels, which possibly reflects the central proserotoninergic activity of these medications; this would decrease the amount of serotonin necessary to be released for a certain effect to be obtained [47].

Beta-Adrenoceptor Blockers

The anti-headache effect of the beta-adrenoceptor blockers was first noted by Rabkin and colleagues in 1966 in a study on the prophylactic efficacy of propranolol HCl (Inderal) in angina pectoris [48]. They noted prompt relief of long-standing vascular headaches by propranolol in a 59-year-old man, with relapse of the headaches during placebo intake. Subsequently, case reports appeared on the prophylactic treatment of migraine with propranolol, and the first double-blind, placebo-controlled study confirming this effect of propranolol was published in 1972 [49]. Many studies have since appeared confirming propranolol's prophylactic effect in migraine and extending it to the beta-

Table 7.1. Characteristics of the Beta-Adrenoceptor Blockers Effective in the Prophylactic Treatment of Migraine

Agent	Partial agonist activity	Membrane-stabilizing activity	Cardio-selectivity	Penetration into central nervous system
Atenolol (Tenormin)	no	no	yes	poor
Metoprolol tartrate (Lopressor)	no	no	yes	good
Nadolol (Corgard)	no	no	no	poor
Propranolol HCl (Inderal)	no	yes	no	good
Timolol maleate (Blocadren)	no	no	no	good

blockers, atenolol (Tenormin), metoprolol tartrate (Lopressor), nadolol (Corgard), and timolol maleate (Blocadren) [50,51].

Other beta-blockers, including acebutolol HCl (Sectral), alprenolol, oxprenolol, and pindolol (Visken) have also been studied by not found to be effective in migraine [52]. As they are all beta-adrenoceptor blockers, apparently beta blockade as such is not sufficient to explain the prophylactic antimigraine effect of these medications; therefore, an additional characteristic must be relevant. When characteristics such as partial agonist activity, membrane-stabilizing activity, cardioselectivity, and penetration into the central nervous system are considered, the beta-blockers with antimigraine efficacy seem to share a lack of partial agonist activity (Table 7.1).

The lack of partial agonist or intrinsic sympathomimetic activity of the beta-blockers effective in migraine indicates that these medications are devoid of stimulatory effect on the beta-adrenoceptors. The beta-blockers that have been shown to be ineffective as migraine prophylactic medications all possess partial agonist activity and thereby have a stimulatory effect on these receptors. Such an effect is relevant in migraine when dilation of blood vessels is important in its pathogenesis, as blood vessels contain beta-adrenoceptors that promote vasodilation. Then, such an effect is not likely to be beneficial, and may even be detrimental, while beta-blockade without stimulation may be beneficial. This is because of the associated vasoconstriction, as evidenced by the increase in peripheral resistance, that is seen with beta-adrenoceptor blockers that lack partial agonist activity [52].

Tricyclic Antidepressants

In 1964, Lance and Curran published an extensive study on the treatment of chronic muscle contraction headache, now called chronic tension-type headache [53]. This is a headache that occurs all day and every day and supposedly is caused by sustained contraction of the head and neck muscles. Little research has been done on this particular variety of headache, although it is very common. An estimated 5% of the population suffers from headache every day, and a large proportion of this may be accounted for by muscle-contraction headache.

It has been demonstrated in a series of experiments by Simons and Wolff that sustained contraction of muscles of the head and neck can cause headache [54,55]. A possible involvement of the vasculature in the generation of the headache was examined by Tunis and Wolff, and the observation was made that vasoconstriction may be an additional process, reducing the total amount and duration of muscle contraction needed to cause headache by inadequate oxygenation of the tissues [56]. However, this was later refuted by Onel and colleagues who studied the clearance of intramuscularly injected radioactive sodium and found it to be increased during headache supposedly caused by muscle contraction [57].

Whatever the involvement of the vasculature, sustained contraction of muscle does cause pain, not due to inadequate oxygenation, as was originally assumed, but due to accumulation in the muscle of a catabolite other than carbon dioxide or lactic acid [58]. The most important aspect may be the balance between the contraction on the one hand and the blood flow on the other; and it is conceivable that pain may arise from sustained muscle contraction even while blood flow is increased as long as the balance is not met. An example of this may be the headache disorder that we know of as muscle-contraction vascular, mixed, or combined headache in which both mechanisms of sustained muscle contraction and vasodilation are involved.

To relieve the pain of muscle-contraction headache, vasodilator medications such as nicotinic acid and amyl nitrite were first used, but for symptomatic treatment only [59,60]. Preventive treatment was attempted for the first time by Lance and Curran who studied a great number of medications, including amobarbital (Amytal), nicotinic acid, ergotamine, methysergide, diazepam (Valium), amitriptyline HCl (Elavil, Endep), imipramine HCl (Tofranil), and placebo [53]. They found that amitriptyline had the highest preventive efficacy in muscle-contraction headache, followed by imipramine, with both medications being about twice as effective as placebo, while the other medications were equally effective as placebo or only slightly superior. Lance and Curran subsequently performed a double-blind, placebo-controlled study of amitriptyline in chronic muscle-contraction headache and established its efficacy, later confirmed by Diamond and Baltes [61].

Amitriptyline was first reported to be effective in the preventive treatment of migraine by Mahloudji in 1969 which was subsequently confirmed in double-blind, placebo-controlled studies [62-64]. Double-blind, placebo-controlled studies using the tricyclic antidepressant, clomipramine HCl, have shown this medication to be ineffective in migraine prevention [65,66].

Amitriptyline, therefore, is the only tricyclic antidepressant adequately studied and found to be effective in headache, and apparently with preventive efficacy in both migraine and muscle-contraction headache. As amitriptyline is effective in both headache disorders, the mechanism involved must relate to an aspect common to both disorders. Obviously pain is such an aspect, and may be that which is relevant in amitriptyline's beneficial effect, as the medication has also been shown to be effective in several other seemingly unrelated pain conditions. Amitriptyline interferes with the uptake of both serotonin and noradrenaline into the presynaptic nerve endings, thereby potentiating the effects of both amines on the postsynaptic receptors. However, its effect on the uptake of serotonin is much more pronounced than that on the uptake of noradrenaline, justifying the characterization of amitriptyline as a proserotoninergic agent.

In discussing the antiserotoninergic medications, I mentioned the possible involvement of the central serotoninergic system in the pathogenesis of migraine and the possible interaction of the antiserotoninergic medications with this system. The central serotoninergic system, however, may also be involved in the pathogenesis of muscle-contraction headache as well as in the pathogenesis of a great variety of other pain conditions. An effect of amitriptyline on this system, potentiating the effects of it in times of relative under-functioning, may therefore be relevant to its efficacy in headache as well as in other pain conditions. Such a central analgesic effect of tricyclic antidepressants, including amitriptyline, has recently been documented in animal experiments [67].

Calcium Entry Blockers

The calcium entry blockers are medications that interfere with the influx of calcium into cells and cell organelles. They have been introduced into the preventive treatment of migraine on the basis of this effect with regard to brain cells and vascular smooth muscle cells. Through their interference with the influx of calcium into brain cells, these medications have a protective effect on the brain against the deleterious effects of hypoxia. The interference with the calcium influx into vascular smooth muscle cells gives the calcium entry blockers an antivasoconstrictor effect that is nonselective, i.e., independent of the nature of the agent causing the vasoconstriction.

It is hypothesized that through the antivasoconstrictive effect the calcium entry blockers prevent the cerebral vasoconstriction, which, according to Wolff's theory, constitutes the initial step in the pathogenesis of the migraine attack [68]. In addition, through their cerebral hypoxia protective effect they further interfere with what was thought to be the essential component of the pathogenesis of migraine, cerebral hypoxia. In migraine with aura, cerebral hypoxia was considered to be the cause of the aura, and through a mechanism of reactive hyperemia that involved not only the cerebral but also the extracranial circulation, it was considered to be the cause of the headache also.

In migraine without aura, Wolff hypothesized that the hypoxia occurred in a so-called clinically silent area of the cerebral cortex [68].

The first calcium entry blocker to be investigated in migraine treatment was flunarizine (not FDA approved in the United States), which in a double-blind, comparative study with its parent compound, cinnarizine, was shown to decrease the frequency, duration, and intensity of the attacks [69]. The preventive effect of the medication in migraine has subsequently been demonstrated in several double-blind, placebo-controlled studies [70]. Also, several other calcium entry blockers have been studied in migraine, and to date nimodipine (Nomotop) and verapamil HCl (Calan, Isoptin) have been shown to be effective [71].

Since the introduction of the calcium entry blockers, Wolff's theory with regard to the pathogenesis of the migraine aura has come under close fire. This resulted from the cerebral blood flow studies performed since the beginning of the 1980s [39,40]. These studies have demonstrated that the cerebrovascular changes of the migraine aura consist of a localized increase in cerebral blood flow in the occipitoparietal area, followed by a decrease and a gradual spreading of the decrease toward the frontal pole. The spreading decrease in cerebral blood flow was calculated to be in the order of magnitude of 25%, which is not sufficient to cause cerebral hypoxia, although there has been recent discussion about this [40,82]. The forward spreading of the decrease progressed at a speed slightly over 2 mm per minute, and it was this rate of propagation that brought back a hypothesis formulated by Milner in 1958 that the migraine aura is caused by Leão's spreading depression [72]. Leão's spreading depression is a neurophysiological phenomenon described in 1944, consisting of a wave of inhibition of the cortical neuronal activity which travels over the cerebral cortex at a rate calculated to be between 2 to 5 mm per minute [73,74].

In 1941, Lashley calculated that the process underlying the scintillating scotoma, a typical symptom of the migraine aura, travels over the occipital cortex at a rate of 3 mm per minute [75]. The similarity in rate of propagation between Leão's spreading depression and the scintillating scotoma made Milner suggest that spreading depression rather than vasoconstriction-induced hypoxia is responsible for the aura. In addition, Milner felt that the nature of the spreading depression, i.e., inhibition of neuronal activity preceded by a short-lasting phase of intense neuronal activity, better fitted that of the scintillating scotoma than did cerebral hypoxia [74].

With regard to the cerebrovascular changes, Leão demonstrated that the spreading depression is accompanied by vasodilation and an increase in blood flow [76]. This was recently confirmed by Lauritzen and colleagues, who also demonstrated that the increase was only short lasting and was followed by a long-lasting decrease in cerebral blood flow [77]. The decrease was calculated to be in the order of 20% to 25%, which is similar to the decrease observed during the development of the migraine aura [40].

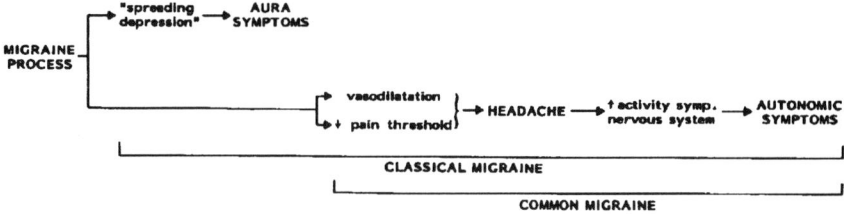

Figure 7.4. Adaptation of Wolff's concept of the pathogenesis of the migraine attack with inclusion of spreading depression as the underlying mechanism of the migraine aura. Note that in this concept the pathogenetic processes underlying the migraine aura and headache are viewed as parallel rather than as sequential, and that the concept also includes an explanation of the autonomic symptoms of migraine.

Of the calcium entry blockers, flunarizine has recently been shown to affect the spreading depression in terms of interfering with its initiation and propagation [78]. It is doubtful, however, that this action, even if applicable to all calcium entry blockers, explains their beneficial effect in migraine. The reason is that it is hard to conceive that spreading depression can occupy the same central position in the pathogenesis of the migraine attack as hypoxia did in Wolff's theory. This is because spreading depression is not followed by an increase in cerebral blood flow but by a decrease, and there is no evidence that spreading depression can be induced by vasoconstriction. The initiation of spreading depression probably needs an excitatory stimulus, as it is actually not a spreading depression but a spreading excitation followed by inhibition of the neuronal activity [74].

One way of incorporating spreading depression into Wolff's theory is by putting it in place of both the vasoconstriction and cerebral hypoxia, and by disconnecting the pathogenesis of the migraine aura from that of the migraine headache, i.e., by looking upon them as parallel rather than as sequential processes (Figure 7.4). This would also better explain the independent occurrence of the different parts of the migraine syndrome, i.e., the headache without aura, as in common migraine, and the aura without headache, as in what has been referred to by Fisher as "transient migrainous accompaniments," and what I have termed "isolated neurological migraine accompaniments" [79,80]. Such an incorporation of the spreading depression in Wolff's theory would, however, still not explain the efficacy of the calcium entry blockers in migraine beyond the aura.

Conclusions

As is evident, the majority of the medications that are not analgesics but still effective in relieving headache have been studied in relation to migraine.

Migraine is the nonstructural or functional headache disorder that has attracted more medical attention than any other headache disorder, probably because of its impressive and often fascinating manifestations. It is also a headache disorder that is common in our society, with an estimated 9% of men, 16% of women, and 3% to 4% of children suffering from it [81]. However, it is probably not the most common headache disorder that affects mankind, which in all likelihood is chronic tension-type headache. Because of its all day and every day occurrence, chronic tension-type headache is a disorder responsible for a great deal of suffering, not so much because of its intensity but because of its unrelenting character.

Regarding medical treatment of chronic tension-type headache, amitriptyline is basically the only medication with a well-established efficacy. The effect of amitriptyline on chronic tension-type headache is, however, probably nonspecific as the medication is also effective in other pain conditions with seemingly unrelated pathogenesis. One of these other pain conditions is migraine, in which amitriptyline is only one of the several medications that have been proven to be effective. The specificity of the other medications is basically unknown, as these medications have not been investigated in other pain conditions; it is, however, my assumption that there is at least some specificity to their effect.

In the above presented modification of Wolff's theory, the antiserotoninergic agents can be hypothesized to act on the mechanism of the migraine headache by hampering vasodilation, as with methysergide, or by potentiating the inhibiting effect of serotonin on the transmission of pain signals in the central nervous system, as with pizotifen and cyproheptadine. This would make the mode of action of the latter medications in migraine basically the same as that of amitriptyline, which raises the question whether these medications are also effective in relieving chronic tension-type headache. In this regard, it is interesting to note that amitriptyline, pizotifen, and cyproheptadine are the only antiheadache medications structurally related, as they all possess a tricyclic structure.

The beta-adrenoceptor blockers in the above concept would probably also have their main effect on the pathogenesis of the migraine headache, hampering vasodilation through an increase in vascular tone secondary to blockade of beta-receptors without agonist activity. The mode of action of the calcium entry blockers, apart from a possible interference with the spreading depression, remains a question. Finally, the vasoconstrictors that are effective in the abortive treatment of migraine seem to have the most straightforward action, i.e., constriction of the painfully dilated extracranial blood vessels causing the migraine headache.

References

1. Eulenburg A. Zur Pathologie des Sympathicus. *Berl Klin Wschr 10*: 169-180, 1873.

2. Moellendorf. Ueber Hemikranie. *Arch Pathol Anat Physiol Klin Med 41*: 385-395, 1867.
3. Berger O. Zur Pathogenese der Hemicranie. *Arch Pathol Anat Physiol Klin Med 59*: 315-340, 1874.
4. du Bois-Reymond E. Zur Kenntniss der Hemikrania. *Arch Anat Physiol 4*: 461-468, 1860.
5. Dale HH. On some physiological actions of ergot. *J Physiol 34*: 163-206. 1906.
6. Rothlin E. Ueber die pharmakologische und therapeutische Wirkung des Ergotamins auf den Sympathicus. *Klin Wschr 4*: 1437-1443, 1925.
7. Maier HW. L'ergotamine inhibiteur du sympathique etudié en clinique comme moyen d'exploration et comme agent therapeutique. *Rev Neurol 33*: 1104-1108, 1926.
8. Lennox WG. The use of ergotamine tartrate in migraine. *N Engl J Med 210*: 1061-1065, 1934.
9. Graham JR, Wolff HG. Mechanism of migraine headache and action of ergotamine tartrate. *Arch Neurol Psychiat 39*: 737-763, 1938.
10. Heyck H. *Neue Beitraege zur Klinik und Pathogenese der Migraene*. Stuttgart, Georg Thieme Verlag, 1956.
11. Heyck H. Pathogenesis of migraine. *Res Clin Stud Headache 2*: 1-28, 1969.
12. Sucquet JP. *D'une Circulation Dérivative dans les Members et dans la Tête chez l'Homme*. Paris, Delahaya, 1862.
13. Rowbotham GF, Little E. New concepts on the aetiology and vascularization of meningiomata; the mechanisms of migraine; the chemical processes of the cerebrospinal fluid; and the formation of collections of blood or fluid in the subdural space. *Br J Surg 52*: 21-24, 1965.
14. Spierings ELH, Saxena PR. The action of ergotamine on the distribution of carotid blood flow: The migraine shunt theory revisited. *Headache 20*: 143-145, 1980.
15. Spierings ELH, Saxena PR. Antimigraine drugs and cranial arteriovenous shunting in the cat. *Neurology 30*: 696-701, 1980.
16. Stolzenburg HJ. Experimentelle Untersuchungen ueber das Verhalten der arterivenoese anastomosen. *Zschr Mikr-Anat Forsch 41*: 348-358, 1937.
17. Mueller-Schweinitzer E, Stuermer E. Investigations on the mode of action of ergotamine in the isolated femoral vein of the dog. *Br J Pharmacol 51*: 441-446, 1974.
18. Mueller-Schweinitzer E, Weidmann H. Regional differences in the responsiveness of isolated arteries from cattle, dog and man. *Agents Actions 7*: 383-389, 1977.
19. Spierings ELH, Saxena PR. Effect of isometheptene on the distribution and shunting of 15 μm microspheres throughout the cephalic circulation of the cat. *Headache 20*: 103-105, 1980.
20. Wolff HG, Tunis MM, Goodell H. Evidence of tissue damage and changes in pain sensitivity in subjects with vascular headaches of the migraine type. *Arch Intern Med 92*: 478-484, 1953.
21. Ostfeld AM, Chapman LF, Goodell H, et al. Summary of evidence concerning a noxious agent active locally during migraine headache. *Psychosom Med 19*: 199-208, 1957.
22. Graham JR. Use of a new compound, UML-491 (1-methyl-d-lysergic acid butanolamide), in the prevention of various types of headache. *N Engl J Med 263*: 1273-1277, 1960.
23. Ostfeld AM. Some aspects of cardiovascular regulation in man. *Angiology 10*: 34-42, 1959.
24. Scuteri F. Prophylactic and therapeutic properties of 1-methyl-lysergic acid butanolamide in migraine. *Int Arch Allergy Appl Immunol 15*: 300-307, 1959.
24a. Doenicke A, Brand J, Perrin VL. Possible benefit of GR 43715, a novel 5-HT1-like receptor agonist, for the acute treatment of severe migraine. *Lancet 1:* 1309-1311, 1988.
24b. Humphrey PPA, Feniuk W, Perrin MJ, et al. GR 43175 – a selective agonist for the functional 5-HT1-like receptors in dog saphenous vein. *Br J Pharmacol 92*: 616, 1987.
24c. Brittain RT, Butina D, Coates IH, et al. GR 43175 selectively constricts the canine arterial bed via stimulation of 5-HT1-like receptors. *Br J Pharmocol 91*: 618, 1987.
24d. Feniuk W, Humphrey PPA, Perren MJ. Selective vasoconstricotr action of GR 43175 on arteriovenous anastomoses (AVAs) in the anaesthetised cat. *Br J Pharmacol 92:* 756, 1987.

24e. Buzzi MG, Moskowitz MA. The antimigraine drug, sumatriptan (GR 43175), selectively blocks neurogenic plasma extravasation from blood vessels in dura mater. *Br J Pharmacol* 99: 202-206, 1990.
25. Sicuteri F, Testi A, Anselmi B. Biochemical investigations in headache: Increase in the hydroxyindoleacetic acid excretion during migraine attacks. *Int Arch Allergy Appl Immunol* 19: 55-58, 1961.
26. Curran DA, Hinterberger H, Lance JW. Total plasma serotonin, 5-hydroxyindoleacetic acid and p-hydroxy-m-methoxymandelic acid excretion in normal and migrainous subjects. *Brain* 88: 997-1010, 1965.
27. Spierings ELH. *The Pathophysiology of the Migraine Attack.* Brussels, Stafleu's Scientific Publishing Company, 1980.
28. Anthony M, Hinterberger H, Lance JW. The possible relationship of serotonin to the migraine syndrome. *Res Clin Stud Headache* 2: 29-59, 1969.
29. Schumacher GA, Wolff HG. Experimental studies in headache: A. Contrast of histamine headache with the headache of migraine and that associated with hypertension. B. Contrast of vascular mechanisms in preheadache and in headache phenomena of migraine. *Arch Neurol Psychiat* 45: 199-214, 1941.
30. Hare EH. Personal observations on the spectral march of migraine. *J Neurol Sci* 3: 259-264, 1966.
31. Marcussen RM, Wolff HG. Studies on headache: 1. Effects of carbon dioxide-oxygen mixtures given during the preheadache phase of the migraine attack. 2. Further analysis of pain mechanisms in headache. *Arch Neurol Psychiat* 63: 42-51, 1950.
32. Lance JW, Anthony M, Gonski A. Serotonin, the carotid body and cranial vessels in migraine. *Arch Neurol* 16: 553-558, 1967.
33. Saxena PR. The effects of antimigraine drugs on the vascular responses by 5-hydroxytryptamine and related biogenic substances on the external carotid bed of dogs: Possible pharmacological implications to their antimigraine action. *Headache* 12: 44-54, 1972.
34. Welch KMA, Spira PJ, Knowled L, et al. Simultaneous measurement of internal and external carotid blood flow in the monkey. *Neurology* 24: 450-457, 1974.
35. Grimson BS, Robinson SC, Danford ET, et al. Effect of serotonin on internal and external carotid artery blood flow in the baboon. *Am J Physiol* 216: 50-55, 1969.
36. Deshmukj VD, Harper AM. The effect of serotonin on cerebral and extracerebral blood flow with possible implications in migraine. *Acta Neurol Scand* 49: 649-658, 1973.
37. Mylecharane EJ, Spira PJ, Misbach J, et al. Effects of methysergide, pizotifen and ergotamine in the monkey cranial circulation. *Eur J Pharmacol* 48: 1-9, 1978.
38. Olesen J. Effect of serotonin on regional cerebral blood flow (rCBF) in man. *Cephalalgia* 1: 1-10, 1981.
39. Olesen J, Larsen B, Lauritzen M. Focal hyperemia followed by spreading oligemia and impaired activation of CBF in classic migraine. *Ann Neurol* 9: 344-352, 1981.
40. Lauritzen M, Olsen TS, Lassen NA, et al. Changes in regional cerebral blood flow during the course of classic migraine attacks. *Ann Neurol* 13: 633-641, 1983.
41. Sicuteri F. Pain syndrome in man following treatment with p-chlorophenylalanine. *Pharmacol Res Commun* 3: 401-407, 1971.
42. Tenen SS. Antagonism of the analgesic effect of morphine and other drugs by p-chlorophenylalanine, a serotonin depletor. *Psychopharmacology* 12: 278-285, 1968.
43. Samanin R, Gumulka W, Valzelli L. Reduced effect of morphine in midbrain raphe lesioned rats. *Eur J Pharmacol* 10: 339-343, 1970.
44. Basbaum AI, Fields HL. Endogenous pain control mechanisms: Review and hypothesis. *Ann Neurol* 4: 451-462, 1978.
45. Anselmi B, Baldi E, Cassacci F, et al. Endogenous opioids in cerebrospinal fluid and blood in idiopathic headache sufferers. *Headache* 20: 294-299, 1980.

46. Hardebo JE, Edvinsson L, Owman CH, et al. Potentiation and antagonism of serotonin effects on intracranial vessels. *Neurology 28*: 64-70, 1978.
47. Hole K. The effects of cyproheptadine, methysergide, BC 105 and reserpine on brain 5-hydroxytryptamine and brain growth. *Eur J Pharmacol 19*: 156-159, 1972.
48. Rabkin R, Stables DP, Levin NW, et al. The prophylactic value of propranolol in angina pectoris. *Am J Cardiol 18*: 370-380, 1966.
49. Weber RB, Reinmuth OM. The treatment of migraine with propranolol. *Neurology 22*: 366-369, 1972.
50. Weerasuriya K, Patel L, Turner P. Beta-adrenoceptor blockade and migraine. *Cephalalgia 2*: 33-45, 1982.
51. Ryan RE, Ryan RE Jr, Sudilovsky A. Nadolol: Its use in the prophylactic treatment of migraine. *Headache 23*: 26-31, 1983.
52. Man in 't Veld AJ, Schalekamp MADH. How intrinsic sympathomimetic activity modulates the haemodynamic responses to beta-adrenoceptor antagonists: A clue to the nature of their antihypertensive mechanism. *Br J Clin Pharmacol 14*: 733-737, 1982.
53. Lance JW, Curran DA. Treatment of chronic tension headache. *Lancet 1*: 1236-1239, 1964.
54. Simons DJ, Day E, Goodell H, et al. Experimental studies on headache: Muscles of the scalp and neck as sources of pain. *Proc Assoc Res Nerve Ment Dis 23*: 228-244, 1943.
55. Simons DJ, Wolff HG. Studies on headache: Mechanisms of chronic post-traumatic headache. *Psychosom Med 8*: 227-242, 1946.
56. Tunis M, Wolff HG. Studies on headache: Cranial artery vasoconstriction and muscle contraction headache. *Arch Neurol Psychiat 71*: 425-434, 1954.
57. Onel Y, Friedman AP, Grossman J. Muscle blood flow studies in muscle-contraction headache. *Neurology 11*: 935-939, 1961.
58. Rodbard S. Pain associated with muscle contraction. *Headache 10*: 105-115, 1970.
59. Brazil P, Friedman AP. Craniovascular studies in headache: A report and analysis of pulse volume tracings. *Neurology 6*: 96-102, 1956.
60. Ostfeld AM, Reis DJ, Wolff HG. Studies in headache: Bulbar conjunctival ischemia and muscle contraction headache. *Arch Neurol Psychiat 77*: 113-119, 1957.
61. Diamond S, Baltes BJ. Chronic tension headache treated with amitriptyline: A double-blind study. *Headache 11*: 110-116, 1971.
62. Mahloudji M. Prevention of migraine. *Br Med J 1*: 182-183, 1969.
63. Gomersall JD, Stuart A. Amitriptyline in migraine prophylaxis. Changes in pattern of attacks during a controlled clinical trial. *J Neurol Neurosurg Psychiat 36*: 684-690, 1973.
64. Couch JR, Hassanein RS. Amitriptyline in migraine prophylaxis. *Arch Neurol 36*: 695-699, 1979.
65. Noone JF. Clomipramine in the prevention of migraine. *J Int Med Res 8 (supp 3)*: 49-52, 1980.
66. Langohr HD, Gerber WD, Koletzki E, et al. Clomipramine and metoprolol in headache prophylaxis: A double-blind crossover study. *Headache 25*: 107-113, 1985.
67. Spiegel K, Kalb R, Pasternak GW. Analgesic activity of tricyclic antidepressants. *Ann Neurol 13*: 462-465, 1983.
68. Wolff HG; Dalessio DJ (eds). *Headache and Other Head Pain*, 4th ed. New York, Oxford University Press, 1980.
69. Drillisch C, Girke W. Ergebnisse der Behandlung von Migraene-Patienten mit Cinnarizin und Flunarizin. *Med Welt 31*: 1870-1872, 1980.
70. Spierings ELH. The efficacy of the calcium entry blocker flunarizine in the prophylactic treatment of migraine. *Int Angio 3 (supp 2)*: 81-87, 1984.
71. Spierings ELH. Clinical and experimental evidence for a role of calcium entry blockers in the treatment of migraine. *Ann NY Acad Sci 522*: 676-689, 1988.
72. Milner PM. Note on a possible correspondence between the scotomas of migraine and spreading depression of Leão. *Electroencephalogr Clin Neurophysiol 10*: 705, 1958.

73. Leão AAP. Spreading depression of activity in the cerebral cortex. *J Neurophysiol 7*: 359-390, 1944.
74. Grafstein B. Mechanism of spreading cortical depression. *J Neurophysiol 19*: 154-171, 1956.
75. Lashley KS. Patterns of cerebral integration indicated by the scotomas of migraine. *Arch Neurol Psychiat 46*: 331-339, 1941.
76. Leão AAP. Pial circulation and spreading depression of activity in the cerebral cortex. *J Neurophysiol 7*: 391-396, 1944.
77. Lauritzen M, Jorgensen MB, Diemer NH, et al. Persistent oligemia of rat cerebral cortex in the wake of spreading depression. *Ann Neurol 12*: 469-474, 1982.
78. Wauquier A, Ashton D, Marrannes R. The effects of flunarizine in experimental models related to the pathogenesis of migraine. *Cephalalgia 5 (supp 2)*: 119-123, 1985.
79. Fisher CM. Late-life migraine accompaniments as a cause of unexplained transient ischemic attacks. *Can J Neurol Sci 7*: 9-17, 1980.
80. Spierings ELH. Migraine: Symptomatology and pathogenesis. *Sandorama (English edition) 2*: 26-34, 1985.
81. Goldstein M, Chen TC. The epidemiology of disabling headache. In: Critchley M, Friedman AP, Goroni S, et al, (eds). *Headache: Physiopathological and Clinical Concepts*. New York, Raven Press, 1982.
82. Olsen TS, Friberg L, Lassen NA. Ischemia may be the primary cause of the neurologic deficits in classic migraine. *Arch Neurol 44*: 156-161, 1987.

Copyright © 1993 PMA Publishing Corp.
Headache: A Clinician's Guide to Diagnosis, Pathophysiology, and Treatment Strategies
Edited by Alan M. Rapoport, M.D. and Fred D. Sheftell, M.D.

8

Migraine: Diagnosis, Pathogenesis, and Treatment

Egilius L.H. Spierings

Introduction

Migraine is a ubiquitous disorder whose prevalence in modern western societies has been estimated to be 9% in men, 16% in women, and 3% to 4% in children [1]. The occurrence of migraine rises sharply during the teens and then stabilizes between the ages of 20 and 40 years, with a decline slowly after the fourth decade of life. Thus, it most severely affects men and women in their years of highest productivity.

Clinically, migraine is characterized by the occurrence of attacks of which headache is the most constant feature. The attacks generally last from a couple of hours to a few days, and they can occur at a greatly varying frequency, up to several times per week. The headache is usually severe in intensity and throbbing in nature with a preference for location in the temple, frequently just on one side of the head. It is often associated with symptoms of gastrointestinal distress such as anorexia, nausea, vomiting, and diarrhea, and with increased sensitivity to light and noises to the extent that exposure to these stimuli may sharply increase the intensity of the pain. In classic migraine (now termed migraine with aura), the headache is preceded by transient focal neurological symptoms, generally known as aura symptoms, making it the most complete

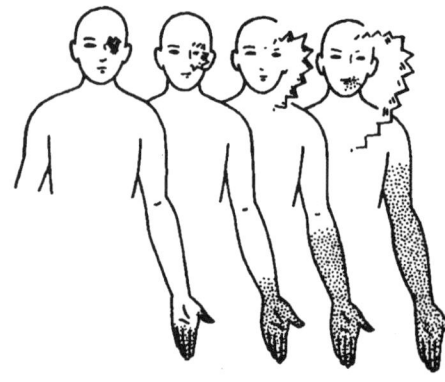

Figure 8.1. The two most characteristic transient focal neurological or aura symptoms of migraine, the scintillating scotoma and digitolingual paresthesias, shown from left to right in their successive stages of development.

migraine syndrome and differentiating it from so-called common migraine (now termed migraine without aura) in which such symptoms do not occur.

Migraine without aura is much more prevalent than migraine with aura and may account for as much as 90% of all migraine. The headache in common migraine is basically the same as in migraine with aura although often more intense and of longer duration. Autonomic symptoms such as pallor, anorexia, nausea, vomiting, diarrhea, cold extremities, and diaphoresis are also generally more prominent.

Migraine Aura

The aura symptoms of classic migraine are almost always visual or somatosensory in nature although a speech disorder can also occur. The two most characteristic examples of the visual and somatosensory disturbances of migraine are the so-called scintillating scotoma and digitolingual paresthesias, shown schematically in Figure 8.1 in their successive stages of development. The scintillating scotoma, also known as teichopsia or fortification spectra, is a visual disturbance that starts off near the center of vision as a small spot surrounded by bright, often flickering and sometimes colorful, zigzag lines. After slight enlargement of the spot, the circle of zigzag lines breaks open on the inner side to take the form of a horseshoe and in that form gradually expands further into the periphery where it ultimately fades away. Vision is usually obscured not only by the zigzag lines but also by a band of dimness that lies against the zigzag lines on the inside of the horseshoe.

The visual disturbance from the moment of its onset near the center of vision to its disappearance in the periphery, generally lasts from 10 minutes to 30 minutes with an average of 20 minutes. This is also the approximate duration of the digitolingual paresthesias. The paresthesias consist of a feeling of numbness or pins-and-needles that starts in the fingers of one hand and gradually extends upward into the arm, ultimately involving the face, especially the nose and mouth area on the same side.

In general, the somatosensory disturbance follows the visual disturbance but can also occur alone, though not as commonly as the visual disturbance. The headache can follow the visual or somatosensory disturbance immediately but can also occur after a certain interval, e.g., up to one hour. The headache can be unilateral and may not necessarily occur on the same side as the visual or somatosensory disturbance, or the headache can be bilateral [2].

The visual disturbance generally affects one side of the visual field only, while the somatosensory disturbance is always limited to one side of the body, distinguishing it from the bilateral numbness of hands and mouth that can occur with hyperventilation, of which headache may also be a symptom. The visual and/or somatosensory disturbance may also occur without being followed by headache, which has been referred to as "transient migrainous accompaniments" (TMAs) and also termed "isolated neurological migraine accompaniments" (INMAs) [3,4]. Among older patients this may present an important differential diagnostic consideration since it must be distinguished from transient ischemic attacks (TIAs) in which transient focal neurological symptoms occur, characteristically not followed by headache, on the basis of a thromboembolic as opposed to a migrainous process.

Sometimes the somatosensory disturbance is so pronounced as to create the impression that the extremity involved is paralyzed; however, examination will disprove this. If a migraine attack is indeed accompanied by paresis or paralysis, it is either hemiplegic or complicated migraine. The former is a condition that occurs almost exclusively in childhood, often with a strong family history, and the latter is an attack of migraine complicated by stroke. In either case, the paresis or paralysis develops during the headache, often at the peak of it, and lasts longer than the attack itself with permanent sequelae common in complicated migraine. However, more frequent in complicated migraine than hemiparesis is a homonymous hemianopia that usually also leads to permanent impairment of vision.

Symptoms of loss of nervous system function in migraine constitute an indication for further examination in order to exclude other pathology, such as arteriovenous malformation in case of hemiplegic migraine and other causes of stroke, such as arteritis associated with collagen vascular disease, infection or granulomatous disease, and coagulation disorder in complicated migraine.

Spreading Depression

The pathogenesis of the migraine aura has long been thought to be that of vasoconstriction-induced cerebral hypoxia (Figure 8.2) [5]. This notion is based on experiments with cerebral vasodilator agents, such as carbon dioxide and amyl nitrite, which showed a transient clearing of the symptoms following inhalation of the respective agents with return of the symptoms afterwards [6-8]. Actual blood flow measurements, performed since the 1970s, however, initially

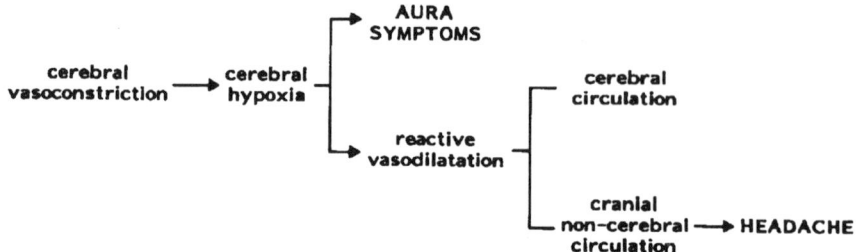

Figure 8.2. Schematic representation of the vasoconstriction – cerebral hypoxia – vasodilation concept of the pathogenesis of the migraine attack as proposed by Wolff in the 1950s [5].

showed a generalized and bilateral decrease in cerebral blood flow despite the focal and lateralized nature of the symptoms, which, in addition, outlasted the duration of the symptoms [9-11]. This generalized decrease in cerebral blood flow has been shown more recently to be but the final step in a series of changes [12,13]. These changes consist of an initial short-lasting increase in cerebral blood flow in the occipitoparietal area, followed by a decrease and a gradual spreading of the decrease toward the frontal pole (Figure 8.3). The decrease is in the order of 25%, not enough to cause neuronal dysfunction by ischemia, which needs a decrease in cerebral flood flow of at least 50%. The decrease was therefore referred to as oligemia rather than ischemia, and the rate of forward spreading of the oligemia was determined to be approximately 2.2 mm/min [13]. It is, however, possible that with the technique used and due to scattered radiation, small areas of hypoxia occur which are currently not being picked up [13a].

The particular nature of the cerebral blood flow changes observed during the migraine aura, as described above, has shed new light on a hypothesis regarding the pathogenesis of these symptoms as formulated by Milner in 1958 [14]. This hypothesis states that the aura symptoms are caused by a primary neuronal process like the one described by Leão in 1944 as "spreading depression" [15]. The suggestion was made on the basis of the observed similarities in features and rate of propagation of the scintillating scotoma and spreading depression. The rate of propagation of the scintillating scotoma had been calculated by Lashley in 1941 to be approximately 3 mm/min [16]. Spreading depression has been described as a wave of inhibition of the "spontaneous" neuronal activity that travels over the cerebral cortex at a rate of 2 mm to 5 mm/min [15,17]. The inhibition of neuronal activity is preceded by a short-lasting phase of intense neuronal activity, which could account for the positive features of the aura symptoms, i.e., the flickering sensations in the visual disturbance and the sensation of pins-and-needles in the somatosensory disturbance [17]. The vascular changes accompanying the spreading depression consist of a short-

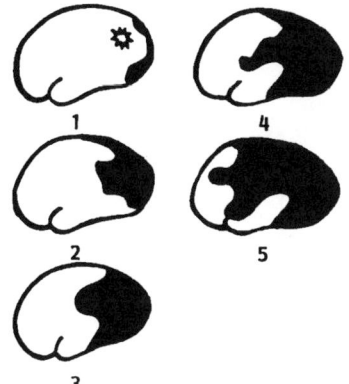

Figure 8.3. Schematic representation of the cerebral blood flow changes of the transient focal neurological or aura symptoms of migraine. These changes have recently been shown to consist of an initial short-lasting increase in cerebral blood flow in the occipito-parietal area (*), followed by a decrease and a gradual spreading of the decrease toward the frontal pole [12,13].

lasting increase in cerebral blood flow followed by a long-lasting decrease of 20% to 25% [18].

Welch et al recently studied energy metabolism in the brain as well as intracellular pH using 31-phosphorus NMR spectroscopy in patients with migraine [18a]. Only in the patients with migraine with aura did they observe a decrease in the brain phosphorylation potential during the attack while intracellular pH was unchanged. The lack of change in intracellular pH during the migraine attack argues against the occurrence of cerebral ischemia as this would be associated with relative acidosis. The decrease in phosphorylation potential indicates decreased energy metabolism in the brain during attacks of migraine with aura. Using the same technique, it was also found that patients with migraine have a decreased intracellular concentration of magnesium in the brain during the attack [18b]. In patients with common migraine, the concentration of magnesium in the erythrocytes has also been observed to be decreased between the attacks [18c]. It is worth noting that magnesium is an important co-factor in energy metabolism and that its deficiency is associated with increased excitability of, among others, brain tissue making it more vulnerable to spreading depression.

MIGRAINE HEADACHE

The migraine headache is presumably caused by dilation of blood vessels in the extracranial circulation, an assumption based on indirect evidence only. This indirect evidence involves the positive response of the headache to the potent vasoconstrictor agent, ergotamine, and the lack of response to dampening of the cerebral vascular pulsations through increasing the cerebrospinal fluid pressure [7,19]. In addition, Graham and Wolff have demonstrated that the effect of ergotamine on the migraine headache occurs very much in parallel to a decrease in pulsation amplitude of the extracranial blood vessels [19]. The superficial temporal artery seems to be preferentially involved in the process of

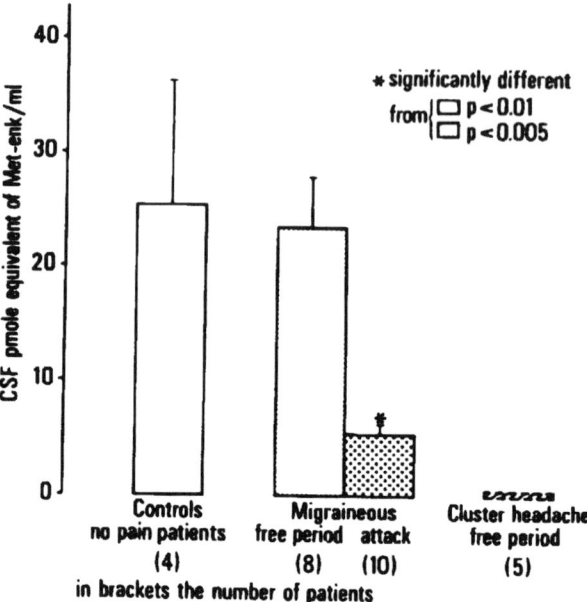

Figure 8.4. Enkephalin level in the cerebrospinal fluid in control patients and in patients with migraine and cluster headache. Note the low level of enkephalin in the migraine patients during attacks and in the cluster headache patients. Reproduced with permission from Anselmi et al [22].

migrainous vasodilation, giving rise to the throbbing pain in the temple so characteristic of migraine.

In the pathogenesis of the migraine headache, apart from dilation of extracranial blood vessels, a decrease in pain threshold may also play a role. This lowering of pain threshold may be due to a peripheral as well as a central mechanism. The peripheral mechanism may include the local release into the tissues of pain-provoking substances, such as substance P and bradykinin. Substance P is the neurotransmitter of the primary sensory nerve fibers that carry pain signals from the periphery of the body to the central nervous system. Upon activation of these fibers, substance P is not only released in the central nervous system but also in the peripheral tissues, causing a decrease in pain threshold locally. The involvement of such a mechanism is suggested by the observation of a decreased pain threshold at the site of the pain as well as of a local accumulation of a pain threshold lowering and vasodilating substance, formerly referred to as "neurokinin" [20,21]. In addition, on the basis of the mode of action of antimigraine medications such as ergotamine and methysergide, it has been suggested that neurogenic inflammation in the dura mater plays a role as well [21a].

The central nervous system mechanism involved in lowering the pain threshold may be a decreased activity of the so-called enkephalinergic interneurons. These neurons secrete enkephalin, an endogenous opiate, as their neurotransmitter, and they have an inhibitory effect on the entry of pain stimuli into

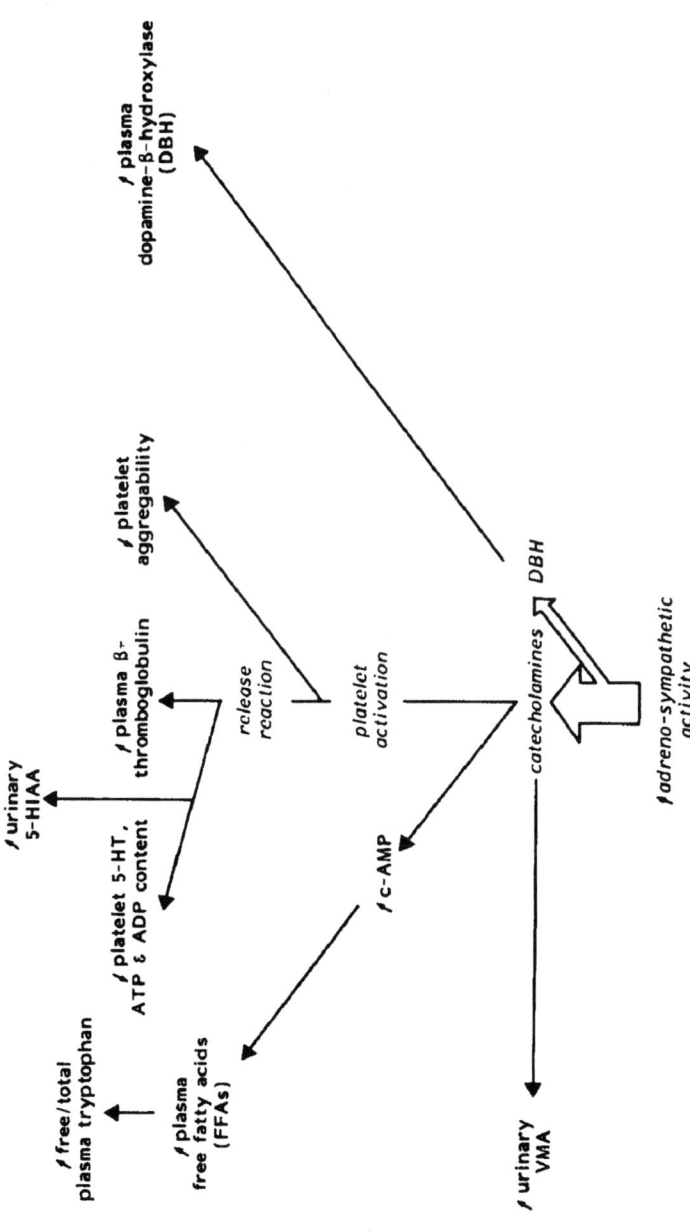

Figure 8.5. Schematic representation of the biochemical changes of the migraine attack, conceived as interrelated consequences of an increased activity of the sympathetic nervous system.

the central nervous system. The finding of a decreased enkephalin level of the cerebrospinal fluid is in support of such a mechanism (Figure 8.4) [22].

AUTONOMIC SYMPTOMS

The autonomic symptoms of migraine are probably due to increased activity of the sympathetic nervous system that has been attributed to the headache, which is generally intense in migraine [23]. This assumption is supported by evidence from biochemical research that has shown several parameters of sympathetic function to be increased during the migraine attack. These parameters include the plasma level of noradrenaline, the neurotransmitter of the postganglionic sympathetic nerve fibers; the plasma activity of dopamine-β-hydroxylase, the enzyme responsible for the conversion of dopamine into noradrenaline and excreted together with the neurotransmitter from the sympathetic nerve fibers; and the urinary excretion of vanillylmandelic acid (VMA), the main metabolite of the catecholamines, noradrenaline and adrenaline [24,25]. Other biochemical changes that have been observed during the migraine attack and that may be linked to the increased activity of the sympathetic nervous system are the increase in plasma cyclic adenosine monophosphate, free fatty acid level, and free to total plasma tryptophan [22,24].

In the schematic summary of the biochemical changes of the migraine attack, as shown in Figure 8.5, I have also linked the platelet activation, which has been documented to occur during migraine, to the increased activity of the sympathetic nervous system, as the catecholamines, noradrenaline and adrenaline, are potent inductors of platelet aggregation. The platelet changes, in particular the fall in platelet serotonin content, the best documented biochemical change of the migraine attack, were once considered of primary importance in the pathogenesis of the attack [25,26]. It was hypothesized that platelet activation constituted the initial event of the migraine attack, possibly due to a change in plasma constitution, among others resulting in a release of serotonin into the plasma [27]. The increase in plasma serotonin level, supposedly resulting from it, was believed to be responsible for the aura symptoms by causing cerebral vasoconstriction leading to hypoxia. The subsequent fall in plasma serotonin due to the rapid metabolism of the serotonin released was considered the cause of the migraine headache by being associated with a loss in tone of the extracranial blood vessels. However, in contrast to the decrease in platelet and plasma serotonin content, an increase in plasma serotonin level preceding the decrease has never been documented [25,28]. Also, it is very doubtful whether the serotonin that is present free in the plasma has any physiological significance, and that the changes in its level as referred to above can have any of the vascular effects claimed. In addition, as reviewed above, a vascular pathogenesis of the migraine aura, as hypothesized by Wolff, has become unlikely on the basis of the recently performed cerebral blood flow studies in favor of a primary neuronal mechanism, such as Leão's spreading depression [5].

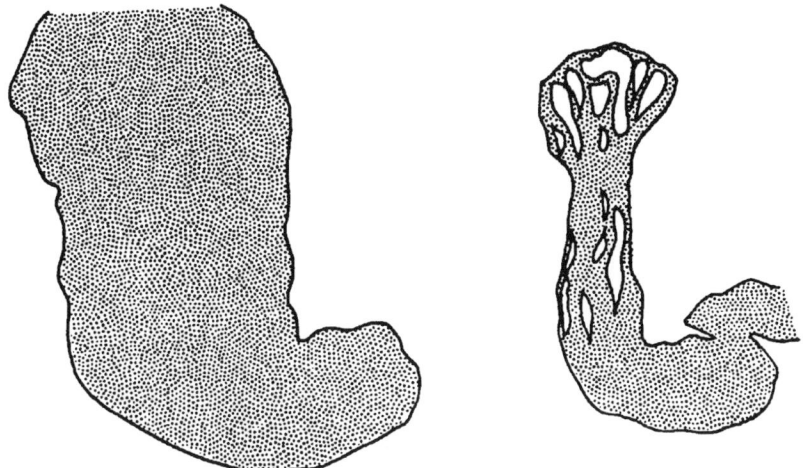

Figure 8.6. Radiographic examination of the stomach during (left) and after (right) the migraine attack. Note the dilation and atony of the stomach with closure of the pyloric sphincter during the attack [30].

TREATMENT OF MIGRAINE

The treatment of migraine, as of headaches in general, can be divided into three categories: abortive, preventive, and causative. The abortive treatment addresses the symptoms and interacts with the underlying mechanisms in a nonspecific or superficial way. It includes the treatment of the migraine headache with analgesic and/or vasoconstrictor medications. The underlying mechanisms of the symptoms are dealt with specifically or in a more profound way with preventive treatment. With regard to migraine, this treatment includes medications like propranolol HCl (Inderal) and amitriptyline HCl (Elavil, Endep) and nonpharmacological techniques such as biofeedback. Preventive treatment, when effective, results in a decrease in frequency, intensity, and duration of the attacks. When attack frequency is high, this kind of treatment is generally indicated next to abortive treatment, as under those circumstances reliance on abortive treatment will result in long-term aggravation of the condition.

The most difficult time- and effort-consuming aspect of the treatment of migraine is that directed toward the causes of the attacks, i.e., causative treatment. Migraine is a condition that often has a hereditary basis, as suggested by a positive family history of migraine in 70-90% of cases, but nevertheless individual attacks usually do not occur without underlying causes [29]. Causative treatment aims at identifying and eliminating these underlying causes.

ABORTIVE TREATMENT

In the abortive treatment of migraine in general only pharmacological approaches are effective. The medications used for treatment of the headache are analgesics and vasoconstrictors. However, before any medication can be effective, it must be absorbed and absorption of oral medications is impaired during the migraine attack due to a dysfunction of the gastrointestinal tract. This dysfunction consists of atony and dilation of the stomach with closure of the pyloric sphincter (Figure 8.6), which is probably due to the activation of the sympathetic nervous system mentioned above [30]. For orally administered medications it signifies a delay in absorption, as has been demonstrated for aspirin and acetaminophen [31-33]. The delay in absorption is probably responsible for the general ineffectiveness of these medications in the treatment of the migraine attack. It can be reversed by metoclopramide (Reglan), which, apart from being an anti-emetic, also has gastrokinetic properties leading to an increase in gastrointestinal motility and gastric emptying [34,35]. Prior administration of metoclopramide has been shown to correct the delayed absorption of aspirin during the attack [32,36]. Also, better symptomatic relief, including relief of headache and nausea, has been shown with the combination of metoclopramide and aspirin than with aspirin alone [37].

However, in general, more potent relief of the migraine headache can be obtained with medications which possess vasoconstrictor properties. One such medication is isometheptene mucate, one of the components of Midrin, which in addition contains acetaminophen and dichloralphenazone, a muscle relaxant. Midrin has been shown to be significantly better than placebo in the treatment of migraine [39]. Another vasoconstrictor agent for the symptomatic treatment of migraine is ergotamine tartrate, which is an ingredient in Cafergot. Ergotamine is a very potent vasoconstrictor that has been used for the treatment of migraine since the 1920s. It is usually administered together with caffeine to enhance its absorption from the gastrointestinal tract [40]. The medication is best administered rectally because of the disturbance in gastrointestinal functioning that occurs during the attack. Half a rectal suppository of Cafergot (1 mg of ergotamine tartrate) has been shown to provide total headache relief within three hours in 73% of patients [41]. Side effects were observed in less than 5% and consisted mainly of nausea and vomiting. These side effects can usually be avoided by using an antiemetic prior to the ergotamine.

However, when used frequently, ergotamine may also cause headache, in this way defeating its purpose. This may already occur when the medication is used as infrequently as once per week. The removal of the ergotamine from the body is then followed by rebound vasodilation that results in headache indistinguishable from migraine. A cycle is thus created of headache occurrence and ergotamine intake with a gradual increase in both over time, ultimately leading to what is often referred to as status migrainosus. This is an intractable situation in which migraine attacks follow each other in rapid succession requiring daily or almost daily intake of ergotamine. At that point the only treatment is the total discontinuation of the ergotamine for which hospitalization may be required. A reduction in headache frequency and intensity usually follows, once withdrawal from the medication has been accomplished [42,43].

Dihydroergotamine mesylate (D.H.E. 45) is a derivative of ergotamine which is available for parenteral administration. In a dose of 0.75 mg intravenously, it has been shown to be effective in the abortive treatment of migraine [43a]. It has also been shown, in a dose of 1 mg intravenously, to be better than either meperidine 50 mg or butorphanol 2 mg intramuscularly in the abortive treatment of vascular headache [43b]. As nausea and vomiting are possible side effects of dihydroergotamine, the medication should always be given together with an antinausea medication such as metaclopramide (Reglan) 10 mg intravenously or orally.

A vasoconstrictor medication like ergotamine and dihydroergotamine which has also been shown to be effective in the abortive treatment of migraine is sumatriptan succinate (Imitrex) [43c]. In a dose of 2 mg intravenously, the medication has been shown to relieve migraine headaches in 71%. [43d]. The efficacy of the medication in a dose of 6 mg subcutaneously has been shown to be 70% in decreasing the intensity of moderate or severe migraine headaches to mild or no headache [43e]. Sumatriptan differs from ergotamine and dihydroergotamine in particular in the fact that it does not cause nausea or vomiting, but instead relieves them.

PREVENTIVE TREATMENT

When frequent occurrence of migraine attacks is not associated with the intake of abortive medication, attack frequency may be reduced with preventive treatment. This treatment may be pharmacological or nonpharmacological, and the latter may include techniques like biofeedback that involves acquiring the ability to voluntarily increase finger temperature, relax the forehead musculature, and/or reduce temporal artery pulsation amplitude [44]. The pharmacological preventive treatment of migraine involves the daily intake of medication, whether a headache is present or not, to reduce the frequency, intensity, and/or duration of the attacks.

The first one introduced and also the most potent of the preventive antimigraine medications is methysergide maleate (Sansert), an antagonist of the type 2 serotoninergic receptors. It was first used for the treatment of migraine in 1959 on the assumption that a liberation of serotonin into the body played a significant role in the pathogenesis of the attack [45]. This assumption was based on the observation that during an attack, patients excrete an increased amount of the serotonin metabolite, 5-hydroxyindoleacetic acid, in their urine (Figure 8.5) [46].

In double-blind, placebo-controlled studies, methysergide has been shown to be an effective antimigraine medication; at a dosage of 6 mg/day, it reduced migraine by more than half in 60% of patients [47-49]. Side effects were mainly of gastrointestinal nature like nausea and stomach ache. However, much more serious side effects have been reported with prolonged use of methysergide, consisting of extra fibrous tissue formation in body cavities like abdomen and chest, known as retroperitoneal and pleuropulmonary fibrosis [50]. To prevent this from occurring in a clinically significant form, methysergide should not be used for longer than four to six months at a time, after which it should be discontinued for at least two to four weeks.

The preventive antimigraine medication most widely used in the United States today is propranolol, a beta-adrenoceptor blocker. Its efficacy in migraine was discovered accidentally in a patient with angina, first described in 1966 [51]. Since then, propranolol has been shown to be effective in a great number of double-blind, placebo-controlled studies [52]. It is usually prescribed in doses of 80 mg to 160 mg/day, and in these dosages it is generally well tolerated. Side effects are loss of energy and fatigue, insomnia, impotence, depression, and cold extremities. The medication is contraindicated in congestive heart failure, obstructive pulmonary disease, and diabetes. Other beta-blockers with demonstrated efficacy in migraine are timolol maleate (Blocadren), atenolol (Tenormin), metoprolol tartrate (Lopressor), and nadolol (Corgard) [52].

Another medication that is effective preventively is amitriptyline. Its efficacy was initially reported in 1969 and has since been confirmed in two double-blind, placebo-controlled studies [53-55]. It had also been shown to be effective in chronic tension-type and mixed (tension-type/vascular) headache [56]. It is an antidepressant, but for the treatment of migraine lower dosages, i.e., 10 mg to 150 mg/day may be effective. Side effects are daytime drowsiness, dry mouth, weight gain, and constipation; contraindications are glaucoma, prostatic hypertrophy, epilepsy, and cardiac arrhythmias.

The latest addition to the group of preventive antimigraine medications is verapamil HCl (Calan, Isoptin), a calcium entry blocker. The calcium entry blockers were introduced into the treatment of migraine on the basis of their ability to antagonize vasoconstriction and to protect the brain against the deleterious effects of hypoxia [57]. These properties were considered relevant against the background of Wolff's hypothesis of the pathogenesis of the migraine attack (Figure 8.2). Of the calcium entry blockers to date, flunarizine (Sibelium), nimodipine (Nimotop), and verapamil (Calan, Isoptin) have been shown in double-blind, placebo-controlled studies to be effective in migraine prevention [58,59]. Verapamil has been investigated in two double-blind, placebo-controlled studies and found effective in dosages of 240 mg and 320 mg/day [60,61]. The most common side effect of verapamil is constipation, and contraindications for its use are congestive heart failure and conduction disorders of the heart. Diltiazem (Cardizem) has so far not been studied in migraine prevention and nifedipine (Procardia), on the basis of its vasodilating effect, actually causes vascular headaches as a side effect.

CAUSATIVE TREATMENT

Ultimate management of migraine can only be achieved by the identification and elimination of the factors that are responsible for the occurrence of the attacks. These factors can be of psychological, physiological, or environmental nature, and can alone or in interaction with each other trigger migraine attacks. The way to identify them is by keeping track of the circumstances under which attacks occur.

Of the factors that can trigger migraine attacks, psychosocial stress is probably the one most frequently implicated. In a prospective study involving 49 patients who registered 121 attacks over a two-month period, more than half of the attacks occurred under situations of stress [62]. However, when migraine attacks are triggered by stress, they usually do not occur during the stress but in the period of relaxation following it [63].

From the physiological factors, the hormonal changes related to the menstrual cycle are particularly important. In women of reproductive age, approximately 30% of all attacks occur during the first four days of the menstrual cycle, i.e., during the menses [64]. The occurrence of attacks during the menses is not related to the absolute levels of the female hormones, estradiol and progesterone, as these are the same in patients with or without menstrually related migraine [65,66]. The timing of the attacks at the menses has been linked to the decrease in plasma estradiol level while that of the menses themselves is related to the decrease in plasma progesterone [65,66]. Dalton has suggested that, as with the premenstrual syndrome, it is the relative deficiency of progesterone that sets the grounds for menstrual migraine. The occurrence of menstrual migraine has been shown to be related to the onset of migraine around menarche and improvement of migraine during pregnancy but not with menopause [68]. Women with menstrual migraine are also particularly susceptible to the detrimental effect of oral contraceptives in terms of increasing headache suffering [64]. This detrimental effect occurs in 40% to 50% of all patients, as has been revealed by a review of the literature [69]. In addition, Kudrow has shown that the frequency of migraine headaches decreases by at least 60% in 70% of women after discontinuing the use of oral contraceptives [69a]. A similar effect was observed in 25% of women after decreasing the dose of estrogen used for menopause therapy by at least 50% and by decreasing the intake of the hormones.

The environmental factor most thoroughly investigated relates migraine and food. The food products most frequently mentioned by migraine patients as trigger factors of their attacks are chocolate (19.2%), cheese (18.2%), citrus fruits (11.1%), and alcohol (29.0%) [70]. The occurrence of attacks following the ingestion of these food products is usually attributed to certain chemicals contained in them, although sometimes also an allergic reaction is implicated. The chemicals that are thought to be migraine-producing are phenylethylamine in chocolate and tyramine in cheese. Both are stimulators of the sympathetic nervous system, and an effect similar to that of stress may be responsible.

Tyramine is also present in certain alcoholic beverages, but alcohol itself probably also triggers migraine attacks by its vasodilator properties. Some alcoholic beverages, particularly red wine, also contain histamine that is a potent vasodilator agent. The offending chemical in the citrus fruits supposedly is octopamine, which depletes the sympathetic nervous system of its neurotransmitter, noradrenaline, by acting as a "false transmitter."

Food additives that have been implicated as trigger factors of migraine attacks are sodium nitrite and monosodium glutamate [71,72]. Sodium nitrite is used in the preparation of cured meat products (hot dogs, bacon, salami, ham) and monosodium glutamate is frequently used as a taste enhancer in Chinese foods. The onset of migraine attacks following the ingestion of sodium nitrite-containing foods is attributed to the vasodilator properties of the chemical. However, not only ingestion of food but also lack of food, as in skipping meals, can trigger migraine attacks. Possibly as much as 50% of migraine patients are sensitive to this effect of skipping a meal [73,74]. This has been attributed to a relatively low or decreased glucose level in the blood, although this has not been confirmed in systematic investigations [74].

Other environmental factors to be considered in relation to the onset of migraine attacks are weather conditions and high altitude. Research in this particular area has revealed that migraine attacks occur less frequently with barometric pressures lower than 1005 mb and with increases in barometric pressure of more than 15 mb in the preceding 24 hours [75]. The less frequent occurrence of attacks with low barometric pressures may be related to the cloudiness that is associated with it, as clouds protect us from sunlight, and sunlight is a trigger factor of migraine attacks in 30% of patients [76].

References

1. Goldstein M, Chen TC. The epidemiology of disabling headache. In: Critchley M, Friedman AP, Goroni S, et al, (eds). *Headache: Physiopathological and Clinical Concepts*, pp 3477-390. New York, Raven Press, 1982.
2. Peatfield RC, Gawel MJ, Rose FC. Asymmetry of the aura and pain in migraine. *J Neurol Neurosurg Psychiat 44*: 846-848, 1981.
3. Fisher CM. Late-life migraine accompaniments as a cause of unexplained transient ischemic attacks. *Can J Neurol Sci 7*: 8-17, 1980.
4. Spierings ELH. Migraine: Symptomatology and pathogenesis. *Sandorama (English edition) 2:* 26-34, 1985.
5. Wolff HG. In: Dalessio DJ, (ed). *Headache and Other Head Pain*, ed 4. New York, Oxford University Press, 1980.
6. Marcussen RM, Wolff HG. Studies on headache: I. Effects of carbon dioxide-oxygen mixtures given during the preheadache phase of the migraine attack. II. Further analysis of pain mechanisms in headache. *Arch Neurol Psychiat 63*: 42-51, 1950.
7. Schumacher GA, Wolff HG. Experimental studies on headache: A. Contrast of histamine headache with the headache of migraine and that associated with hypertension. B. Contrast

of vascular mechanisms in pre-headache and in headache phenomena of migraine. *Arch Neurol Psychiat 45*: 199-214, 1941.
8. Hare EH. Personal observation on the spectral march of migraine. *J Neurol Sci 3*: 259-264, 1966.
9. O'Brien MD. Cerebral blood flow changes in migraine. *Headache 10*: 139-143, 1971.
10. O'Brien MD. The relationship between aura symptoms and cerebral blood flow changes in the prodrome of migraine. In: Dalessio DJ, Dalsgaard-Nielsen T, Diamond S, (eds). *Proc Int Headache Symp*, Elsinore, Denmark, pp 141-143. Basel, Sandoz, 1971.
11. Mathew NT, Hrastnik F, Meyer JS. Regional cerebral blood flow in the diagnosis of vascular headache. *Headache 15*: 252-260, 1976.
12. Olesen J, Larsen B, Lauritzen M. Focal hyperemia followed by spreading oligemia and impaired activation of rCBF in classic migraine. *Ann Neurol 9*: 344-352, 1981.
13. Lauritzen M, Olsen TS, Lassen NA, et al. Changes in regional cerebral blood flow during the course of classic migraine attacks. *Ann Neurol 13*: 633-641, 1983.
13a. Olsen TS. Friberg L, Lassen NA. Ischemia may be the primary cause of the neurologic deficits in classic migraine. *Arch Neurol 44*: 156-161, 1987.
14. Milner PM. Note on a possible correspondence between the scotomas of migraine and spreading depression of Leão. *EEG Clin Neurophysiol 10*: 705, 1958.
15. Leão, AAP. Spreading depression of activity in the cerebral cortex. *J Neurophysiol 7*: 359-390, 1944.
16. Lashley KS. Patterns of cerebral integration indicated by the scotomas of migraine. *Arch Neurol Psychiat 46*: 331-339, 1941.
17. Grafstein B. Mechanism of spreading cortical depression. *J Neurophysiol 19*: 154-171, 1956.
18. Lauritzen M, Jorgensen MB, Diemer NH, et al. Persistent oligemia of rat cerebral cortex in the wake of spreading depression. *Ann Neurol 12*: 469-474, 1982.
18a. Welch KMA, Levine SR, D'Andrea G, et al. Preliminary observations on brain energy metabolism in migraine studied by in vivo phosphorus 31 NMR spectroscopy. *Neurology 39*: 538-541, 1989.
18b. Ramadan NM, Halvorson H, Vande-Linde A, et al. Low brain magnesium in migraine. *Headache 29*: 416-419, 1989.
18c. Schoenen J, Sianard-Gainko J, Lenearts M. Blood magnesium levels in migraine. *Cephalagia 11*: 97-99, 1991.
19. Graham JR, Wolff HG. Mechanism of migraine headache and action of ergotamine tartrate. *Arch Neurol Psychiat 39*: 737-763, 1938.
20. Wolff HG, Tunis MM, Goodell H. Studies on headache: Evidence of tissue damage and changes in pain sensitivity in subjects with vascular headaches of the migraine type. *Arch Intern Med 92*: 478-484, 1953.
21. Chapman LF, Ramos AO, Goodell H, et al. A humoral agent implicated in vascular headache of the migraine type. *Arch Neurol 3*: 223-229, 1960.
21a. Saito K, Markowitz S, Moslowitz MA. Ergot alkaloids block neurogenic extravasation in dura mater: propposed action in vascular headaches. *Ann Neurol 24*: 732-737, 1988.
22. Anselmi B, Baldi E, Cassacci F, et al. Endogenous opioids in cerebrospinal fluid and blood in idiopathic headache sufferers. *Headache 20*: 294-299, 1980.
23. Spierings ELH. Migraene und sympathisches Nervensystem. In: Pfaffenrath V, Schrader A, Neu IS, (eds). *Primaere Kopfschmerzen: Pathogenese, Diagnostik und Therapie*, pp 53-66. Muenchen, Medizine Verlag, 1984.
24. Anthony M. Biochemical indices of sympathetic activity in migraine. *Cephalalgia 1*: 83-89, 1981.
25. Curran DA, Hinterberger H, Lance JW. Total plasma serotonin, 5-hydroxyindoleacetic acid and p-hydroxy-m-methoxymandelic acid excretion in normal and migrainous subjects. *Brain 88*: 997-1010, 1965.

26. Spierings ELH. *The Pathophysiology of the Migraine Attack*. Brussels, Stafleu's Scientific Publishing Company, 1980.
27. Anthony M, Hinterberger H, Lance JW. The possible relationship of serotonin to the migraine syndrome. *Res Clin Study Headache* 2: 29-59, 1969.
28. Somerville BW. Platelet-bound and free serotonin levels in jugular and forearm venous blood during migraine. *Neurology* 26: 41-45, 1976.
29. Lance JW, Anthony M. Some clinical aspects of migraine: A prospective survey of 500 patients. *Arch Neurol* 15: 356-361, 1966.
30. Kaufman J, Levine I. Acute gastric dilatation of stomach during attack of migraine. *Radiology* 27: 301-302, 1936.
31. Volans GN. Absorption of effervescent aspirin during migraine. *Br Med J* 4: 264-269, 1974.
32. Volans GN. The effect of metoclopramide on the absorption of effervescent aspirin in migraine. *Br J Clin Pharmacol* 2: 57-63, 1975.
33. Tokola RA, Neuvonen PJ. Absorption of effervescent paracetamol during migraine. *Acta Pharmacol Tox (supp 1)*: 78, 1981.
34. Johnson AF. Gastroduodenal motility and synchronization. *Postgr Med J 49 (July supp)*: 29-33, 1973.
35. Howard FA, Sharp DS. The effect of intra-muscular metoclopramide on gastric emptying during labour. *Postgr Med J 49 (July supp)*: 53-56, 1973.
36. Ross-Lee LM, Eadie MJ, Heazlewood V, et al. Aspirin pharmacokinetics in migraine: The effect of metoclopramide. *Eur J Clin Pharmacol* 24: 777-785, 1983.
37. Tfelt-Hansen P, Olesen J. Effervescent metoclopramide and aspirin (Migravess) versus effervescent aspirin or placebo for migraine attacks: A double blind study. *Cephalalgia* 4: 107-111, 1984.
38. Spierings ELH, Saxena PR. Effect of isometheptene on the distribution and shunting of 15 μm microspheres throughout the cephalic circulation of the cat. *Headache* 20: 103-106, 1980.
39. Diamond S. Treatment of migraine with isometheptene, acetaminophen, and dichloralphenazone combination: A double blind, crossover trial. *Headache* 15: 282-287, 1976.
40. Schmidt R, Fanchamps A. Effect of caffeine on intestinal absorption of ergotamine in man. *Eur J Clin Pharmacol* 7: 213-216, 1974.
41. Graham JR. Rectal use of ergotamine tartrate and caffeine alkaloid for the relief of migraine. *N Engl J Med* 250: 936-938, 1954.
42. Tfelt-Hansen P, Aebelholt Krabbe A. Ergotamine abuse. Do patients benefit from withdrawal? *Cephalalgia* 1: 29-32, 1981.
43. Ala-Hurula V, Myllylä V, Hokkanen E. Ergotamine abuse: Results of ergotamine discontinuation, with special reference to plasma concentrations. *Cephalalgia* 2: 189-195, 1982.
43a. Callaham M, Raskin N. A controlled study of dihydroergotamine in the treatment of acute migraine headache. *Headache* 26: 168-171, 1986.
43b. Belgrade MJ, Ling LJ, Schleevogt MB, et al. Comparison of single dose meperidine, butorphanol, and dihydroergotamine in the treatment of vascular headache. *Neurology* 39: 590-592, 1989.
43c. Humphrey PPA, Feniuk W, Perren MJ, et al. GR 43175, a selective agonist for the 5-HT$_1$-like receptor in dog isolated saphenous vein. *Br J Pharmacol* 94: 1123-1132, 1988.
43d. Doenicke A, Brand J, Perrin VL. Possible benefit of GR 43175, a novel 5-HT$_1$-like receptor agonist, for the acute treatment of severe migraine. *Lancet* 1: 1309-1311, 1988.
43e. Cady RK, Wendt JK, Kirchner JR, et al. Treatment of acute migraine with subcutaneous sumatriptan. *JAMA* 21: 2831-2835, 1991.
44. Jessup BA, Neufeld RWJ, Merskey H. Biofeedback therapy for headache and other pain: An evaluation review. *Pain* 7: 225-270, 1979.
45. Sicuteri F. Prophylactic and therapeutic properties of 1-methyl-lysergic acid butanolamide in migraine. *Int Arch Allergy* 15: 300-307, 1959.

46. Sicuteri F, Testi A, Anselmi B. Biochemical investigations in headache: Increase in the hydroxyindoleacetic acid excretion during migraine attacks. *Int Arch Allergy 19*: 55-58, 1961.
47. Shekelle RB, Ostfeld AM. Methysergide in the migraine syndrome. *Clin Pharmacol Ther 5*: 201-204, 1964.
48. Southwell N, Williams JD, Mackenzie I. Methysergide in the prophylaxis of migraine. *Lancet 1*: 523-524, 1964.
49. Pedersen E, Moller CE. Methysergide in migraine prophylaxis. *Clin Pharmacol Ther 7*: 520-526, 1966.
50. Graham JR, Suby HI, LeCompte PR, et al. Fibrotic disorders associated with methysergide therapy for headache. *N Engl J Med 274*: 359-368, 1966.
51. Rabkin R, Stables DP, Levin NW, et al. The prophylactic value of propranolol in angina pectoris. *Am J Cardiol 18*: 370-380, 1966.
52. Weerasuriya K, Patel L, Turner P. Beta-adrenoceptor blockade and migraine. *Cephalalgia 2*: 33-45, 1982.
53. Mahloudji M. Prevention of migraine. *Br Med J 1*: 182-183, 1969.
54. Gomersall JD, Stuart A. Amitriptyline in migraine prophylaxis: Changes in pattern of attacks during a controlled clinical trial. *J Neurol Neurosurg Psychiat 36*: 684-690, 1973.
55. Couch JR, Hassanein RS. Amitriptyline in migraine prophylaxis. *Arch Neurol 36*: 695-699, 1979.
56. Lance JW, Curran DA. Treatment of chronic tension headache. *Lancet 1*: 1236-1239, 1964.
57. Amery WK, Wauquier A, Van Neuten GM, et al. The anti-migrainous pharmacology of flunarizine (R 14950), a calcium antagonist. *Drugs Exptl Clin Res 7*: 1-10, 1981.
58. Spierings ELH. Clinical evaluation of calcium entry blockers in migraine. In: Godfraind T, Herman AG, Wellens D, (eds). *Calcium Entry Blockers in Cardiovascular and Cerebral Dysfunctions*, pp 271-281. The Hague, Martinus Nijhoff, 1984.
59. Spierings ELH. Calcium entry blockers in the treatment of migraine. In: Godfraind T, Vanhoutte PM, Govoni S, (eds). *Calcium Entry Blockers and Tissue Protection*, pp 245-254. New York, Raven Press, 1985.
60. Solomon GD, Steel JG, Spaccavento LJ. Verapamil prophylaxis of migraine: A double-blind, placebo-controlled study. *JAMA 250*: 2500-2502, 1983.
61. Markley HG, Cheroms JCD, Piepho RW. Verapamil in prophylactic therapy of migraine. *Neurology 34*: 973-976, 1984.
62. Rees WL. Stress, distress and disease. *Br J Psychiat 128*: 3-18, 1976.
63. Dalkvist J, Ekbom K, Waldenlind E. Headache and mood: A time-series analysis of self-ratings. *Cephalalgia 4*: 45-52, 1984.
64. Dalton K. Migraine and oral contraceptives. *Headache 15*: 247-251, 1976.
65. Somerville BW. The role of progesterone in menstrual migraine. *Neurology 21*: 853-859, 1971.
66. Somerville BW. The role of estradiol withdrawal in the etiology of menstrual migraine. *Neurology 22*: 355-365, 1972.
67. Dalton K. *The Premenstrual Syndrome and Progesterone Therapy*. London, William Heinemann Medical Books, 1977.
68. Epstein MT, Hockaday JM, Hockaday TDR. Migraine and reproductive hormones throughout the menstrual cycle. *Lancet 1*: 543-548, 1975.
69. Spierings ELH. Migraine and "the pill." *J Drug Res 5 (Nov supp)*: 67-71, 1980.
69a. Kudrow L. The relationship of headache frequency to hormone use in migraine. *Headache 15*: 36-40, 1975.
70. Peatfield RC, Glover V, Littlewood JT, et al. The prevalence of diet-induced migraine. *Cephalalgia 4*: 179-183, 1984.
71. Henderson WR, Raskin NH. "Hot dog" headache: Individual susceptibility to nitrite. *Lancet 2*: 1162-1163, 1972.
72. Gore ME, Salmon PR. Chinese restaurant syndrome: Fact or fiction? *Lancet 1*: 251-252, 1980.

73. Blau JN, Cummings JN. Method of precipitating and preventing some migraine attacks. *Br Med J 2*: 1242-1243, 1966.
74. Hockaday JM, Williamson R, Whitty CWM. Blood-glucose levels and fatty-acid metabolism in migraine related to fasting. *Lancet 1*: 1153-1156, 1971.
75. Cull RE. Barometric pressure and other factors in migraine. *Headache 21*: 102-103, 1981.
76. Vijayan N, Gould S, Watson C. Exposure to sun and precipitation of migraine. *Headache 20*: 42-43, 1980.

Copyright © 1993 PMA Publishing Corp.
Headache: A Clinician's Guide to Diagnosis, Pathophysiology, and Treatment Strategies
Edited by Alan M. Rapoport, M.D. and Fred D. Sheftell, M.D.

9

Tension-Type Headache

Seymour Diamond and Glen D. Solomon

Introduction

In the common classification of headache, the category of nonvascular headache usually includes muscle contraction headache as well as the mixed headache syndrome. Acute muscle contraction headache is the typical, episodic tension headache, related to contraction of the head and neck muscles. It is usually relieved by over-the-counter analgesics and is associated with fatigue, excesses of food and drink, and temporary stress situations. Chronic muscle contraction or tension headaches may be a part of a headache symptom complex, partly due to psychological problems. This complex often presents in persons subject to depression. If episodic muscle contraction headache occurs more than several times weekly, or is unresponsive to over-the-counter analgesics, it is imperative that the patient seek medical management. The focus of this chapter will be the treatment of chronic muscle contraction headache (chronic tension-type headache).

Tension or Muscle Contraction Headache (Chronic Tension-Type Headache)

Chronic tension or muscle contraction headache may be defined as a daily or almost daily headache. It usually occurs bilaterally and exhibits a steady and non-pulsatile ache. In contrast to migraine, it is not associated with neurological symptoms or gastrointestinal distress. Chronic muscle contraction headache is characterized by the absence of periodicity or a headache-free interval, and usually manifests as a daily, or almost daily headache, frequently lasting all day, and is unresponsive to progressively increasing amounts of analgesics. This pattern contrasts to acute muscle contraction headaches that are generally infrequent, of short duration, and responsive to simple analgesics. Tension headache is described as a steady, non-throbbing ache occurring bi-temporally, occipitally, or in a hatband distribution. The muscles of the head, neck, jaw, or upper back may be contracted and tender, and they may contain localized nodules that are tender on palpation.

Although more frequent in women, muscle contraction headache does occur in men. When these headaches occur in families, some experts consider this a learned pattern of behavior.

One key to the overall management of chronic muscle contraction headache is the realization that a serious emotional disorder, such as depression, may be concealed. Depressive headaches occur at regular intervals, often presenting on weekends, holidays, vacations, or following stressful situations, such as exams [1]. Characteristically, these headaches are more severe in the morning, and often occur from 4:00 to 8:00 pm and from 4:00 to 8:00 am, periods that are frequently the times of great, although sometimes silent, family discord. Although depressive headaches do not awaken the patients, these patients are plagued with early awakening (late insomnia). Those early morning hours may then be spent anguishing over conflicts at home or work.

The depressed patient often presents with a wide variety of complaints that can be categorized as physical, emotional, and psychic. The physical complaints include chronic pain, headaches, sleep disturbances, severe insomnia, early awakening, appetite changes, anorexia, rapid weight loss, and a decrease in sexual activity, which may manifest as impotence in males and amenorrhea or frigidity in females. Emotional complaints range from feeling blue to feelings of anxiety, as well as rumination over the past, present, and future. Psychic complaints may include statements such as morning is the worst time of day, as well as suicidal thoughts and death wishes.

The physician must obtain a thorough history that includes a detailed psychiatric inventory describing the patient's marital relations, occupation, social relationships, life stresses, personality traits, habits, methods of handling tension situations, and sexual problems. Two basic questions often provide insight into a possible depression. First, inquiries should be made regarding a past family or personal history of depression, or if the patient has had similar symptoms previously. Many patients will describe similar complaints occurring years ago, or will provide some obscure symptoms that are actually depressive equivalents. Second, the patients should be questioned about a possible relationship between the onset of symptoms and any precipitating event. Depressive attacks often succeed a wide variety of events that the patient perceives as traumatic or considers a personal loss, frequently out of proportion to the severity of the resultant depression. A patient may indicate that the illness started after some form of bodily injury, an infection, receiving an injection, a surgical procedure, or a diagnostic examination. The event that precipitated the headache or other depressive equivalent would not be sufficient to cause the problem nor is it compatible with the depression. The patient usually feels weakened or maimed by the event.

Of 423 patients who suffered from various types of depression, Diamond reported 84% had headache as one of their complaints or as a single complaint [2]. The most frequent symptom associated with depression is sleep disturbance. Ninety-seven percent of the patients that were examined had this symptom as one of their presenting complaints. As a rule, the younger patient has less variation in sleep. Older individuals experienced more difficulty with sleep disturbances. Sleep disturbances may manifest as hypersomnia, insomnia, early awakening, or disturbing dreams. Early awakening is probably the most common of the sleep disturbances.

For many patients, the physical symptoms of headache are more socially acceptable than the diagnosis of anxiety or depression. Biochemically, depression may be considered an illness involving both the depletion of biogenic amines and defects of neurotransmitters. Headache investigators have theorized that chronic muscle contraction headache results from disturbances of the monoaminergic, serotoninergic, and endorphin function, possibly involving the hypothalamus, brain stem, and spinal cord. These disturbances may be due to a referred or central pain phenomena from the intermingling of major circuits of the brain and spinal cord.

The pain pathway attributed to both the depressive equivalent and neurohumoral hypotheses of chronic muscle contraction headache includes alterations in biogenic amines. Therefore, drugs that affect synthesis or uptake of serotonin and/or norepinephrine have been utilized in the pharmacologic therapy of muscle contraction headache. This therapy encompasses all antidepressant agents, including the tricyclics and monoamine oxidase inhibitors (MAOIs).

The patient with chronic tension headache is often habituated or addicted to over-the-counter analgesics, barbiturates, benzodiazepines, and narcotics. The habituated patient requires detoxification before treatment can be initiated, and thus may only be resolved on an inpatient basis. To avoid habituation, clinicians should not prescribe medications that possess addictive properties, but utilize nonaddictive drugs for tension headache relief (Table 9.1). Daily use of any analgesic should be avoided.

The treatment of depressive headache and muscle contraction headache focuses on the use of antidepressant agents. The tricyclics are usually the drugs of choice and include amitriptyline HCl (Elavil, Endep), imipramine HCl (Tofranil), protriptyline HCl (Vivactil), trimipramine maleate (Surmontil), dox-

Table 9.1. Non-Habituating Analgesics
Naproxen sodium (Anaprox)
Meclofenamate sodium (Meclomen)
Ibuprofen (Motrin, Rufen)
Fenoprofen calcium (Nalfon)
Mefenamic acid (Ponstel)
Diflunisal (Dolobid)
Chlorzoxazone and Acetaminophen (Parafon Forte)
Orphenadrine citrate
Carisoprodol (Norflex, Soma)
Cyclobenzaprine HCl (Flexeril)
Methocarbamol (Robaxin)

epin HCl (Sinequan), nortriptyline HCl (Pamelor), and desipramine (Norpramin, Pertofrane). Amoxapine (Asendin), an antidepressant distinct from the tricyclics, has not been demonstrated as useful in headache management and is replete with side effects. Maprotiline HCl (Ludiomil), a tetracyclic with similar action to the tricyclics, is considered beneficial. Trazodone HCl (Desyrel), a non-tricyclic antidepressant, is sedating, has a decreased anticholinergic effect, and may be beneficial for patients in whom tricyclics are contraindicated. The usual dosage of trazodone is 50 mg to 100 mg at bedtime, gradually increasing to 200 mg to 250 mg. If daytime sedation is indicated because of agitation or anxiety, a 50 mg dose may be added in the morning and increased if indicated. The efficacy of these agents has been demonstrated in numerous studies.

The choice of antidepressant is dependent on the unique characteristics of each agent (Table 9.2). In reviewing the tricyclics, amitriptyline is the most sedating and possesses the highest anticholinergic effect. Despite its side effects, amitriptyline is probably the most widely used antidepressant in outpatient practice. Studies dating back to the early 1960s chronicle the efficacy and safety of this drug. Amitriptyline rarely needs to be discontinued because of its side effects, as most of the symptoms gradually subside. Dosage is based on the age and size of the patient, with therapy usually initiated at 25 mg to 50 mg at bedtime, increasing the nightly dose by increments of 25 mg every third or fourth night until achieving the general therapeutic range (50 mg to 300 mg/d) unless limited by side effects. Full doses should be maintained for at least four weeks before determining treatment failure. In the patient without a sleep disturbance, protriptyline may be the drug of choice. Therapy is initiated at 5 mg daily, increasing as necessary to 30 mg/day.

Doxepin is equally as sedating as amitriptyline but has fewer anticholinergic side effects than other tricyclics. Imipramine is more sedating than desipramine, and nortriptyline's sedating effect is in a range between the other two agents. Usually protriptyline and desipramine have minimal sedating effect. Because

Table 9.2. Effects of Tricyclic Antidepressants

Drug	Serotonin Inhibition	Norepinephrine Inhibition	Dopamine Inhibition	Sedative Effects	Anticholinergic Effects
Amitriptyline	Moderate	Weak	Inactive	Strong	Strong
Desipramine	Weak	Potent	Inactive	Mild	Moderate
Doxepin	Moderate	Moderate	Inactive	Strong	Strong
Imipramine	Fairly potent	Moderate	Inactive	Moderate	Strong
Nortriptyline	Weak	Fairly potent	Inactive	Mild	Moderate
Protriptyline	Weak	Fairly potent	Inactive	None	Strong
Trimipramine	Uncertain	Uncertain	Inactive	Strong	Strong
Amoxapine*	Weak	Strong	Inactive	Mild	Mild
Maprotiline*	Weak	Strong	Inactive	Strong	Mild
Trazodone*	Strong	Weak	Inactive	Strong	Mild

*May not be true tricyclic.

protriptyline is non-sedating, most of the daily dosage should be given in the morning.

Combination products of tricyclics and phenothiazines, such as amitriptyline and perphenazine (Triavil), are only indicated when depression is associated with marked anxiety, agitation, or hostility. Cautious use of these combination drugs is important because the dose of perphenazine is difficult to titrate if used in this manner. Frequently, in patients with agitation or marked early insomnia, a combination of chlordiazepoxide and amitriptyline (Limbitrol) may provide may provide additional sedation.

The onset of activity for tricyclic antidepressants is five days to two weeks. Treatment failures with tricyclics are primarily due to a short-term drug trial or inadequate dosage. A single dose at bedtime is compatible with known pharmacokinetics and may diminish both insomnia and the anticholinergic effects which often present during the day. Patient compliance may be improved by a single daily dose.

Adverse effects and drug interactions with tricyclic and non-tricyclic antidepressants may occur and include dry mouth, constipation, tachycardia, blurred vision, and urinary retention. For the patient with marked anticholinergic effects, such as dry mouth and constipation, bethanechol chloride (Urecholine), 25 mg t.i.d. may alleviate the side effects. Cardiac arrhythmias and exacerbation of problems of congestive heart failure may also rarely occur. The drugs that can potentiate the side effects of tricyclics include phenytoin sodium (Dilantin), phenothiazines, and aspirin. Tricyclic agents inhibit the antihypertensive effects of both clonidine HCl (Catapres) and guanethidine sulfate (Ismelin).

The MAOIs are generally considered the second line of drugs for depression, and often are effective in muscle contraction headache if the tricyclics fail. Adverse effects seen with MAOIs include muscle twitching, insomnia, hypoten-

Table 9.3. Foods to Avoid During Therapy with Monoamine Oxidase Inhibitors

Liquor

Wine

Cheese, except cottage cheese

Herring

Nuts

Excessive amounts of caffeine and chocolate

Vinegar, except white vinegar

Yogurt

Sour cream

Fresh baked breads

Pods of broad beans

Chicken livers

Marinated foods

Fermented foods and drinks

Do not take any medications without advice, including Contac, Dristan, Sinutabs, nose drips, and other cold remedies or diet aids.

Tranquilizers may be used concomitantly with MAOIs.

Narcotics, especially meperidine HCl (Demerol), are known to produce hypotensive episodes when given in association with MAOIs and should be avoided.

sion, dizziness, nausea, fatigue, and weight gain. All patients taking MAOIs must be carefully instructed on the necessity of avoiding foods containing tyramine and dopamine (Table 9.3), and cautioned to avoid medications, both prescription and over-the-counter, which contain sympathomimetic agents. These agents include decongestants, diet aids, and a variety of cough and cold remedies. Additionally, a potentially fatal hypotensive reaction has been reported with the combined use of meperidine HCl (Demerol) and an MAOI.

The MAOIs block the oxidative deamination of numerous monoamines, including epinephrine, norepinephrine, serotonin, and dopamine. The amounts of these substances are increased in the brain and other tissues, and the depression created by their deficiency is ameliorated. The most commonly used MAOI is phenelzine sulfate (Nardil). Phenelzine is usually prescribed in doses of 15 mg t.i.d. An alternative to phenelzine is isocarboxazid (Marplan), usually prescribed at 10 mg q.i.d.

In a review of 33 recidivist headache patients treated with MAOIs at the Diamond Headache Clinic [3], five patients became essentially headache free. Thirteen patients had at least a 50% reduction in the frequency and/or severity of their headaches, and an additional seven patients demonstrated a partial response. Only eight patients failed to demonstrate any improvement. Side effects were common, occurring in 29 patients, but were transient in two thirds of the patients.

The combined use of MAOIs and tricyclic antidepressants has created controversy among authorities. Concomitant use of an MAOI and tricyclic was previously contraindicated. In 1971, Schuckit and his associates reviewed 25 reported cases of morbidity secondary to combined MAOI and tricyclic therapy [4]. They reported that the risks of combination therapy had been greatly exaggerated, as many of the complications could be attributed to drug overdose. Other cases were related to the concomitant use of drugs that act on the central nervous system. In the remaining cases, the tricyclic involved was imipramine, and the MAOIs included isoniazid (INH), tranylcypromine sulfate (Parnate), isocarboxazid (Marplan), pargyline HCl (Eutonyl), and phenelzine sulfate (Nardil). At our clinic, the use of imipramine with an MAOI is prohibited. A recent study has shown that combination therapy with amitriptyline and an MAOI prevents a hypertensive crisis caused by ingestion of tyramine-containing foods [5].

In a recent review by the Diamond Headache Clinic of 14 recidivist patients treated with the combination of an MAOI and a tricyclic antidepressant [6], 78.5% obtained a significant improvement in reducing the frequency and severity of their headaches. Six of these patients had nearly complete amelioration of their headaches, and another five patients had at least a 50% reduction in the frequency and severity of their headaches. Side effects were common but transient and rarely caused discontinuation of the drugs. The adverse effects were intensified because of the synergism of the agents. Concomitant therapy with an MAOI and tricyclic antidepressant should only be initiated under close supervision by physicians familiar with this therapy and is best achieved in an inpatient setting.

Propranolol HCl (Inderal), a drug used in the prophylaxis of migraine, has also been employed in the management of chronic tension headache. It often has been used concomitantly with amitriptyline or other tricyclics with good results. Propranolol's mechanism of action in tension headache is uncertain, but may be related to either its anxiolytic action or its ability to stabilize the extracranial vasculature. The usual starting dose of propranolol is 80 mg once daily, with possible increases as tolerated to 120 mg or 160 mg a day. A once-daily, long-acting form may encourage patient compliance. Because propranolol has some tranquilizing effects, we prefer its use to minor tranquilizers. Other beta blockers can also be used.

Minor tranquilizers, including diazepam (Valium), chlordiazepoxide (Librium), meprobamate (Equanil, Miltown, Meprospan), oxazepam (Serax), and prazepam (Centrax), have been demonstrated as somewhat effective in the acute treatment of muscle contraction headache. The problems of drug dependency without significant resolution of headache further limit the value of these agents. Other potentially habituating drugs frequently used for headache relief

Table 9.4. Nonsteroidal Anti-Inflammatory Agents Useful in Muscle Contraction Headache

Meclofenamate sodium (Meclomen)

Fenoprofen calcium (Nalfon)

Naproxen (Naprosyn)

Naproxen sodium (Anaprox)

Mefenamic acid (Ponstel)

Ibuprofen (Motrin)

Indomethacin (Indocin)

include combinations of analgesics with codeine, propoxyphene (Darvon, Darvocet), and butalbital (Esgic, Fiorinal, Phrenilin).

Muscle relaxants, such as carisoprodol (Soma), cyclobenzaprine HCl (Flexeril), chlorzoxazone (Paraflex, Parafon Forte), and orphenadrine citrate (Norflex, Norgesic, Norgesic Forte) are of limited value in the treatment of chronic tension headache. For adjunctive therapy of acute muscle contraction headache, these drugs may be extremely beneficial.

In patients with muscle contraction headache associated with cervical arthritis (spondylosis), anti-inflammatory agents are frequently effective (Table 9.4). Nonsteroidal anti-inflammatory drugs (NSAIDs) are frequently prescribed on a short-term daily basis, often in combination with a muscle relaxant. Physical therapy, primarily heat and massage to the neck and shoulders with stimulation of both the skin and subcutaneous tissue, should be considered the treatment of choice in this condition. A cervical orthopedic pillow should be used to maintain the cervical lordotic curve during sleep. Additional non-drug therapy, including biofeedback and transcutaneous electrical stimulation (TENS), may also be helpful.

Non-drug therapy for chronic muscle contraction headache may be of great value. Psychotherapy, counseling, and supportive care by the primary physician, psychiatrist, psychologist, or therapist may help resolve psychological problems and lead to a resolution of the headache disorder. Biofeedback is a useful tool for many resistant headache patients. It offers patients a direct role in their headache management and has few contraindications or side effects.

A four-year retrospective study on the value of biofeedback in the treatment of chronic headache was performed at the Diamond Headache Clinic [7]. Of almost 400 patients surveyed, 83% indicated that they experienced improvement in their headaches. Age appeared to be an important factor in predicting the success of biofeedback training. Fifty percent of the patients were between the ages of six and 21 years and had excellent improvement, while 37% had slight improvement. Patients undergoing intensive biofeedback training improved during the initial training period, but were not successful in maintaining their gains. However, over 65% of the patients were able to utilize biofeedback training techniques and maintain gains for several years.

Mixed Headache

The mixed headache syndrome is a combination of vascular and nonvascular headaches. This type of headache pattern is most frequently seen by the headache specialist. It is comprised of the following symptomatology: daily, continuous headache, a sick headache (migraine) occurring one to ten times monthly, and easy susceptibility to habituation to over-the-counter or prescribed analgesics and/or ergotamine tartrate.

When the diagnosis of mixed headache has been made, the use of sedatives, tranquilizers, habituating analgesics, and narcotics must be discontinued to prevent the addiction that perpetuates the headache problem. Detoxification is best achieved in an inpatient setting. The use of ergotamine should be limited to relief of the sick headache and restricted to avoid the rebound phenomena.

Inpatient Treatment

For the patients with chronic muscle contraction headache or mixed headache who are habituated, unable to be monitored for complications arising from complex therapies, or just not improving in outpatient therapy, see Chapter 23 on inpatient units.

References

1. Diamond S, Dalessio DJ. *The Practicing Physician's Approach to Headache*, ed 4. Baltimore, Williams & Wilkins, 1986.
2. Diamond S. Depressive headaches. *Headache 4*: 255-259, 1964.
3. Diamond S. The rationale and use of antidepressants in the treatment of pain. Proc Symp Update on Antidepressants: Pharmacology and Clinical Use. *Fam Pract Recert 5 (supp)*: 19-28, 1983.
4. Schuckit M, Robins E, Feighner J. Tricyclic antidepressants and monoamine oxidase inhibitors. *Arch Gen Psychiat 24*: 509-514, 1971.
5. Pare CMB, Hallstrom C, Kline N, et al. Will amitriptyline prevent the cheese reaction of monoamine oxidase inhibitors? *Lancet 2*: 183-186, 1982.
6. Freitag FG, Diamond S, Solomon GD. Antidepressants in the treatment of mixed headache: MAO inhibitors and combined use of MAO inhibitors and tricyclic antidepressants in the recidivist headache patient. In: Rose FC, (ed). *Advances in Headache Research*, pp 271-275. London, John Libbey and Co, 1987.
7. Diamond S, Montrose D. The value of biofeedback in the treatment of chronic headache: A four-year retrospective study. *Schmertz*: 106-119, 1984.
8. Diamond S, Freitag FG, Maliszewski M. Inpatient treatment of headache: long-term results. *Headache 26*: 189-197, 1986.

10

Cluster Headache: Diagnosis, Pathogenesis, and Treatment

Lee Kudrow

Cluster headache has the dubious distinction of being the most painful primary headache disorder. Despite its ferocity and stereotypical presentation, cluster headache is frequently misdiagnosed. It is hoped that this presentation will provide the clinician with pertinent data to diagnose this syndrome accurately and effectively.

Classification

Excluding rarely encountered variants, there are three major types of cluster headache, each characterized by length of remission (headache-free period). *Episodic cluster headache* is defined by a period of attack-susceptibility (cluster period or cycle) followed by a remission period greater than five months. *Subchronic cluster headache* is characterized by remission periods of less than six months. As defined by Ekbom, the absence of remission for one year or more defines *chronic cluster headache*.

Approximately 80% of cluster headaches are of the episodic type. The remainder is almost equally distributed between subchronic and chronic groups.

Clinical Features

INCIDENCE, AGE, AND SEX DISTRIBUTION

The estimated incidence of cluster headache is approximately 1%. The sex distribution is predominantly male, having a 5-6:1 ratio to females. The incidence appears to be greatest among black populations where the sex ratio has been reported to be between 3.3 and 3.5 to 1, male to female. Cluster headache may begin at any age. The mean age of onset, however, is approximately 30 years. After age 29, the incidence of onset decreases linearly.

THE CLUSTER PERIOD

The cluster period is defined as an attack-susceptible cycle. The mean length of this cycle is approximately two months. The usual range is one to three months. Remissions vary from two to 24 months, with a mean of one year. At the other end of the spectrum, chronic cluster headache cycles are, by definition, at least 12 months.

Episodic cluster patients often experience their cycle onset at the same time of the year. In a recent study concerning the monthly distribution of cluster periods in a population of approximately 400 patients (900 cycles over a ten-year period), we found peak frequencies in July and January, beginning seven to ten days following the longest and shortest day of the year, respectively. As daylight (photoperiods) lengthened and shortened over the year, the frequency of cluster period onsets increased. The frequency curve was interrupted twice per year, seven to ten days following resetting of clocks for Daylight Savings and Standard times. These results suggest that photoperiodic cues may fail to stimulate circannual pacemakers, and in some way may contribute to the onset of the cluster period.

CLUSTER ATTACK

The following is a first-hand account of the cluster headache attack. It should provide the reader with an insight into the often unexpressed anguish experienced by the patient during an attack:

> Following a period of perhaps several hours of feeling quite elated and energetic, I experience a fullness in my ears somewhat more on the right side than the left, and having a character similar to that which occurs during rapid descent in an airplane or elevator. I then become aware of a dull discomfort, an extension over the entire head on both sides, although somewhat more on the right. At this point, two or three minutes have elapsed, seemingly short but long enough for me to know that a cluster has indeed begun and will ultimately get worse. Such anticipation causes me considerable consternation regarding any decision to continue my activities or cancel plans, and find a place to be alone, giving way to a slowly increasing anxiety, fear, panic, and with-

drawal. I become aware of myself listening for changes in my head. Is the cluster prematurely aborting itself, progressing further, or unchanging? A sudden stab, only fleeting, strikes my temple, then again, somewhere near the apex of my skull and upper molars in my face, always on the right side. It strikes me again, deep into the skull base, and as quickly, changes location to a small area above my eyebrow. Ny nose is stuffed and yet runs simultaneously. If I could sneeze, I feel the attack would end. Yet in spite of all tricks, I find myself unable to induce sneezing. While the sharp stabs continue in this fashion, a slow crescendo of dull pain presents itself in an area of a hand's length and breadth over the eye and temporal region. The pain area narrows into a smaller are, and yet, as if magnified, enlarges in intensity. I find myself bending my neck downward, though slightly, as if my head is being gently pushed from behind. My neck, up to the base of my skull, is tight and feels as if I were wearing a neck collar. I feel compelled to remove my tie and loosen my shirt collar, even though I know that it will not offer me even a modicum of relief.

In an effort to alter this persistent discomfort, I drop my head between my legs while seated. My face and eyes seem to fill with fluid, but the pain remains unchanged. Despite my suntan, as I look into the mirror, a gaunt, sickly, pale face peers back. My right lid is only slightly drooping and the white of my eye is charted with many red vessels, giving the eye an overall color of pink. Right and left pupils appear equal and constricted as is usual for light-eyed people. Having difficulty standing in one place too long, I leave the mirror to continue alternating my pacing and sitting.

As usual, I am struck with the additional fear that the pain will never end, but dismiss it as impossible since even if that were the case, I would surely kill myself.

The pain, now located somewhere behind my eye and slightly above it, worsens. The pain is best described as a force pushing with such incredible power through my eye that my head appears to be moving backward, yielding to its resistance. The force wanes and waxes, but the duration of successive exacerbations seems to increase. The cluster attack is at its peak, which is celebrated by an outpouring of tears from only my right eye. I have now been in cluster for thirty-five minutes, ten minutes at its peak.

My wife peeks into the room where I hold forth. I look up and see her expression of pity, frustration, and helplessness. She sees my tortured face as I have seen it in the mirror at this stage before: a drooling mouth, agape, gray face wet on one side, an almost closed eyelid, and smelling of pain and anguish. She closes the door and leaves, feeling hurt for me, anger for the stupidity of medical science, and guilt since deep within her mind is the suspicion that she is the cause for my suffering.

I cry for her, but cry more for myself. The pain is so incredible. Suddenly I am overwhelmed by a fury. I lift a chair high over my head and crash it to the floor. With doubled fist, I strike the wall. The pain persists.

Waning periods soon become longer in duration and I allow myself to suspect that the peak is behind me, but cautiously, since I have been too often disappointed.

Indeed, the pain is ending. The descent from the mountain of pain is rapid. The force is gone. Only severe pain remains. My nose and eye continue to run. The road back, as with all travel, covers the same territory, but faster. Stabbing, easily tolerated pain is felt, then gone. Dull, aching fullness, neck stiffness, all disappear, replaced in turn by a welcome sensation of pins and needles over the right scalp area, similar to the way one's legs feel after they have been asleep. Thus, my head has awakened after a nightmare of torment.

Eye and nose dry, I let out a sigh. I collect my pile of wet tissues that are strewn all over the floor and deposit them into a wastepaper basket. The innocent chair is now uprighted, and I rub my slightly bruised fist.

Thus, having ended the battle and cleaned up its field, I open the door and enter my pain-free world until tomorrow.

FREQUENCY AND DURATION

The attack frequency in episodic cluster headache ranges from two attacks per week to ten per day, with a mean of 1.7 attacks per day, and 2.5 attacks per day for chronic and subchronic types. The mean duration of attacks for all cluster headache types is approximately 60 minutes, with a range of 20 minutes to 180 minutes.

LOCATION AND INTENSITY

The site of pain is always unilateral and most often oculotemporal, oculofrontal, or frontotemporal. It may be limited to the lower face and dental regions solely or occur in combination with upper facial regions. Not infrequently, an ipsilateral suboccipital area may be involved. Misdiagnosis of cluster headache is often encountered when patients present with lower facial pain, often confused with trigeminal neuralgia or dental disease.

The unrelenting exquisite intensity of cluster headache pain appears to have no parallel. Since quantitative measures of pain are unavailable, we have queried a large cluster-headache population who had experienced other painful disorders. Pain intensity of these disorders were compared to that of cluster headache. In no case was the pain of ureteral colic, complicated childbirth, accidental amputation, or trigeminal neuralgia said to be worse than that of cluster headache. Because of this intensity, suicide ideation among cluster-headache patients is common. Fortunately, attacks are short-lived and followed by completely headache-free intervals. Of 600 cluster patients followed at our clinic for a period of one to 15 years, one suicide occurred unrelated to his cluster disorder and during a remission period.

The quality of cluster pain is boring, as if a blunt instrument is being pushed through the eye or temple region. The pain is non-throbbing in approximately 70% of cases.

Associated Symptoms and Signs

The cluster attack is associated with mild-to-profuse ipsilateral lacrimation, rhinorrhea or nasal stuffiness, conjunctival suffusion, miosis, and ptosis. Sweating, or lack of sweating, is quite variable. Ipsilateral facial pallor, orbital swelling, and photophobia are common features during the attack. Less commonly, facial and scalp hyperalgesia, nausea, and temporal artery swelling may occur.

Timing of Attacks

Daily attacks often occur with circadian rhythmicity. Attacks occurring twice a day may be 12 hours apart. Most commonly, headaches occur between 6:00 pm and 8:00 pm, after working hours have ended and the patient has relaxed. The next common time for attacks is 90 minutes after sleep onset associated with the first REM-sleep stage, and to a lesser extent, during other REM sleep. Not infrequently, the patient may be awakened with a headache immediately before his usual wake-up time; and finally, it may occur upon or after awakening. Although cluster headaches may occur at any time of the day, they infrequently occur during working hours.

Provocation of Attacks

Spontaneous attacks may be expected during air travel or during vacations at high altitudes. Alcohol commonly provokes attacks, even when small quantities are ingested. Experimentally, other vasodilators have been shown to induce attacks. These include histamine injected subcutaneously or intravenously, alcohol ingestion, and sublingual nitroglycerin. It should be noted that cluster headaches may be induced by these agents only during the cluster period.

Behavior during Attacks

Not unlike the behavior of patients experiencing ureteral colic, the cluster headache sufferer writhes with pain when attempting to lie still. Usually, he must sit in a chair, often rocking forward and back, or he may pace around the room at a rate commensurate with the pain intensity. The inability to lie still during a cluster headache attack is pathognomonic of this condition.

Habits and Personality Factors

While there appears to be no cause and effect relationship of cigarette smoking or alcohol use to cluster headache, in general, a significantly greater use of these substances is found in cluster-headache populations when compared to controls. Approximately 80% of patients smoke cigarettes and drink alcohol. Between 40% and 50% of alcohol users drink more than the equivalent of two drinks a day. These findings persist throughout the various types of cluster headache. Further, cessation of these habits has little affect on the course of this disorder.

Abuse of prescription or street drugs was found in 12% of episodic patients, 17% of the chronic group, and 46% of subchronic patients. These findings were partially consistent with scores for addiction-proneness on evaluation by the Minnesota Multiphasic Personality Inventory (MMPI). The addiction-proneness score was elevated in one third of episodic groups, and in almost half of the subchronic and chronic groups. Neurotic characteristics were also found in these groups by MMPI examination. However, with all groups combined, including the larger population of episodic cluster headache patients, the MMPI patterns differ little from those of controls.

Family History of Cluster Headache

It has been reported that less than 2% of a cluster population has a parental history of cluster headache; yet, approximately 10% claim that one or more relatives have this disorder. Thus, genetic factors are not ruled out in this condition and, if present, may have low expression.

Differential Diagnosis

CHRONIC PAROXYSMAL HEMICRANIA

Some disorders resemble cluster headache by one or more features (Table 10.1). The clinical condition closest to cluster headache is chronic paroxysmal hemicrania (CPH), first described by Sjaastad and Dale in 1974. Since then approximately 20 case reports have appeared in the medical literature substantiating this entity. Indeed, in his review in 1987, Sjaastad reported having been informed of approximately 80 cases of CPH throughout the international medical community.

CPH is similar to chronic cluster headache in that attacks, often REM-related, are quite severe, almost always retro-orbital in location, and associated with ipsilateral lacrimation, rhinorrhea, conjunctival suffusion, miosis and ptosis. Clinically, CPH differs from cluster headache by (1) an increased attack frequency, (2) shorter attack duration, (3) less restlessness during attacks, (4) a total response to indomethacin and lack of response to anti-cluster prophylactic medications, and (5) provocation of attacks by neck flexion, in some cases.

Russell in 1984, reported that CPH attacks occur at a frequency of 4 to 18 per day with a mean of approximately 14. The duration of attacks were found to range from 3 to 46 minutes with a mean of 13 minutes.

While it was initially reported that CPH occurred solely in females, subsequent publications by Price and Posner in 1978 and Rapoport et al in 1981 demonstrated that males were not exempt from this disorder. Indeed, a new publication by Kudrow et al, in which an episodic type of paroxysmal hemicrania was reported, three of six patients were male.

The etiology and pathogenesis of CPH is unknown. Some pathophysiologic parameters, however, have been defined. Ipsilateral intraocular pressure and indentation pulse amplitudes, as well as corneal temperatures, were found to be increased during attack periods as demonstrated by Broch et al in 1970 and Hørven and Sjaastad in 1977, respectively. While similar findings have been noted in cluster headache, magnitudes were found to be greater in CPH.

Further, autonomic dysfunction was noted in regard to forehead sweating which was greater on the symptomatic side during attacks in some patients. This finding, however, was more consistently seen in cluster headache patients, as reported by Sjaastad in 1987. While in cluster headache, sweating could be increased following pilocarpine administration and decreased by heat induction, such responses could not be demonstrated in CPH. In either case, however, mechanisms responsible for pain and autonomic symptoms and signs remain unclear.

The treatment of choice for CPH is prophylactic administration of indomethacin. Response is generally complete and considered to be diagnostic of CPH.

Sjaastad suggests that initially a patient should receive 200 mg to 250 mg per day to ensure a therapeutic response. In our own experience, 75 mg to 100 mg per day, in divided doses, has been successful in all cases. The dosage of indomethacin may be decreased to lowest maintenance levels, not infrequently to 25 mg per day. An episodic form has been described.

RAEDER'S PARATRIGEMINAL NEURALGIA

Raeder's Paratrigeminal Neuralgia resembles cluster headache in that the pain of this condition is also unilateral having an ocular or frontal location, and it is associated with a partial Horner's syndrome (ptosis and miosis). It also awakens the patient from sleep. These similarities may suggest shared pathways with cluster headache. The headache of Raeder's syndrome, however, is persistent throughout most of its course of several weeks to months, during which the pain is only moderate to moderately severe in intensity.

Table 10.1. Differential Diagnosis of Cluster Headache

Conditions Resembling Cluster	Timing of Attacks	Frequency	Duration	Location	Intensity	Character	Associated Signs and Symptoms
Cluster headache	Occurs with regularity, often awakens from sleep	1-3 per day	30-90 min	Unilateral, oculofrontal, temporal	Excruciating	Nonthrobbing, boring	Unilateral lacrimation, rhinorrhea, conjunctival injection, partial Horner's, Cannot lie down
Chronic paroxysmal hemicrania (CPH)	Paroxysms around the clock	15 per day or more	5-20 min	same as above	same as above	same as above	same as above
Raedere's syndrome (paratrigeminal neuralgia)	Often awakens from sleep	persistent	persistent	Unilateral, supraocular	Severe	Burning, throbbing, nonthrobbing	Partial Horner's syndrome
Trigeminal neuralgia	Related to facial trigger zones	Many per day	Intermittent, seconds to four min	Unilateral distribution of cranial nerve V, usually and/or 3rd division	Severe	Lancinating, lightning-like	Stimulation of trigger areas starts pain
Temporal arteritis	No consistent pattern	Daily	Persistent	Unilateral, temporal	Moderate to severe	Burning, nonthrobbing	Tortuosity and tenderness of affected artery, elevated ESR loss of vision

Trigeminal Neuralgia

Trigeminal neuralgia shares a few characteristics with cluster headache. Attacks result from stimulation of facial trigger zones, usually in the second or third division of the fifth cranial nerve. The pain is sharp, lightninglike, or lancinating, only seconds to four minutes in duration, repeatedly for several minutes. No autonomic signs are present. Dilantin and Tegretol are helpful.

Temporal Arteritis and Post-herpetic Neuralgia

The headache of temporal arteritis and post-herpetic neuralgia is constant with no consistent pattern and having a burning quality. The patient is usually female and over 60. In temporal arteritis, the affected artery is often tender, tortuous, and pulseless. There may be an ipsilateral decrease in vision. A recent history of herpes zoster infection is diagnostic of post-herpetic neuralgia.

Pathogenesis of Cluster Headache

Neither the etiology nor the pathogenesis of cluster headache has been established. Several pathways, however, have been elucidated, affording at least a partial understanding of this disorder.

The following is an account of a pathogenetic model in abbreviated form that attempts to collate fragments of experimental and clinical data (Figure 10.1).

Oxygen inhalation was reported to be effective in the symptomatic treatment of cluster headache attacks. Its rapid action suggests a direct effect on hypoxemia and implies that hypoxemia may play a role in the pathogenesis of cluster headache. The relationship of hypoxemia to attacks is further supported by the provocation of attacks during altitude hypoxia; further, agents known to induce cluster attacks, such as alcohol, nitroglycerin, and histamine may affect a hypoxemic state where compensatory circulatory reflexes are impaired.

Cluster headache attacks have been temporally associated with the REM stage of sleep. A recent sleep study also showed that cluster attacks often occur with moderate decreases of oxygen saturation (65% to 90%) in association with, or independently of, REM stage of sleep. Indeed, sleep apnea was found in five out of five episodic cluster headache subjects and one out of five chronic patients.

Since the carotid body functions as the most sensitive chemoreceptor of hypoxemia, impaired carotid body activity may play a major role in the pathogenesis of this disorder. The carotid body dysfunction may be the consequence of periodic failure of hypothalamic regulation.

There is evidence to suggest involvement of the hypothalamus in cluster headache. As mentioned earlier, there appears to be a relationship between onset of cycles and photoperiods, indicating that the circannual pacemakers are unable to respond to environmental cues. Chronobiological pacemakers are thought to reside in the hypothalamus. Dysrhythmic circadian activity of

Figure 10.1 Suggested pathways of the cluster period, induction, and symptoms of attack

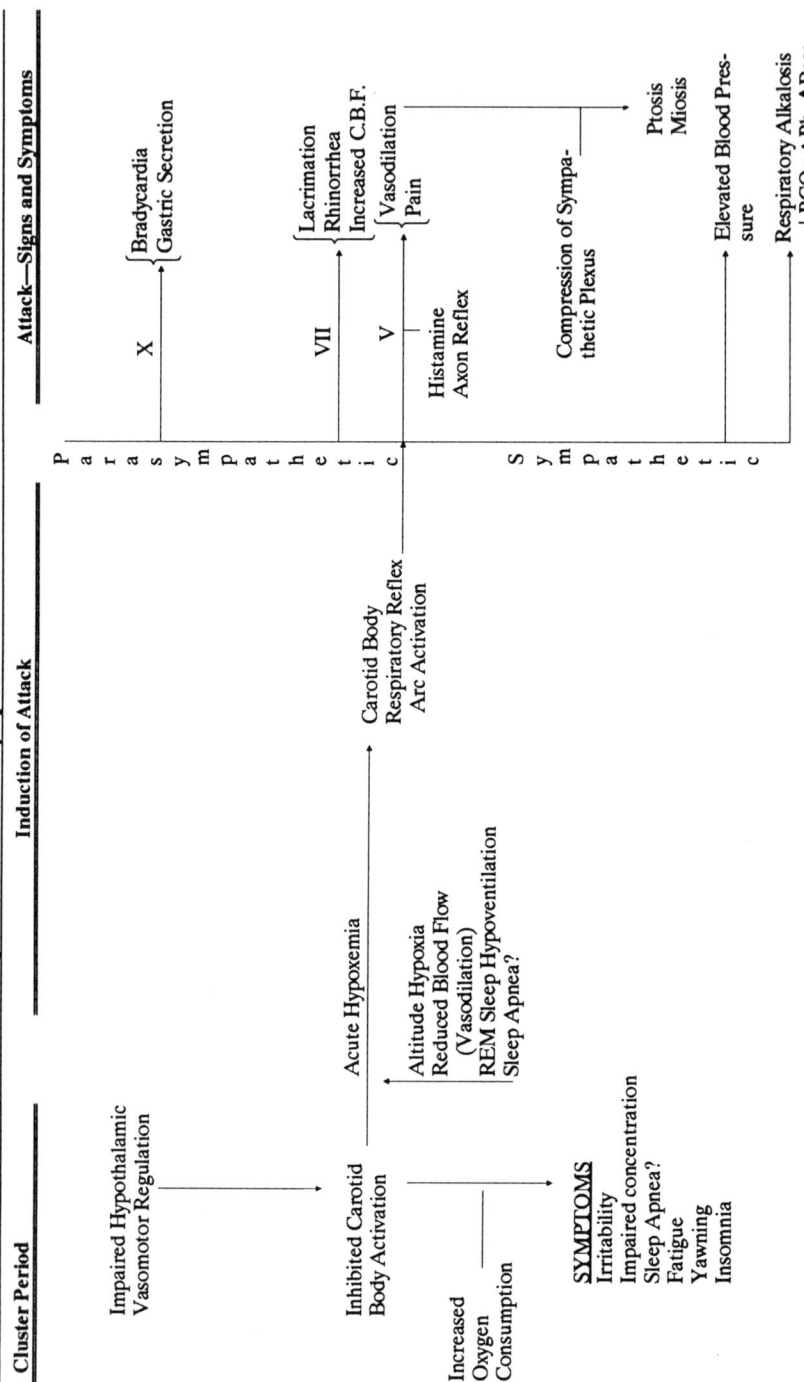

temperature and hormonal changes, such as luteinizing hormone (LH), testosterone, prolactin, and melatonin, have been reported to occur during cluster periods.

It should be noted that the hypothalamus helps regulate carotid body activity via sympathetic connections. Several investigations demonstrated decreased sympathetic activity during the cluster period.

It is suggested that only when critical levels of hypoxemia are reached, the partially denervated chemoreceptors may be activated in the manner of a hypersensitivity denervation response to stimulate the nuclei of the seventh and tenth cranial nerves and the respiratory centers via interconnections with the nucleus solitarius. Thus induction of the cluster headache attack.

The final pathway, as noted in Figure 10.1, involves the stimulation of peripheral secretory receptors innervated by the seventh and tenth cranial nerves. A surgical section at various levels of the seventh cranial nerve pathway has been shown to be at least partially successful in abolishing this disorder. These sites include the nervus intermedius, greater superficial petrosal nerve, and the sphenopalatine ganglion.

During an attack in one case, cerebral angiography demonstrated a decrease in the flow of dye in the ipsilateral osseous portion of the internal carotid artery, and dilation of the ophthalmic artery. This finding suggested that dilation of the internal carotid artery in its bony canal may compress the surrounding sympathetic plexus, including the oculosympathetic nerve, which may result in the partial Horner's syndrome associated with the cluster attack.

Mast cell changes in cluster headache has lead Appenzeller to conclude that histamine may play a role in the production of pain in cluster headache via a histamine axon reflex.

Lastly, the sensory appreciation of pain is mediated by the fifth cranial nerve; cluster headaches have been abolished by injections of glycerol into the trigeminal cistern. A somewhat higher success rate was reported following gasserian ganglion radiofrequency lesions.

Treatment of Cluster Headache

At the California Medical Clinic for Headache, several guidelines govern management of cluster headache. These include providing information and follow-up, avoidance therapy, and prophylactic and symptomatic treatment.

INFORMATION AND FOLLOW-UP

Patients should be instructed in the current medical knowledge of cluster headache. This affords a better doctor-patient relationship, alleviates the patient's anxiety regarding serious complications, dispels misinformation, and allows him to participate in his treatment program with greater awareness. Patient cooperation is a prerequisite for a successful management.

Not all patients respond to first-line selection of medications. Follow-up visits, in person or by telephone, are necessary to reevaluate progress and change medications, where indicated. Hence, patients are instructed to keep accurate records of their attacks.

Avoidance

In all cases, patients are instructed to avoid afternoon naps and alcoholic beverages, including wine and beer. As noted earlier, alcohol will in most instances induce acute attacks during an active period, but not during remissions. Dietary influences, with the exception of alcohol, appear to have little importance in cluster headache.

Short sleep periods during the afternoon or early evening may induce acute cluster attacks. The pain may awaken the patient or begin soon after he awakens. Cluster attacks occurring during sleep are likely to be associated with the REM state. It is possible that the latency of REM-onset is shorter during naps.

Bursts of anger, prolonged anticipation, excitement, and excessive physical activity are to be avoided, since cluster headaches are apt to occur in the relaxation period that follows. We have also observed that prolonged or sustained periods (two weeks or more) of anger, rage, or frustration experienced during remission periods are often associated with a cluster period onset.

Not infrequently, cluster periods begin after alterations in sleep-wake cycles. Vacation trips, work shift changes, new occupations, postsurgical periods, completion of university studies, etc., are conditions commonly associated with the cluster period onset. Although there are many variables associated with such life-style changes, alteration of sleep-wake patterns, which often accompany these changes, may be the most significant.

Prophylactic Medications

The selection of particular drugs depends upon compatibility with other medications, history of untoward reaction or poor responsiveness, and the health of the patient. Drug selection will also depend on cluster headache type, frequency, timing of attacks, and the patient's age.

The following recommended treatment guide is outlined in Table 10.2. Criteria for selection of medication, other than those mentioned above, include patient's personality, behavior pattern, life style, and reliability. These data may alter the choice of drug as recommended in the table. it should also be noted that the site of action of beneficial cluster headache medications is unknown.

Episodic Cluster Headache in Patients Under 30 Years

Ergotamine tartrate is the prophylactic treatment of choice in patients who experience one predictable attack daily. A 2 mg dose administered two hours before the expected headache generally prevents the attack. For the attack that awakens the patient at any time during sleep, ergotamine tartrate, 2 mg at

Table 10.2. Guide for Prophylactic Treatment of Cluster Headache

	Episodic Type			Chronic or Subchronic
	Under 30 years of age			
	One attack/day	>1 attack/day	>30 years of age	Any age or frequency
First choice	Ergotamine tartrate 2 mg, two hours before expected attack	Lithium carbonate 300 mg b.i.d.	Verapamil 80 mg q.i.d.	Verapamil 80 mg q.i.d.
If resistant	Methysergide maleate (Sansert) 2 mg q.i.d.	Add ergotamine tartrate 2 mg HS	Add ergotamine tartrate 2 mg HS	Add ergotamine tartrate 2 mg HS
If resistant	Prednisone (Table 10.3)	Add verapamil 80 mg q.i.d.	Add lithium carbonate 300 mg b.i.d.	Add lithium carbonate 300 mg b.i.d.

bedtime, is recommended. Ergotamine appears to provide an excellent preventative effect only after hours following administration, in contrast to symptomatic treatment that requires immediate use. This disparity suggests that ergotamine may have two sites of action.

In our experience 2 mg/day of ergotamine tartrate is not likely to cause ergotamine rebound, as seen in migraine headache. Nor have we seen complications resulting from the use of this amount in a rather large population of patients treated for extended periods.

Methysergide maleate (Sansert) is recommended in the event of ergotamine resistance in episodic cluster headache patients. It may be used safely and effectively for short periods (not longer than three months). The usefulness of methysergide is usually limited to the first few cluster periods in the course of the disorder, since resistance increases with subsequent cycles. It is to be noted that ergotamine and methysergide are contraindicated in the presence of pregnancy, hepatitis, severe infection, and cardiovascular and peripheral vascular disease.

If the young patient does not adequately respond to ergotamine or methysergide, a course of Prednisone should be considered (Table 10.3). Steroids are highly effective in episodic cluster headache. One must be cautioned, however, that prolonged use of steroids may cause a patient to become steroid-fast. In our experience, this can be avoided if the course of treatment is limited to a three-week period. When the dosage of Prednisone has been reduced to 15 mg/day, attacks may reappear. Ergotamine tartrate, 2 mg at bedtime, may be added to the remaining Prednisone regimen.

When attack frequency exceeds one per day, lithium carbonate (Eskalith, Lithobid) is the treatment of choice. The dosage schedule should not exceed 600 mg/day (in divided doses) since few patients are helped more by greater

Table 10.3. Recommended 21 Day Schedule of Prophylactic Prednisone in Cluster Headache

Daily dosage	Duration
10 mg q.i.d.	5 days
10 mg t.i.d.	5 days
10 mg b.i.d.	4 days
5 mg t.e.d.	3 days
5 mg b.i.d.	2 days
5 mg daily	2 days

amounts. It is unnecessary to obtain frequent blood levels since, unlike treatment of bipolar disease, the therapeutic level range is quite low and usually achieved by a daily dose of 600 mg. The most common side effect of lithium is hand tremor, more evident when the daily dose exceeds 600 mg. Lithium is not recommended for patients who are maintained on diuretics or low salt diets since toxicity may result as a consequence of competition between intracellular lithium and sodium.

In the category of frequent attacks in young episodic cluster patients, failure to respond to lithium should indicate the need to use ergotamine. Ergotamine tartrate, 2 mg at bedtime, may be added to the lithium for better results. Adverse effects of this combination have not been noted at our clinic. If the response remains poor, verapamil HCl (Calan, Isoptin) should be added to the above combination. In our experience, verapamil is the single most effective prophylactic agent in cluster headache. At our clinic it is reserved for young patients who are unresponsive to other medications, but used as a first-choice prophylactic agent for all others. Verapamil is contraindicated in certain cardiac arrhythmias, hypotension, and left ventricular failure. The most common side effects are constipation, myalgias, and fluid retention.

Episodic Cluster Headache in Patients Over 30 Years and All Chronic and Subchronic Types

The prophylactic treatment of choice for all other cluster patients is verapamil, 80 mg q.i.d. for men and t.i.d. for women. Ergotamine, 2 mg at bedtime should be added to the verapamil regimen in the event of an inadequate response to verapamil alone. Resistance to this combination indicates the need for lithium carbonate, 300 mg b.i.d.

In the event a patient remains resistant to all treatment attempts, it is imperative to rule out the presence of intracranial abnormalities such as arterio-venous malformation, aneurysm, or tumor. Several case reports have demonstrated an association of such lesions with cluster headache, although this is a rare finding. Narcotic addiction should also be ruled out. Finally, unresponsiveness or contraindication to all medical treatment may indicate the need for hospitalization or surgical intervention. In this author's opinion, the surgical approach should be decided in consultation with a surgeon experienced in the treatment of this disorder. The most promising and least hazardous procedure appears to be radiofrequency lesions of the trigeminal ganglion.

SYMPTOMATIC TREATMENT

Oxygen inhalation is the most effective and safest symptomatic treatment of the cluster headache attack. At onset of the attack, the patient should breathe 100% oxygen at 7 L/min through a facial mask for not more than 15 to 20 minutes. Our data show that 70% of attacks may be aborted within 10 minutes, and an additional 15% to 20% of attacks within 15 to 20 minutes. Patients who experience infrequent attacks often resist the use of prophylactic medication and prefer the sole use of oxygen inhalation symptomatically. When oxygen inhalation is inconvenient (during travel), rapidly acting preparations of ergotamine is recommended. These include sublingual or inhalation preparations. These agents are nearly as effective as oxygen inhalation. Finally, recent experimental studies by Ekbom, et al suggest symptomatic efficacy of a 5-HT$_1$ receptor agonist called sumatriptan (Imitrex). Further studies of and experience in the symptomatic treatment of cluster headache attacks should be forthcoming.

Summary

The cluster headache syndrome is divided into three types: episodic, subchronic, and chronic. It is a male-dominant disorder having an incidence of approximately 1% in a general population.

The mean duration of cluster periods is approximately two months with a mean remission duration of approximately one year. Frequency of attacks during the cluster period is from one to three per day, each lasting 45 minutes to an hour and a half. The pain is exceedingly intense, unilateral, located around the eye and temporal region, and it is associated with ipsilateral lacrimation, rhinorrhea, conjunctival suffusion, partial Horner's syndrome, and an inability to lie still. Attacks are likely to occur in the evenings, including during sleep periods.

The frequency of smoking and drinking is high in cluster headache populations. Neuroses, drug abuse, and addiction-proneness occur frequently in subchronic and chronic headache types.

In this presentation, cluster headache has been differentiated from several other conditions that share some common characteristics. These include CPH, Raeder's paratrigeminal neuralgia, trigeminal neuralgia, temporal arteritis, and post-herpetic neuralgia.

A hypothetical model of pathogenesis was presented to collate fragments of experimental and clinical data. It suggests that inhibition of hypothalamic regulation of the autonomic nervous system activity affects chemoreceptor function, allowing hypoxemic states to occur. Under certain conditions, a low critical value of PO_2 finally stimulates chemoreceptor activity in a denervation hypersensitivity response. Via interconnecting central nuclei, the seventh cranial nerve is stimulated, resulting in the signs and symptoms of the cluster headache.

Bibliography

Appenzeller O, Becker WJ, Ragaz A. Cluster headache: Ultra-structural aspects and pathogenetic mechanisms. *Arch Neurol 18*: 302-306, 1981

Broch A, Hørven I, Nornes H, Sjaastad O, Tønjum A. Studies of cerebral and ocular circulation in a patient with cluster headache. *Headache 10*: 1-8, 1970.

Ekbom K. Nitroglycerin as a provocative agent in cluster headache. *Arch Neurol 19*: 487-493, 1969.

Ekbom K. A clinical comparison of cluster headache and migraine. *Acta Neurol Scand 4146 (supp)*: 1-48, 1970.

Ekbom K, Greitz T. Carotid angiography in cluster headache. *Acta Radiol Diagnosis 10*: 177-186, 1970.

Ekbom K, Lindgren L, Nilsson BY, et al. Chronic migrainous neuralgia treated by retrogasserian injection of glycerol. *Fifth International Migraine Symposium*, London, September 19-20, 1984.

Ekbom, et al. Treatment of acute cluster headache with sumatriptan. *N Engl J Med 325*: 322-326, 1991.

Friedman AP, Mikropoulos HE. Cluster headache. *Neurology 8*: 653-663, 1958.

Gardner WJ, Stowell A, Dutlinger R. Resection of the greater superficial petrosal nerve in the treatment of unilateral headache. *J Neurosurg 4*: 105-114, 1947.

Horton BT, MacLean AR, Craig WM. A new syndrome of vascular headache: Results of treatment with histamine"Preliminary report. *Mayo Clin Proc 14*: 257-260, 1939.

Hørven I, Sjaastad O. Cluster headache syndrome and migraine: Ophthalmological support for a two-entity theory. *Acta Ophthalmol (Kobenh) 55*: 35-51, 1977.

Kudrow L. *Cluster Headache: Mechanisms and Management*, pp 99-126. London, Oxford University Press, 1980.

Kudrow L. Response of cluster headache attacks to oxygen inhalation. *Headache 21*: 1-4, 1981.

Kudrow L. A possible role of the carotid body in the pathogenesis of cluster headache. *Cephalalgia 3*: 242-247, 1983.

Kudrow L, McGinty DJ, Phillips ER, et al. Sleep apnea in cluster headache. *Cephalalgia 4*: 33-38, 1984.

Kudrow L. Subchronic cluster headache. *Headache 27*: 197-200, 1987.

Kudrow L. The cyclic relationship of natural illumination to cluster period frequency. Procedures of Third International Congress, Florence. *Headache*, September 1987.

Kudrow L, Esperanca P, Vijayan N. Episodic paroxysmal hemicrania? *Cephalalgia 7*: 197-201, 1987.

Kunkle EC, Pfeiffer JB Jr, Wilhoit WM, et al. Recurrent brief headache in cluster pattern. *Trans Am Neurol Assoc 77*: 240, 1954.

Lance JW. *Mechanism and Management of Headache*, ed 3. London, Butterworths, 1978.

Mathew NT, Hurt W. Radiofrequency trigeminal gangliolysis in the treatment of chronic intractable cluster headache. *Headache 25*: 166, 1985.

Meyer JS, Hardenberg J. Clinical effectiveness of calcium entry blockers in prophylactic treatment of migraine and cluster headache. *Headache 23*: 266-277, 1983.

Price RV, Posner JB. Chronic paroxysmal hemicrania: A disabling headache syndrome responding to indomethacin. *Ann Neurol 3*: 183-184, 1978.

Rapoport AM, Sheftell FD, Baskin SM. Chronic paroxysmal hemicrania: Case report of the second known definite occurrence in a male. *Cephalalgia 1*: 67-69, 1981.

Russell D, von der Lippe A. Cluster headache: Heart rate and blood pressure changes during spontaneous attacks. *Cephalalgia 2*: 62-70, 1982.

Russell D. Chronic paroxysmal hemicrania: Severity, duration and time of occurrences of attacks. *Cephalalgia 4*: 53-56, 1984.

Saunte C. *Cluster headache syndrome: Studies on autonomic dysfunction*. University of Trondheim publication. Faculty of Medicine, Dept. of Neurology, Trondheim, Norway, 1984.

Sjaastad O, Dale I. Evidence for a new (?) treatable headache entity. *Headache 14*: 105-108, 1974.

Sjaastad O. Chronic paroxysmal hemicrania: Clinical aspects and controversies. In: Blau JN, (ed). *Migraine: Clinical, Therapeutic, Conceptual and Research Aspects*, pp 135-152. London, Chapman and Hall, 1987.

Sweet WH, Poletti CE, Macon JB. Treatment of trigeminal neuralgia and other facial pains by retrogasserian injection of glycerol. *Neurosurgery 9*: 647-653, 1981.

Waltz TA, Dalessio DJ, Ott KH, et al. Trigeminal cistern glycerol injections for facial pain. *Headache 25*: 354-357, 1985.

Watson CP, Morley TP, Richardson JC, et al. The surgical treatment of chronic cluster headache. *Headache 23*: 289-295, 1983.

11

Headache Due to Pain Sensitive Structures Within the Head

Seymour Solomon

Intracranial Pain-Sensitive Structures

The brain and most blood vessels within the head are relatively insensitive to pain; therefore, intracranial pathology evokes the sensation of headache by stimulating only certain pain-sensitive structures [1]. Pain impulses are carried by cranial nerves V, VII, IX, and X, as well as by all of the posterior nerve roots of the spinal cord. With regard to headache, the trigeminal nerve and the first three cervical nerves are most relevant.

Stimulation of the dura mater at the base of the skull and the tentorium of the cerebellum causes pain [2,3]. The superior surface of the tentorium and the dura of the floor of the anterior fossa are innervated by the ophthalmic division of the trigeminal nerve, which refers pain to the anterior half of the head, including the orbits. The inferior surface of the tentorium and the dura of the floor of the posterior fossa are supplied by the upper three cervical nerves which refer pain to the posterior half of the head and the back of the neck. The floor of the middle fossa is insensitive to pain, as is the dura over the convexity of the cerebrum. The pia-arachnoid is similarly insensitive to pain.

The main trunks of the dural arteries are sensitive to pain [1]. The branches of the middle meningeal artery, but not those of the anterior or posterior meningeal arteries, are pain-sensitive. The major, if not the sole, nociceptive innervation of the middle meningeal artery and its branches is the trigeminal nerve. The site of pain roughly corresponds to the site overlying the area of stimulation.

The proximal trunks of the intracranial carotid artery and the middle and anterior cerebral arteries are innervated by the trigeminal nerve and stimulation of these vessels causes pain in the area of the orbit [4]. Stimulation of the vertebral and posterior inferior cerebellar arteries causes occipital and suboccipital pains. The pial arteries and veins are insensitive to pain.

The walls of the superior sagittal sinus are sensitive to pain, but the degree of pain is slight to moderate [1,2]. Pain is referred primarily to the frontal and orbital areas, but also to the parietal and vertex regions. Tributary veins are sensitive only at their junction with the sinus. The tentorial branches of the trigeminal nerve supply these venous structures. Unilateral stimulation of the superior surface of the transverse sinus, torcula herophili, and straight sinus causes ipsilateral pain in the forehead and eye. Stimulation of the infratentorial surfaces of these sinuses causes pain behind the ipsilateral ear. Major veins under the temporal lobe that drain into the transverse, superior, and petrosal sinuses are sensitive and transmit pain to the temporal areas on the side of the stimulus. Stimulation of the occipital sinus causes pain behind the ear or occipital area; this sinus is innervated by the upper cervical nerves. The inferior sagittal sinus and other venous channels are insensitive to pain.

In the early experiments that mapped these pain-sensitive structures within the cranium, not all vessels or areas were stimulated because of their inaccessibility [1]. It was noted, however, that traction on arteries at the base of the brain during tumor removal evoked widespread pain. Headaches associated with ventricular dilation and intracranial hypertension are probably due to traction on blood vessels, whereas the headache of meningitis is due to irritation of meninges, blood vessel walls, and cranial and cervical nerve roots.

With few exceptions, headaches caused by intracranial disease do not have pathognomonic features. Nevertheless, certain qualities of headaches may raise the suspicion of underlying disease and greatly aid in diagnosis.

Brain Tumors

The word tumor, used in its broadest sense, incorporates all mass lesions, not only neoplasms but also abscesses, hematomas, and cysts. The headache associated with a brain tumor is usually caused by stretch of basal blood vessels. However, brain tumors often fail to cause headaches because the intracranial dynamics may change very gradually.

NEOPLASMS

In the 1950s and 1960s, headache was the first symptom of a brain tumor in 80% of patients [5]. In subsequent decades, the incidence decreased to approximately 30% and, with the advent of new imaging techniques, the number will undoubtedly continue to shrink. Neoplasms in the posterior fossa, those affecting midline structures, and those causing cerebral edema tend to produce early increased intracranial pressure and generalized headaches. Posterior fossa tumors may cause headache by several mechanisms. Obstructing cerebrospinal fluid (CSF) outflow causes increased intracranial pressure and generalized headache. Pressure on pain-sensitive cranial nerves (trigeminal, facial, glossopharyngeal, or vagus nerves) refers pain to the face, ear, or throat. Pain may be due to irritation of the dura or stretch of the basal blood vessels with or without tonsillar herniation; if tonsillar herniation occurs, there may be traction on upper cervical nerve roots [6]. The headache is usually occipito-nuchal and neck pain may cause contraction of neck muscles with head tilt. Traction on the tentorium (innervated by the trigeminal nerve) causes pain referred to the forehead and eyes [3]. Mass lesions of the anterior or middle fossa are usually associated with a consistently ipsilateral headache, often frontal or frontotemporal and roughly overlying the area of the tumor.

As with other symptoms of a brain neoplasm, the headache tends to be progressive, increasing in severity, duration, and frequency, eventually becoming continuous [7]. The headache may awaken the patient toward the end of sleep. Unless the neoplasm is benign, the headache is of relatively recent onset, i.e., weeks or months. A slowly infiltrating glioma or meningioma may reach a large size without causing headache, either because basal vessels are not affected or the vessels and the meninges are not acutely stretched. In these cases, other signs of brain tumor will occur before the onset of headache. Because the density of the neoplasm is different from that of the parenchyma, slight shift of the mass relative to normal tissue may occur on head movements and headache may be precipitated or briefly increased. Similarly, transient increase in the volume of intracranial venous blood causes or adds to intracranial hypertension and evokes or aggravates headaches during the valsalva phenomenon that occurs while coughing or straining.

In most cases, the clinical diagnosis of brain tumor is made not by the headache characteristics but by associated neurological features. These may be generalized (depression of consciousness, impairment of mentation, change in personality, or seizures) or focal (hemiparesis, hemisensory impairment, hemianopsia, aphasia, cranial nerve signs, or cerebellar defects).

INTRACRANIAL ABSCESS

Headache and other features of brain abscess are generally indistinguishable from that of neoplasm [8]; fever, often thought to be present with abscess, is usually conspicuous by its absence. Abscess or granuloma may be suspected when a septic source is present in some area of the body such as the heart, lungs, or ear, or in patients with AIDS and, much less commonly, when signs of brief cerebritis with fever occur prior to the more indolent course of a mass lesion.

Epidural abscesses usually arise from extension of infections of the paranasal sinuses or middle ear or after intracranial surgery [9]. In addition to headache, fever may accompany early focal or generalized cerebral signs.

INTRACRANIAL HEMATOMA

Headache due to increased intracranial pressure is usually an accompanying feature of dural hematomas, but it is not a necessary diagnostic symptom. *Chronic subdural hematoma* is a common intracranial mass [10]. Most cases do not present with a classic picture of depressed consciousness following head injury. In contrast to *acute subdural hematoma*, a history of head injury is often absent in these patients, especially the elderly. Presentation is likely to simulate a stroke with focal signs of hemiparesis and generalized signs of cognitive impairment or drowsiness; headache may or may not be present. *Epidural hematomas* are typically acute with initial brief loss of consciousness, followed by progressive drowsiness with focal cerebral signs. These hematomas usually follow obvious head trauma with temporal bone fracture rupturing the middle meningeal artery.

An *intracerebral hematoma* typically presents with the sudden onset of focal signs and generalized brain dysfunction [11]. Severe headache occurs in the majority of these patients and may be generalized or on the side of the cerebral lesion [12]. A premonitory headache (sentinel headache) occurs in 10% to 15% of patients and is most common prior to *subarachnoid hemorrhage* secondary to a ruptured aneurysm. Cerebral hemorrhage usually occurs in patients who have experienced many years of hypertension. In addition, a large number of hemorrhages are due to clinically silent amyloid angiopathy. A vascular anomaly may also rupture into the brain parenchyma and a small number of cerebral hemorrhages are due to vasculitis or blood dyscrasia. With the advent of computed tomography (CT) and magnetic resonance imaging (MRI), small hemorrhages are being visualized in patients without headache and with only minor cerebral signs.

A *cerebellar hematoma* usually manifests itself by sudden, severe occipital headache and vertigo, nausea, and vomiting [13]. Examination reveals ataxia, nystagmus, and other oculomotor signs. Accompanying depression of consciousness may progress to coma and death unless the diagnosis is promptly made and the hematoma surgically evacuated. Small cerebellar hemorrhages present in a less dramatic fashion and may be treated conservatively.

ARACHNOID CYSTS

Arachnoid cysts produce a mass effect very slowly [14]. The brain is displaced so gradually that headache and focal signs occur late in the course, if at all. An exception to that general rule is the *colloid cyst* of the third ventricle. Movement or change in position may cause the cyst to obstruct the foramen of Monro or the aqueduct of Sylvius with rapid development of severe generalized headache, sometimes with loss of consciousness and/or alteration in respiration.

Changes in Intracranial Pressure

Intracranial hypertension, regardless of the cause, will precipitate generalized headache, usually due to a stretch of blood vessels at the base of the skull [15]. When cerebellar tonsillar herniation occurs, occipito-nuchal pain is associated. The qualities of the headache are not specific and the clinical diagnosis must rest on associated neurological features (focal or generalized, as noted above), as well as systemic signs, particularly projectile vomiting. In both *obstructive* and *communicating hydrocephalus*, the triad of impaired mentation, gait difficulty (especially gait apraxia), and urinary incontinence are typical. These symptoms usually develop rapidly in patients with disease (especially a mass lesion) that obstructs ventricular CSF outflow at the aqueduct of Sylvius or at the foramina of Luschka and Magendie. Communicating hydrocephalus is usually due to impairment of absorption of CSF over the convexity of the cerebrum or obstruction of basal cisterns and may occur with arachnoiditis following subarachnoid hemorrhage. The symptoms in these patients develop insidiously and headache is often absent. Headache is also a late development in patients with aqueductal stenosis and is usually not seen with normal pressure hydrocephalus.

Cerebral edema often causes intracranial hypertension. Edema commonly accompanies primary cerebral neoplasms, metastatic carcinoma, lymphoma, and encephalitis. The headache of encephalitis is usually generalized, but in the early stage of herpes simplex encephalitis, the pain is often localized to the side of the lesion. In herpes simplex encephalitis, the acute onset of focal signs, including seizures, implicates a temporal or orbito-frontal lobe [16]. With most other forms of encephalitis, including the increasingly prevalent AIDS encephalitis, generalized signs of cerebral disease occurs [17].

Pseudotumor cerebri or *benign intracranial hypertension* is due to cerebral edema of uncertain mechanism [18,19]. This condition is usually manifested only by generalized headache and papilledema. Occasionally, false localizing signs occur, such as sixth nerve palsy, and visual obscurations may be caused by long-standing increased intracranial pressure. Pseudotumor cerebri most typically occurs in adolescent or young women; obesity or menstrual abnormalities or both are frequently noted. Other organic disease must always be excluded before the diagnosis is made. Imaging techniques reveal edema of the parenchyma and small ventricles. In past decades, pseudotumor cerebri was thought to be due to impaired CSF absorption following otitis and associated dural sinus thrombosis, but since the advent of the antibiotic era, these causes have been eliminated. The underlying mechanism in most cases is obscure.

There are many rare causes of cerebral edema with papilledema and headache [20]. Increased intracranial pressure may be due to an excess of intracranial blood volume resulting from elevated pCO_2 and arterial dilation. Cardiovascular diseases may cause cerebral edema by passive congestion or high cardiac output. Hypertensive encephalopathy due to the malignant phase of essential hypertension or as a manifestation of a pheochromocytoma will cause cerebral edema and associated headache; generalized or focal cerebral signs may also occur. The symptoms and signs respond promptly to intravenous antihypertensive therapy. Anemia and other blood dyscrasias; endocrinopathies affecting the thyroid, parathyroid, or adrenal glands; and many toxins including hypervitaminosis A and D, tetracycline and other antibiotics, and heavy metals will produce cerebral edema with papilledema and headache.

Plateau waves of extreme increased intracranial pressure reach levels of 60 mm to 80 mm mercury (800 mm to 1,000 mm water) from baselines of intracranial hypertension in the range of 20 mm mercury (220 mm to 280 mm water) [21]. These plateau waves, which last two to 20 minutes, may occur spontaneously or may be precipitated by movement or coughing. Severe headache is the most prominent clinical feature. Other symptoms are pains in the neck due to tonsillar herniation, numbness of the face or upper extremities due to traction of the trigeminal nerve or upper cervical nerve roots, obscuration of vision due to decreased retinal perfusion, extra-ocular muscle paresis or pupillary abnormalities due to traction on the oculomotor nerve, and generalized cerebral symptoms (impaired mentation, change of consciousness, or agitation). Tremors or change in tone of the extremities may occur, as well as autonomic symptoms including vomiting, hiccupping, thirst, blush or pallor, sweating or shivering, increase in blood pressure, decrease in pulse, and alteration in respiration. Coma and death may ensue when the rise in intracranial pressure approaches the mean arterial blood pressure.

Intracranial hypotension also causes headache [22]. This occurs when CSF leaks into the soft tissues through the tract made by a lumbar puncture (LP), with a break in the arachnoid after surgery or other trauma, or rarely after a spontaneous tear of the arachnoid. Under these circumstances, a negative pressure within the cranium develops when the patient assumes the erect position. Loss of the hydraulic support of the brain puts traction on the meninges and the basal blood vessels. The resultant severe headache clears when the intracranial pressure is raised by resuming a horizontal position. The post LP headache usually lasts several days but may last two weeks, clearing with the healing of the puncture wound. On rare occasions, an epidural blood patch is needed to correct the arachnoid leak.

Meningeal Irritation

Headache invariably accompanies *purulent meningitis* [23]. The headache is acute and is generalized or in the occipito-nuchal region. Accompanying features include fever, nausea, vomiting, severe malaise, and other signs of toxicity plus nuchal rigidity and positive Kernig's and Brudzinski signs. *Chronic meningitis* due to fungi or other organisms may or may not present with headache, fever, or nuchal rigidity. Noninfectious meningitides due to sarcoidosis or carcinomatosis usually follow a chronic course. The more insidious the course, the less likely headache will be present until obstructive hydrocephalus ensues. In subacute meningitis due to tuberculosis, headache and nuchal rigidity are common. The clinical diagnosis is supported by the development of cerebral infarction secondary to tuberculous arteritis. The diagnosis of meningitis is confirmed by examination of the CSF, which may show cloudy fluid under raised pressure, pleocytosis, elevated protein, depressed glucose, and positive cultures with elevated antigen levels.

Blood in the subarachnoid space is usually due to an acute event [24]. Blood causes a meningeal inflammatory response, probably due to platelet breakdown and the release of serotonin, which activates a plasma kinin-forming cascade. The chemical stimulation of nociceptive nerve endings in the meninges evokes contraction of the neck extensor muscles with associated nuchal rigidity and Kernig's sign. Subarachnoid hemorrhage due to a ruptured aneurysm typically presents with a sudden, excruciating, generalized, often throbbing headache — the worst headache ever experienced by the patient. Exertion or the valsalva maneuver is a precipitating mechanism in about one third of all cases. Loss or alteration of consciousness and vomiting often accompanies the onset; and, depending upon the site of the aneurysm and the direction of the blood flow, there may be signs of dysfunction of an extraocular nerve or brain parenchyma. Blood in the spinal subarachnoid space may irritate nerve roots and cause pain in the back or extremities. The sudden rise of intracranial pressure may evoke a sub-hyaloid hemorrhage or papilledema. Other systemic features may include an initial rise in blood pressure, lowering of pulse, low grade fever, and changes in the electrocardiogram. The initial headache is due to the sudden change in intracranial dynamics. The persistent headache, occipito-nuchal or generalized, is due to continued increased intracranial pressure with traction on blood vessels at the base of the brain or sterile meningeal inflammation. A sentinel headache, usually lasting more than 24 hours, precedes the subarachnoid hemorrhage by days or weeks in 20% to 30% of cases. The diagnosis must always be suspected when patients present with sudden excruciating headache, even when there are no other symptoms or signs. If the CT of the head does not reveal blood in the subarachnoid cisterns, an LP is mandatory in search of blood. Xanthochromia develops within four to 12 hours and persists for two to four weeks. There may be a CSF lymphocytic response, as well as elevated protein and, rarely, depression of glucose. In rare cases, arteriography may be warranted even if the CT or MRI and LP are normal. Subarachnoid hemorrhage due to a ruptured arteriovenous malformation is less acute in presentation and headache is less severe. Seizures and parenchymal hemorrhage are more likely than with a ruptured aneurysm. The symptoms of subarachnoid hemorrhage following intracerebral hemorrhage are usually overshadowed by the signs of the parenchymal lesions. Trauma, blood dyscrasia, arteritis, and brain tumor are other causes of subarachnoid hemorrhage. Cerebral arteritis is often associated with headache unrelated to subarachnoid hemorrhage.

A history of migraine is reported in 5% to 30% of patients with subarachnoid hemorrhage following a ruptured anomaly [24,25]. The relationship may be coincidental, for the side of migraine headache does not necessarily correspond to the side of the aneurysm. On the other hand, about half of these patients no longer experience migraine after the subarachnoid hemorrhage, suggesting a relationship that is more than a matter of chance. The recurrence of migraine invariably over the same side of the head on repeated occasions does not in itself warrant angiography unless there is reason to suspect a vascular anomaly by a history of seizures or the finding of a bruit; but it should raise the index of suspicion of structural disease.

Cerebrovascular Disease

Headache is a prominent symptom of cerebrovascular disease [12,26-30]. When hemorrhage or edema or both accompany stroke, headache can be attributed to mechanisms noted before. The mechanism of headache with ischemic cerebrovascular disease is unknown, but it may be related to the pathophysiology of migraine. Intracerebral and extracerebral arteries have a network of perivascular nerves that contain not only adrenalin, acetylcholine, and serotonin, but many other peptide neurotransmitters: neuropeptide Y, calcitonin gene-related peptide (CGRP), substance P, vasoactive intestinal polypeptide (VIP), and neurokinin A. Several of these substances evoke neurogenic inflammation due to their chemotactic, macrophage-stimulating, and histamine-liberating actions. The pain of migraine and perhaps headache associated with ischemic cerebrovascular disease is probably due to the liberation of these perivascular peptides. The peptide release may be mediated by neural stimuli, but circulating biochemicals may also be an important factor. The neuropeptides are vasoactive and induce or enhance vasoconstriction or vasodilation. Substance P, for example, is not only a nociceptive neurotransmitter but also a vasodilator. Nerve fibers containing substance P originate in the trigeminal ganglion [4]. Vasodilation may be a response to an impending or present ischemic event. The distension of arteries may initiate a cascade of events leading to headache or may be an epiphenomenon.

Another explanation for headache in patients with ischemic cerebral disease has to do with increased platelet activity. Increased platelet aggregability, noted during migraine and cerebral ischemia, leads to release of serotonin and prostaglandins, which may play roles in headache production [26].

In prospective studies of stroke (hemorrhagic as well as ischemic), headache occurred in approximately one third of all cases [29,30]. Headache was noted in 23% to 57% of patients with parenchymal hemorrhage, 19% to 29% with bland infarcts, 6% to 36% with transient ischemic attacks, and 6% to 17% with lacunar infarcts. The incidence of headache with disease of the anterior circulation was the same as that in the posterior circulation.

Ten percent of patients experience a headache prior to the stroke; the headaches are usually episodic and throbbing [29]. A sentinel headache may occur days to weeks before a stroke but is more likely to occur before a subarachnoid hemorrhage. These headaches often last for more than 24 hours and have been reported in 10% to 15% of patients with parenchymal ischemia or hemorrhage [30].

Headaches during a stroke occur in women more often than in men; the headache is usually throbbing in nature. In two prospective studies, 50% to 74% of headaches were unilateral; of these, 50% and 67% were ipsilateral to the lesion (25% and 7% were contralateral) [29,30]. Disease of the carotid artery is often associated with pain in the ipsilateral forehead or eye. In some studies, bifrontal headaches were associated with lesions in the anterior circulation while strokes in the posterior circulation caused occipital headache, but there has not been consistent correlation between site of headache and location of the lesion.

References

1. Ray BS, Wolff HG. Experimental studies on headache: Pain sensitive structures of the head and their significance in headache. *Arch Surg 41*: 813-8566, 1940.
2. Penfield W, McNaughton F. Dural headache and innervation of the dura mater. *Arch Neurol Psychiat 44*: 43-75, 1940.
3. Feindal W, Penfield W, McNaughton F. The tentorial nerves and localization of intracranial pain in man. *Neurology 10*: 555-565, 1960.
4. Moskowitz MA. The visceral organ brain: implications for the pathophysiology of vascular head pain. *Neurology 31*: 182-186, 1991.
5. Rushton JG, Rooke ED. Brain tumor headache. *Headache 2*: 147-152, 1962.
6. Kerr FWL. A mechanism to account for frontal headache in cases of posterior fossa tumors. *J Neurosurg 18*: 605-109, 1961.
7. Alksne JF. Headache and brain tumor. In: Dalessio DJ, (ed). *Wolff's Headache and Other Head Pain*, 5th ed, pp 288-300. New York, Oxford University Press, 1980.
8. Brewer NS, MacCarty CS, Wellman WE. Brain abscess: A review of recent experience. *Ann Intern Med 82*: 571-576, 1975.
9. Coonrad JD, Dans PE. Subdural empyema. *Am J Med 53*: 85-91, 1972.
10. Rowland LP, Sciarra D. Head injury. In: Rowland LP, (ed). *Merritt's Textbook of Neurology*, 8th ed, pp 369-392. Philadelphia, Lea & Febiger, 1989.
11. Ropper AH, Davis KR. Lobar cerebral hemorrhages: Acute clinical syndromes in 26 cases. *Ann Neurol 8*: 141-147, 1980.
12. Edmeads J. Headache in cerebrovascular disease. In Rose FC, (ed). Headache. In: Vinken PJ, Bruyn GW, Klawans HL, (eds). *Handbook of Clinical Neurology*, Vol 4(49), pp 273-290. New York, Elsevier Science Publishing Co, 1986.
13. Ott KH, Kawe CS, Ojemann RG, et al. Cerebellar hemorrhage diagnosis and treatment,, A review of 56 cases. *Arch Neurol 31*: 160-167, 1974.
14. Adams RA, Victor M. *Principles of Neurology*, 4th ed, p 533. New York, McGraw Hill, 1989.

15. Alksne JF. Headaches associated with changes in intracranial pressure. In: Dalessio DJ, (ed). *Wolff's Headache and Other Head Pains*, 5th ed, pp 301-313. New York, Oxford University Press, 1980.
16. Adams H, Miller D. Herpes simplex encephalitis: A clinical and pathological analysis of twenty-two cases. *Postgrad Med J 49*: 393-397, 1973.
17. Navia BA, Jordan BD, Price RW. The AIDS dementia complex I: Clinical features. *Ann Neurol 19*: 517-524, 1986.
18. Corbett JJ, Thompson HS. The rational management of idiopathic intracranial hypertension. *Arch Neurol 46*: 1049-1051, 1989.
19. Welsberg LA. Benign forms of intracranial hypertension. *Medicine 54*: 197-207, 1975.
20. Bucheit WA, Burton C. Bwirott H, Shaw D. Papilledema and idiopathic intracranial hypertension. *N Engl J Med 280*: 938-942, 1969.
21. Lundberg N. Continuous recording and control of ventricular fluid pressure in neurosurgical practice. *Acta Psychiatr Scand 36 (Supp 149)*: 1-193, 1960.
22. Kunkle EC, Ray BS, Wolff HH. Experimental studies on headache: Analysis of the headache associated with changes in intracranial pressure. *Arch Neurol Psychiat 49*: 323-358, 1943.
23. O'Connell JEA. The clinical signs of meningeal irritation. *Brain 69*: 9-21, 1946.
24. Lance JW. Intracranial causes of headache. In: *Mechanisms and Management of Headache*, 4th ed, pp 86-99. Boston, Butterworth Scientific, 1982.
25. Bruyn GW. Intracranial arteriovenous malformation and migraine. *Cephalalgia 4*: 191-207, 1984.
26. Edmeads J. The headaches of ischemic cerebrovascular disease. *Headache 19*: 345-349, 1979.
27. Fisher CM. Headache in acute cerebrovascular disease. In: Vinken PJ, Bruyn GW, (eds). *Headache and Cranial Neuralgias. Handbook of Clinical Neurology*, Vol 5. pp 124-156. New York, Elsevier Science Publishing Co, 1968.
28. Mohr JP, Caplan LR, Melski JW, et al. The Harvard Cooperative Stroke Registry: A prospective registry. *Neurology 28*: 754-762, 1978.
29. Portenoy RK, Abissi CJ, Lipton RB, et al. Headache in cerebrovascular disease. *Stroke 15*: 1009-1012, 1984.
30. Gorelick PB,, Hier DB, Caplan LR, et al. Headache in acute cerebrovascular disease. *Neurology 36*: 1445-1450, 1986.

12

Miscellaneous Headache: More Unusual Types

Arthur H. Elkind and Mitchell S. Elkind

Many patients who present with acute and chronic headache symptoms cannot be diagnosed as having migraine, tension-type, cluster, or any of the other more commonly described headache disorders. Physicians who encounter more unusual symptoms will find it useful to review the less common causes of headache.

While some of the disorders in this category are quite rare, others occur with a much more significant frequency; several of these disorders, moreover, are very controversial. In some instances, in fact, the primary disease entity, which has headache as a leading or significant symptom, may itself be in doubt. Fibromyalgia and chronic mononucleosis syndrome (chronic active Epstein-Barr virus infection), for example, are disorders with headache as a symptom, and around which there is still controversy surrounding definition, diagnosis, and frequency of the illness.

The physician encountering these less common causes of headache should, first of all, recognize that a thorough history is especially critical. The history should include all aspects of the headache's characteristics and also associated illnesses.

Concomitant diseases such as diabetes mellitus and the presence of ocular nerve palsies, for instance, can help in the diagnosis of patients with these diseases who suffer with headache [1]. Headache may also be present with third cranial nerve palsy in pituitary adenoma, pituitary apoplexy, and posterior communicating artery aneurysms [2]. Because many of the miscellaneous causes of headache are associated with the ingestion, regular use, or abuse of certain foods, medications, or other substances, it is particularly important that the history be as complete as possible in areas relevant to these items. Similarly, because some headaches occur in relation to weather, altitude, or environmental change, the physician will want to be aware of any direct relationships or recurrent patterns among such causes and the onset of headaches.

Physical examination may also be important in dental, sinus, and temporomandibular joint disorders. Patients presenting with acute onset of headache related to effort, cough, or other activities must also be carefully screened for intracranial disease. The rare bregmatic headache, in which the headache is an anginal referred symptom, is associated with ischemic heart disease. Neck pain, however, is the usual referred symptom in this disease, with facial pain presenting slightly more often than headache.

Dental Disease

Dental problems may cause headache. In such cases, the patient will often present to the physician because of pain radiating to the jaw, facial regions, or head. Pain may originate in the pulp area of a diseased tooth or be an indication of periodontal disease. Referral to a dentist is necessary if it is suspected that the origin of the pain is dental.

An incomplete tooth fracture, also referred to as "cracked tooth syndrome," may be responsible for unexplained head pain. Pain usually occurs after biting on food and it may be sudden in onset as well as severe; the patient may not localize the origin of the pain to the affected tooth. Mandibular second molars are most commonly involved in cracked tooth syndrome; first molars, both mandibular and maxillary, are next in frequency. If this disorder is suspected, prompt referral to a dentist is in order.

Temporomandibular Disorders

Temporomandibular (TM) and temporomandibular joint (TMJ) disorders have been increasingly recognized as a prominent cause of head and face pain. These disorders are also referred to as "myofascial pain dysfunction disorders." Solberg has recently classified temporomandibular disorders into seven groups:[3]

1. acute masticatory muscle disorders
2. TMJ derangements
3. TMJ inflammatory disorders
4. degenerative diseases
5. extrinsic trauma
6. chronic hypomotility

7. growth disorders

These disorders seem more prevalent in women than men, and the symptoms are usually present in younger age groups. Underlying emotional problems frequently accentuate the symptoms. Symptoms, moreover, may mask the underlying disorder so that care must be taken in establishing the diagnosis; it is also important to remember that TMJ dysfunction is not a diagnosis but a group of disorders. A synovitis of the TMJ may be part of a systemic disorder and it may mimic or be confused with disease of the surrounding structures. Diseases of the parotid gland and the ear, as well as facial neuralgias, may be confused with TMJ disease.

Physicians are often first to see temporomandibular disorders because the patient may present with headache or earache.

Palpation of the TMJ may help identify inflammation and clicking. Tenderness of the masticatory muscles and the TMJ may also be present. Therapy includes nonsteroidal anti-inflammatory drugs (NSAIDs), biofeedback, dental bite appliances, muscle relaxants, and/or tricyclic antidepressants. Supportive therapy by the physician or dentist is also important.

A recent report by Reïk reviewed 100 consecutive headache patients and found that only four satisfied the requirements for TMJ pain dysfunction syndrome [4]. Sixteen patients, however, had been treated previously for TMJ disorders and had not improved with dental treatment. The author concluded that unnecessary dental treatment may be common due to incorrect diagnosis. He further concluded that therapy should be medical at the onset and mechanical only if the individual is edentulous when starting treatment.

Although temporomandibular disorders are not commonly responsible for non migrainous headache, the physician will want to avoid overlooking the diagnosis when it is appropriate. The diagnosis of a temporomandibular disorder is most often incorrectly made when the physician mistakenly concentrates on the isolated problem of the temporomandibular area, failing to adequately account for stress-related factors and other aspects of the personality of the patient.

Sinus Headache

Paranasal sinus disease is, perhaps, one of the medical terms most frequently misused by the layman. The over-the-counter drug market is replete with analgesics and sympathomimetic amines used for the reduction of headache and facial pain. Sinus disorders, however, are an infrequent cause of chronic headache, although acute sinus disease may be associated with headache and facial pain.

In acute sinus headache disorders, there are usually accompanying symptoms and signs: nasal discharge and/or stuffiness, epistaxis, ear symptoms, and occasional facial fullness. Fever and tenderness of the affected maxillary or ethmoid sinuses may also be present. The headache can usually be diagnosed in circumstances where these signs and symptoms are present. The headache of acute disease is usually a deep, dull ache exaggerated by head movements or straining.

Otolaryngologists and other physicians interested in headache disorders mostly agree that the paranasal sinuses and related nasal structures are less often the cause of chronic headache than is generally believed. Patients with headache but otherwise asymptomatic infrequently have disease of the ear, nose, or sinus structures. Only occasionally will a chronic disease such as a tumor or a fungal infection persist for months and present with pain.

The relationship between chronic headache and sinus disease remains controversial, however. Faleck reports finding subacute sinusitis in 15 of 150 patients with chronic daily headache [5]. The patients all had histories and clinical signs which were indistinguishable from those of patients with stress headache, and, other than headache, they were all asymptomatic for sinus disease. Radiologic investigation was required for diagnosis. Successful therapy included antibiotic and decongestant therapy. The author concludes that further study is needed to better determine the differences between patients with headache due to subacute sinusitis and those with headache due to muscle contraction.

Pain from the paranasal sinus structures is often referred to the overlying structures, but may also be referred to the teeth. Sphenoid sinus pain may cause retro-orbital and retronasal pain. Pain can also be referred to the temporal, occipital, and shoulder areas in sphenoid sinus disease. Ethmoid and frontal sinus pain may be referred to the temporal and occipital areas.

Examination with close inspection of ocular, oral, nasal, and aural structures is indicated. Most diseases of the sinuses will be detected in the middle meatus since the openings of the frontal, maxillary, and anterior ethmoids occur here, making this area the most accessible to examination. Diagnostic work-up should include a culture when infection is suspected. Chronic infections and fungal disease may be difficult to diagnose and demonstration of organisms may be extremely important. Routine sinus roentgenograms, tomography, computed tomograph (CT) scanning, and magnetic resonance imaging (MRI) may be needed for diagnosis in sinus disease. It is also very important to remember that the presence on X-ray of clouding of the sinuses in chronic headache patients may be unrelated to the cause of the headache. The investigation of etiology should not stop once evidence of an infection is found. If a patient does have headache symptoms due to chronic sinus infection, then the patient will also have nasal symptoms and inflammation.

When the ostia of a sinus becomes permanently blocked, a mucocoele may result. The mucus secretion without free access to drainage will result in a cystic lesion which expands slowly over a prolonged period of time. Bone may be eroded and a dull headache may result. The only symptom of a sphenoid mucocoele may be headache; visual field defects may be the only sign. CT scanning may be essential for proper diagnosis and surgery may be indicated. Ethmoid and sphenoid sinusitis may present as a medical emergency because of the possibility of complicating cavernous sinus thrombosis.

Two fungal infections involving the paranasal sinuses that may produce serious complications and are often fatal ought to be considered in patients presenting with chronic headache. Aspergillosis is the most common fungal infection affecting normal paranasal sinuses in immunocompromised hosts. Roentgenograms may show opacification, bony erosion, and air-fluid levels. Infection may spread to the cranial cavity directly from the paranasal sinuses to meninges, and headache may be present; amphotericin B (Fungizone) is the treatment of choice.

Rhinocerebral mucormycosis may also invade the central nervous system from the paranasal sinuses and produce a rapidly fatal infection [6,7]. Patients with diabetic ketoacidosis are at risk although those who are immunocompromised or malnourished are also susceptible to a much lesser degree. Early symptoms may include severe headache overlying the affected sinus and nasal discharge. Signs are dirty red or black necrotic turbinates with extension to the ethmoid or frontal sinuses. Absence of air-fluid levels is noted on X-ray with nodular thickening of the mucous membranes and destruction of the bony walls. An orbital apex syndrome may result with destruction of cranial nerves III, IV, and VI, and the ophthalmic branch of V. Blindness results from obstruction of the central retinal artery, and further intracranial spread may be rapidly fatal. Prompt and aggressive amphotericin B or ketoconazole (Nizoral) therapy should be instituted, as well as surgical removal of necrotic tissue.

Chronic headache is infrequently due to disease of the mastoid sinuses. Acute infections, however, may result in head pain over the mastoid and surrounding regions.

Rapid changes in atmospheric pressure may result in sinus headache with negative pressure developing within the sinuses. Hemorrhage may occur on the mucosal linings. "Vacuum headache" is the name given by otorhinolaryngologists to the resulting symptoms, although some authorities still dispute the existence of such a disorder. The distress may be due to the effects of altitude change on the nasal structures and ostia of the sinuses rather than due to a primary sinus disturbance.

Disease of Internal Medicine and Endocrine Disorders

Numerous diseases are associated with headache, but usually the headache presents as a minor symptom and diagnosis of the disorder is more readily established by other signs and symptoms, or by abnormal laboratory tests. We will describe some of the more unusual cases in which headache is reported as a major symptom of a medical disorder.

BREGMATIC HEADACHE

Lefkowitz and Biller described a 62-year-old man with headache and chest pain produced by effort and stress [8]. Treatment with sublingual nitroglycerin relieved both symptoms. Following angiography to determine arterial disease, coronary artery bypass surgery was performed and definitively relieved headache and chest pain. This type of headache, a very rare presentation of ischemic heart disease, is also called bregmatic headache.

HYPERPARATHYROIDISM

Blair and Fekety report an unusual case of fever and unremitting headache resulting from a parathyroid adenoma [9]. Headache was present for over a year before hyperparathyroidism was diagnosed; it was a significant symptom in hyperparathyroidism in five of 57 patients, according to another recent study [10].

HYPOGLYCEMIA

Headache may be a symptom, though not a prominent one, in diabetics with hypoglycemia secondary to excess insulin administration. Other characteristic acute symptoms of hypoglycemia are hyperepinephrinemia, including tachycardia, sweating, and tremulousness; mental changes may follow. Many patients with reactive hypoglycemia may have abnormalities on personality testing. Headache has also been reported as a symptom in functional hypoglycemia (idiopathic functional hypoglycemia); however, functional hypoglycemia is not adequately explained in the majority of patients. Rebound hypoglycemia may occur after eating, usually three to four hours later.

The headache associated with hypoglycemia is usually generalized and may persist after correction of the hypoglycemia. To establish a relationship between the headache and the hypoglycemia, an attempt should be made to obtain blood glucose levels during episodes of headache. An eight-hour glucose tolerance test may be required to rule out hypoglycemia with attendant headache.

Migraine may also be triggered by missing meals or by ingestion of a high carbohydrate meal resulting in a postprandial relative hypoglycemia with blood sugars between 40 and 60 mg. Migrainous individuals may prevent such attacks by eating at regular intervals and avoiding high carbohydrate binges.

Patients with chronic headache of a non migrainous type may have had a previous diagnosis of hypoglycemia. Other neurasthenic symptoms may be reported, including fatigue, depression, and sleepiness. To correct the misleading diagnosis, an adequate glucose tolerance test should be performed. Patients with prominent fatigue and headache should be considered for the diagnosis of one of the chronic fatigue syndromes discussed later in this chapter.

HYPERPROLACTINEMIA

Hyperprolactinemia has been associated with headache in women lacking evidence of significant pituitary enlargement [11]. A study of 46 women with hyperprolactinemia determined that 27 (58%) had headache occurring one or more times per week. Six percent of the patients had daily headaches.

Patients with sella abnormalities or microadenomas greater than 1 cm were excluded. A control group of patients had significantly fewer headaches. No relation could be demonstrated between level of serum prolactin and headache severity or presence of headache. The authors conceded that microadenoma of the pituitary could not be excluded using the polytomographic evaluations they relied upon. In the future, upon further improvement on the technique for evaluating the pituitary, it may be established that there is a relationship between headache and microadenoma, though no relationship has yet been determined.

In explaining their headaches, patients gave a description most similar to tension-type headache. Headaches were typically of one hour or longer duration; there were no prodromata and headache location was variable. Many patients had a previous diagnosis of migraine, tension-type, or sinus headache.

The authors noted that treatment with bromocriptine mesylate (Parlodel) was effective for some of their patients. The mechanism for headache production was not clear, but somehow serotonin-mediated changes resulted in the hyperprolactinemia and the headaches. Women with menstrual abnormalities and chronic headache similar to tension-type headache should have prolactin levels determined. Even the absence of microadenoma over 1 cm may warrant a trial with bromocriptine, although the response to the drug is not clear-cut.

A later report based on a multicenter study included women 17 to 41 years of age presenting with secondary amenorrhea and/or galactorrhea [12]. Three groups were described and the incidence of headache in the hyperprolactinemia group without adenoma was 6%, while in the hyperprolactinemia group with adenoma the incidence of headache was 23% — significantly higher (p = 0.0001). The authors suggest that the space occupying prolactinoma is responsible for the headache. They further add that chronic headache in women with amenorrhea and/or galactorrhea warrants investigation for a prolactinoma.

Diet-Related Headache

CAFFEINE

Caffeine is often overlooked as an abused substance. Many beverages and foods, including coffee, tea, cola, and chocolate, contain caffeine in significant amounts. Although conclusive evidence of its efficacy is lacking, caffeine is useful in preparations for migraine and may potentiate the effects of analgesic agents in tension-type headaches. It is used in combination with analgesic agents in over-the-counter headache medications. Caffeine is the most potent CNS and skeletal muscle stimulant of the three methylxanthines. Small doses may stimulate the cerebral cortex while larger doses stimulate lower brain stem functions. Mental acuity is increased by 50-200 mg doses. Caffeine may also counteract the sedative influence of barbiturates, and it has potent effects on the cardiovascular system. The constrictor effects on cerebral vessels may be the mechanism that produces headache relief in caffeine users.

One may enjoy the benefits of caffeine if total daily consumption is kept below 200-300 mg. There are many individuals, however, who consume excessive amounts of caffeine from one or more sources, The pharmacologically active dose of caffeine is 50-200 mg, while a large dose is 500 mg. It should be further recognized that coffee, chocolate, and cola contain not only caffeine, but also other methylxanthines with similar, if not as potent, effects.

Caffeine has been shown to increase work endurance. The short-term effect on work capacity, however, may be negated by the side effects of insomnia, restlessness, and irritability. The effects of caffeine also vary, apparently, with personality type [13]. Introverts and extroverts given caffeine in differing doses exhibited varying responses when tested on verbal performance. Excess caffeine use is associated with psychological and psychophysiological effects.

Caffeine dependence develops after continued excessive use; headache is one of the symptoms noted after withdrawal for 12 to 16 hours. The amount of caffeine used in compounds for headache relief as well as in caffeine-containing beverages may produce a vasoconstriction followed by a rebound dilation hours later which results in so-called "caffeine withdrawal headache. " Chronic excessive use may cause a degree of stimulation that is later followed by both a let-down and onset of headache during the withdrawal period. Patients with chronic headache should be questioned about the amount of caffeine consumed both in drugs and in foods and beverages. Some patients who use caffeine excessively may be suffering from morning withdrawal headache: these individuals require coffee in the morning to relieve the pain of headache. Some patients may consume other medications in excess because of the negative effects of caffeine.

It has been suggested that those individuals consuming 500 mg or more of caffeine each day evaluate their dependence as well as their possible psychological impairment and work efficiency. The exact daily intake required for dependence, side effects, and optimum efficiency depends to a great extent on the individual's tolerance. Therapeutic techniques have been suggested to reduce one's dependence on caffeine. Behavior modification, combined with an awareness of the implications of caffeine abuse, has been used with success. Monitoring consumption can aid a patient in the reduction of dependency.

Caffeine abuse should certainly be considered when treating the daily headache sufferer who frequently uses over-the-counter remedies or caffeine-containing prescription drugs while continuing to drink caffeine-laden beverages. The effects on personality and performance, and the production of headaches following transient headache relief are readily apparent. Caffeine withdrawal headache should also be considered in all patients with daily morning headache, in the group with chronic continuous headache. and those with weekend headaches

Alcohol

Most people are familiar with the "hangover headache." The exact cause of such headaches, however, is not clear. It occurs many hours after excessive ingestion of alcoholic beverages. Whether it is due to the impurities in alcoholic beverages or a direct effect of the metabolic products of the alcohol is not clear. The discomfort is probably due to vasodilation; evidence for this includes the throbbing quality of the pain and the decrease during carotid artery compression. Other less obvious circumstances, including emotional and social conditions, may play a role. The subject's lack of sleep or social excitement may intensify the headache's effects.

Dalessio maintains fructose as a prophylactic and therapeutic agent in modifying hangover headache [14]. Fructose accelerates the metabolism of alcohol and thereby modifies the symptoms of the headache. Kaivola and colleagues cite tolfenamic acid as an effective prophylactic treatment of hangover headache as well as other symptoms associated with alcohol use [15]. Because tolfenamic acid is known to inhibit prostaglandin biosynthesis, they also suggest that prostaglandin may play a role in provoking hangover symptoms, including headache.

Monosodium Glutamate

Glutamate headaches, or "the Chinese restaurant syndrome," first came to the attention of physicians in the 1960's when a letter to the editor was published in the New England Journal of Medicine [16]. The letter described symptoms that occurred after eating in certain Chinese restaurants. Within several weeks more letters followed, and eventually monosodium glutamate (MSG) was implicated in the pathogenesis of this headache syndrome . Individuals vary in their susceptibility to MSG, and presenting symptoms include burning and tightness in the face and headache with a tightness or throbbing over the temporal areas. Bandlike sensations around the head may also occur. All or some of these symptoms, as well as trunk and extremity distress and anxiety, may be present.

Symptoms of this headache may begin several minutes after consuming foods with large amounts of MSG added. The symptoms usually abate after an hour. The mechanism may be generalized vasomotor reaction, but this is not certain.

"Liver Lovers' Headache"

"Liver lovers' headache," associated with excessive dietary liver ingestion, is believed to be caused by vitamin A toxicity [17]. Vitamin A is present in large amounts in liver. Excessive vitamin A intake is associated with pseudotumor cerebri (PTC), a condition in which cerebrospinal fluid pressure increases without the presence of any demonstrable lesion such as a tumor or obstruction. PTC almost always presents with headache as a symptom, and in the great majority of cases it is the most prominent symptom. Selhorst and colleagues report that the ingestion of beef liver, as well as the liver of less commonly consumed meats like bear and shark, can lead to PTC [18].

"ICE CREAM HEADACHE"

"Ice cream headache" can occur in sensitive individuals after the exposure of the palate to cold [18]. Intense pain may appear on top of the head between and behand the eyes, or behind the ears. The pain may last 20 to 30 seconds, and it is common and severe in patients with migraine. The mechanism may be vascular and/or secondary to glossopharyngeal nerve stimulation; it is thought to be due to the sudden cooling of the mouth or pharynx. Cooling of the esophagus or stomach, however, does not produce headache.

"HOT DOG HEADACHE"

Headache may occur after exposure to nitrites in food or in a working environment. The headache is usually dull, aching, and accompanied by facial flushing. Symptoms occur in susceptible individuals, and there is great variation in tolerance to the nitrite substances. Migraine sufferers may be more likely to have a nitrite headache, which has been nicknamed "hot dog" headache. It would thus be wise for such individuals to avoid meat and other foods cured with nitrites such as bologna, salami, ham and bacon.

Isobutyl nitrite, a volatile liquid also known as "Rush," is frequently sold as a "room deodorizer," but more often used for the feelings of euphoria to which it gives rise in those who inhale it. Schwartz and Peary report that 34% of subjects aged 13 to 22 years experienced a pulsatile headache as a result of Rush inhalation [30]. Chemically similar to amyl nitrite, isobutyl nitrite induces a rapid and extreme vasodilation that results in a rush of blood to the head.

Amyl nitrite has been noted in experiments to induce a headache following a fall in systolic and diastolic blood pressure [20]. There is an increased pulsation of the extracranial blood vessels accompanying the headache. Subsequent diminution of the pulsation is accompanied by disappearance of the headache.

TYRAMINE

Tyramine and other pressor amines have been implicated in producing hypertensive crises in patients receiving monoamine oxidase inhibitors (MAOIs) and ingesting foods, particularly cheeses, containing significant amounts of pressor amines. Hanington suggested in 1967 that tyramine may also be responsible for the migraine attack that follows the ingestion of cheese [21]. She was able to induce headache 78% of the time in those patients who developed migraine after eating cheese by giving them 100 mg of tyramine [22]. Other investigators, however, were either unable to reproduce these results or found a less clear cut response to tyramine [23]. Sandler found a deficiency of platelet MAO activity during migraine [24]. This deficiency was more often found in male than female patients.

Conflicting data has left the relationship of tyramine and headache in doubt. Headache does not appear to be related to a pressor effect of tyramine and occurs only after a substantial period of time. In headache sufferers who find that their migraine is triggered by tyramine-containing foods, the relationship is not straightforward.

For migrainous individuals, present knowledge and clinical experience would warrant the avoidance of foods rich in tyramine and also of the excessive ingestion of foods that contain lower amounts of tyramine. Patients receiving MAOIs should absolutely avoid tyramine-rich foods because of the dangers of a hypertensive crisis with a precipitous rise in blood pressure. Foods to avoid include cheese, except cottage and cream cheese, dark beer, red wine, sherry, liqueurs, yeast and protein extracts, fava or broad beans, smoked or pickled foods, chicken livers, fermented sausages, figs, usually canned or ripe, and bananas. Chocolate and cream in excess have also been implicated in hypertensive crises in patients receiving MAOI drugs, as well as in the production of migraine in some sufferers. Over the counter cold preparations containing sympathomimetic amines should also be avoided.

Drugs and Other Foreign Substances as a Cause of Headache

Some foreign substances may result in migraine headache in susceptible individuals. They may also produce a vascular headache of the non-migrainous type in other individuals. Nitroglycerin and related substances such as isosorbide dinitrate (Isordil, Sorbitrate), hydralazine HCl (Apresoline), other vasodilatory drugs, phenylpropranolamine, and numerous other agents can provoke headache [30]. (See Chapter 18).

PHENYLPROPANOLAMINE

Several physicians report cases of children or young adults with severe CNS complications associated with phenylpropranolamine, which is used in over-the-counter diet pills and cold remedies [25]. Symptoms are usually transient and include severe headache, grand mal seizures, and hypertensive crises. Bale and colleagues, however, reported that one seventeen-year-old boy went into a coma and died as a result of 100 mg dose of the substance; massive intracerebral and intraventricular hemorrhages were found on autopsy.

Phenylpropranolamine has amphetamine-like, sympathomimetic effects on the CNS, accounting for the hypertension, headache, and intracranial hemorrhage, as well as tremor, agitation, and hallucinations. Phentolamine (Regitine) is suggested as a treatment of choice for persistent hypertension. Several substances, including caffeine and alcohol, may potentiate the effects of phenylpropanolamine. The Food and Drug Administration has recently concluded that products that combine phenylpropanolamine and caffeine are too dangerous to be marketed over the counter. It should be remembered, however, that even in recommended doses phenylpropanolamine poses the threat of severe CNS complications. Because phenylpropanolamine may be related to intracranial hemorrhage, CT scans of the head should be obtained in patients with neurological deficiencies or evidence of meningeal irritation.

In a recent report, there are claims that the interaction between MAOI and substance ingestion resulting in adverse effects has been exaggerated [27]. The drugs are useful in depressive disorders and at times in chronic headache disorders, but the prescribing physician should be aware of interactions and advise the patient accordingly.

Aspartame and Carbohydrates

Aspartame, particularly in combination with carbohydrates, causes an elevation in the amount of tyrosine in the brain [28]. The increased tyrosine levels can lead to headache symptoms. Ferguson described an interaction between aspartame and carbohydrates that led to serious headache symptoms in a young woman being treated with an MAOI for an eating disorder and depression [29]. The 22-year-old woman, while on a regimen of 10 mg/day of tranylcypromine sulfate (Parnate), found that a severe and throbbing headache followed her binges in which she would consume the artificial sweetener aspartame and large amounts of carbohydrates. Saccharin did not produce the headaches, however. The author concluded that this interaction between aspartame and carbohydrates is important to remember when using MAOIs to treat patients with depression and/or eating disorders. Certain individuals seem to be susceptible to ingestion of aspartame containing foods and beverages and develop headaches even when not on MAOIs.

Carbon Monoxide

Dalessio reports that carbon monoxide (CO) inhalation may also result in a form of toxic vascular headache with severe symptoms [31]. CO poisoning may be the result of environmental hazard – such as the incomplete burning of fossil fuels or wood, or the improper ventilation of automobile, exhaust. But cigarette smoking is the most common factor associated with elevated serum levels of CO. The most prominent symptom of CO poisoning is headache, strongly resembling migraine, and associated with nausea, vomiting, and fatigue. Less frequent symptomatic complaints include dyspnea on exertion, lethargy, and muscular weakness. When the patient's history includes smoking, particularly heavy smoking, diagnosis of CO poisoning may be aided by the simple and precise laboratory measurement of carboxyhemoglobin.

"Spousal Headache"

One of the more unusual cases of drug-related headache is associated with transdermal nitroglycerin (Transderm Nitro) as reported by Talley and Crawley [32]. It is known that topical nitroglycerin preparations, very effective in the treatment of coronary atherosclerotic heart disease, can cause headache as a side effect. A man who had been using nitrate for heart disease, having recognized that his usual nitrate headache did not occur when he applied the preparation to his legs, decided to experiment to determine if distance from his head was an important factor in provoking headache. He applied the preparation to his penis; he quickly had an erection and became sexually aroused. Shortly thereafter, he had sexual intercourse with his wife. She then reported having "the worst headache she ever had in her life. " The authors concluded that such "spousal headache" was due to the absorption of nitrate through the mucous membranes of the vaginal lining.

Environmental Headache

ALTITUDINAL HEADACHE

This type of headache normally occurs at altitudes above 8,000 feet, and it is almost universal above 12,000 feet in unacclimatized individuals. The headache is usually throbbing and generalized but may be mostly frontal. It occurs after many hours at the higher elevations and may be increased by effort. Although the mechanism is unknown, high-altitude headache is associated with vasodilation, increased intracranial pressure, and/or cerebral edema. Reeves and colleagues, in a recent study that involved a simulated high altitude, reported that altitudinal headache is not definitively related to internal carotid arterial blood velocity. Individuals who experienced headache symptoms at high altitude failed to show increased blood velocity, while others who showed increased blood velocity did not have headaches [33].

High-altitude headache may also be associated with other symptoms such as nausea, dizziness, palpitations, and dyspnea. There may be impairment of different cognitive functions with the hypoxia, as demonstrated in one study at a simulated altitude of 10,000 feet. There is some evidence for increased cerebrospinal fluid pressure. Papilledema and retinal hemorrhages have been observed at high altitudes — usually at approximately 12,000 feet, but occasionally at lower elevations.

Therapy for this form of headache, as reported by Meehan, has included increased fluid intake, increased carbohydrate consumption, and the use of 250 - 500 mg of acetazolamide (Diamox) (a carbonic anhydrase inhibitor) to ameliorate the headache [34]. Rapid descent may be necessary in the more serious forms of acute high-altitude illness. Steroids and 100% oxygen may also be helpful.

Cluster headache patients and some migraineurs get headaches on a plane with the cabin pressurized to 7,000-8,000 feet.

TIME ZONE-CHANGE HEADACHE

Individuals who travel across many time zones may note headache as a symptom, along with fatigue, weakness, irritability and sleepiness [35]. The mechanism of the headache, a symptom of what is generally known as "jet lag," is not clear but may be related to changes in the sleep cycle and is probably of hypothalamic origin. Other travel-related changes in the individual's environment, however, may compound the symptoms. The headache, if not all of the other symptoms, usually terminates after several days.

LOW BAROMETRIC PRESSURE HEADACHE

Many headache sufferers relate their symptoms to a fall in barometric pressure, claiming that they can even predict inclement weather by the onset of symptoms. Two studies have been published recently dealing with this subject. Whether a low barometric pressure headache entity exists or individuals with existing migraine are susceptible to changes in barometric pressure is still not certain, however.

In the first of these studies, Wilkinson and Woodrow reported no correlation between adverse weather conditions and onset of migraine or number of attacks [36]. Cull, however, found that the frequency of attacks decreased with a low barometric pressure [37]. Most migraine sufferers, however, as Cull notes, believe their headaches increase with stormy weather and a corresponding low barometric pressure. Both studies, therefore, seem to contradict what patients reveal anecdotally. Further studies may resolve the question of whether a low barometric pressure headache exists or are the headache symptoms a mere reflection of the patient's anxiety and emotional state during stormy weather? Many patients are able to determine the type of change in weather which consistently causes their headache.

Allergy and Headache

The current status of allergy as a causative agent in migraine and non migrainous headache remains unclear. Recent studies using elimination diets in adults and children with migraine lend support to the notion of an allergic role in migraine provocation. The natural history of migraine is to remit spontaneously for variable lengths of time. Prolonged studies are therefore needed to determine conclusively the effect of diet alteration on the course of the migraine disorder.

Episodes of non migrainous headache may also decrease in frequency for unexplained reasons. If placing a patient on an elimination diet or keeping the patient from other allergens is followed by an alteration in the course of the illness, the observing physician may too quickly conclude that allergy is responsible for the illness. But serum levels of IgE do not appear to differ between types of headache patients or between headache sufferers and nonsufferers [38]. A history of allergies is as common in headache populations as in nonheadache populations. Clinicians should be alert to the possibility of allergic causes in chronic headache patients because an occasional patient may respond to the avoidance of an offending allergen, dietary or environmental. The vast majority of headache sufferers, however, probably do not have an allergic basis for their chronic headaches. Future investigations may shed light on the relationship between allergy and headache disorders.

Several points should be kept in mind when investigating the possibility of an allergy headache. Firstly, it should be remembered that the avoidance of substances to which a susceptible individual is allergic infrequently results in a complete disappearance of headache. Secondly, migraine may be provoked by the ingestion of certain substances which affect blood vessels — foods containing large amounts of tyramine and nitroglycerin and other nitrates — but the physician must be careful to differentiate these migraine headaches from allergic headaches. A true antigen-antibody reaction provoking a headache can occur but is rare.

Vaughan described a group of 4 patients with the diagnosis of migraine referred from a neurology clinic to an allergy clinic [39]. Sixteen of the patients had positive skin-test results and 25 had no positive reactions. After all 41 patients were placed on elimination diets, 13 had a reduction in migraine frequency of two thirds or more. Ten of these successful patients were from the group who had positive skin-test results. Twelve percent of the patients who had negative results on all skin tests still had successful elimination-diet trials; their diets were free of eggs, corn, wheat, and milk. Vaughan then did double-blind trials with foods. He demonstrated that nine patients reacted to the double-blind challenge with headache. He believed it was the first time in a double-blind study that a relationship between food ingestion and migraine was demonstrated. The same author believed conventional foods were implicated, including wheat, corn, chocolate, cinnamon, and cola.

Egger and colleagues suggested that food sensitivity may contribute to migraine in children [40]. A statistical analysis in a double-blind, placebo-controlled group demonstrated a significant difference in response between groups. When foods that were suspect were avoided, the children did well; an occasional break in diet, however, resulted in headache. The authors further suggested that standard allergy testing is only moderately useful. It is suggested that IgE-mediated allergy was not a factor in food sensitivity in most of the patients. Diamond and Medina similarly concluded that migraine was not an IgE-mediated hypersensitivity disorder [41].

Headache other than migraine may also be triggered by ingestion of foods to which one is allergic. A vascular headache is probably the type produced, but it may have nonspecific features and mimic mixed type (tension-type and vascular) headaches.

Seasonal allergy may trigger headache symptoms in susceptible individuals. Often it is associated with nasal and ocular symptoms, as well. Rarely will it occur without other accompanying symptoms.

I would conclude that allergy may result in headache in susceptible individuals. It may at times be responsible for migraine and non migrainous vascular headaches. The incidence is certainly not known and often exaggerated as a cause of headache. Much investigative work remains to be done to clarify the role of allergy in headache causation.*

Recently Described Syndromes

Two recently described syndromes are chronic active Epstein-Barr virus (CEBV) infection, also known as chronic mononucleosis, and the fibromyalgia syndrome with headache as a significant symptom.

One investigator prefers to call the former "chronic viral fatigue syndrome" because fatigue is always present in patients with this syndrome [42]. Usually young adults are affected and women are affected more often than men. Headache may occur in 35% to 85% of sufferers; there is discrepancy among different studies. Other symptoms include low-grade fever, myalgias, and depression. Many patients manifest recurrent sore throat, sleep disorders, and arthralgias. Some patients also manifest high titers of Epstein-Barr virus (EBV) antibodies. The viral capsid antigen-IgG (VCA-IgG) and early antigen Antibody (EA-Ab) titers are elevated in some individuals suffering from the syndrome. The disorder may be common in a general care practice and many of the symptoms overlap those of individuals suffering from chronic anxiety and depression. The recurrent pharyngitis, adenopathy, arthralgias, and rash are not common in anxiety or depression.

The disorder still requires further research to establish its existence. Treatment at present remains symptomatic; the headaches are most often treated with nonaddictive analgesics.

The fibromyalgia syndrome bears many similarities to the CEBV syndrome [43]. Fatigue, myalgias, and arthralgias, however, predominate in fibromyalgia. Obligatory criteria include chronic generalized aches, pains, or stiffness in at least three anatomic sites for three months or longer. There are also characteristic tender points. Chronic headache is one of the minor criteria [44]. Many of the patients are women between 20 and 50 years of age with a history of tension-type headache. The headache is more characteristic of tension-type headache, and treatment of fibromyalgia is similar to treatment of chronic tension-type headaches. Amitriptyline HCl (Elavil, Endep) and naproxen sodium (Anaprox) have been associated with significant improvement in both symptoms of fibromyalgia and tension-type headache.

One author considers CEBV syndrome and fibromyalgia part of the chronic viral fatigue syndrome although antibody levels in fibromyalgia are normal [45]. Because headache symptoms are common in both groups, physicians should consider both disorders when examining patients with chronic fatigue and headache.

---

* Editor's note: The great majority of researchers agree that true allergy with IgE mediated hypersensitivity is not usually the cause of headache

The more usual as well as the less common miscellaneous causes of headache have been described. Some of the types mentioned are relatively uncommon, but recent interest in them and, at times, overdiagnosis has exaggerated their importance. Allergic, dietary and hypoglycemic causes are probably responsible for a smaller percentage of chronic headaches than is generally thought. Temporomandibular disorders are similarly overdiagnosed; the diagnosis, however, may also be missed if not considered.

References

1. Jackson WP. Ocular nerve palsy with severe headache in diabetics. *Brit Med J 2:* 408-9, 1955.
2. Saul RF, Hilliker JK. Third nerve palsy: the presenting signs of a pituitary adenoma in five patients and the only neurological sign in four patients. *J Clin Neuro-ophthalmol 5:*185-93, 1985.
3. Solberg WK. Temporomandibular disorders: background and the clinical problems. *Br Dent J 160:*157-61, 1986.
4. Reik LJr. Unnecessary dental treatment of headache patients for temporomandibular joint disorders. *Headache 25:* 246-8, 1985.
5. Faleck H, Rothner AD, Erenberg G, Cruse RP. Headaches in subacute sinusitis. Unpublished poster exhibit. American Association for the Study of Headache Meeting, New York 1985.
6. Oakley LA, Fisher JF, Dennison JH, Bread mold infection in diabetes: the life-threatening condition of rhinocerebral mucormycosis. *Postgrad Med 80:* 93-6, 99, 102, 1986.
7. Reich H, Behr W, Barnert J. Rhinocerebral mucormycosis in a diabetic ketoacidotic patient. *J Neurol 232:* 115-7, 1985.
8. Lefkowitz D, Biller J. Bregmatic headache as a manifestation of myocardial ischemia. *Arch Neuro 39:* 130, 1982.
9. Blair DC, Fekety FR. Primary hyperparathyroidism presenting as fever of unknown origin with unremitting headache. *Ann Intern Med 91:* 575-6, 1979.
10. Aurback GD, Mallette LE, Patten BM, et al. Hyperparathyroidism: recent studies. *Ann Intern Med 79:* 566-81, 1973.
11. Kemman E, Jones JR. Hyperprolactinemia and headaches. *Am J Obstet Gyn 145:* 668-71, 1983.
12. Strebel PM, Zacur HA, Gold EB. Headache, hyperprolactinemia and prolactinomas. *Obstet Gynecol 68:* 195-9, 1986.
13. Gilliland K, Bullock W. Caffeine: a potential drug of abuse. *Adv Alcohol Substance Abuse 3:* 53-73, 1983-4.
14. Dalessio DJ, ed. *Wolff's Headache And Other Head Pain.* p 214. New York, Oxford University Press, 1980.
15. Kaivola S, Parantainen J, Oseerman T, et al. Hangover headache and prostaglandins: prophylactic treatment with tolfenamic acid. *Cephalalgia 3:* 31-6, 1983.
16. Schaumberg HH, Byck R, Gerstl R, et al. Monosodium L-glutamate: Its pharmacology and role in Chinese restaurant syndrome. *Science 163:* 826-8, 1969.
17. Muenter MD, Perry HO, Ludwig J. Chronic vitamin A intoxication in adults. *Am J Med 50:* 129-36, 1971.
18. Selhorst JB, Waybright EA, Jennings S, et al. Liver lover's headache: pseudotumor cerebri and vitamin A toxicity. *JAMA 252:* 3365, 1984.
19. Raskin NH, Knittle SC. Ice cream headache: Orthostatic symptoms in patients with migraine. *Headache 16:* 222-5, 1976.
20. Dalessio DJ, ed. *Wolff's Headache And Other Head Pain.* pp 215-6. New York, Oxford University Press, 1980.

21. Hanington E. Preliminary report on tyramine headache. *Br Med J 2:* 550-1, 1967.
22. Hanington E, Horn M, Wilkinson M. Further observations on the effect of tyramine. In: Cochrane AL, ed. *Background To Migraine.*. pp 113-9. London, Heinemann, 1970.
23. Moffett A, Swash M, Scott DF. Effect of tyramine in migraine, a double-blind study. *J Neurol Neurosurg Psychiatry 35:* 496-9, 1972.
24. Sandler M, Peatfield R, Glover V, et al. Tyramine response and platelet monoamine oxidase activity in migraine. In: Rose FC, ed. *Advances In Migraine-research And Therapy.* pp 133-6. NewYork, RavenPress, 1982.
25. Bale JF, Fountain MT, Shaddy R. Phenylpropanolamine-associated CNS complications in children and adolescents. *Am J Dis Child 138:* 683-5, 1984.
26. Bernstein E, Diskant BM. Phenopropanolamine: a potentially dangerous drug. *Ann Emerg Med 11:* 311-5, 1982.
27. Folks DG. Monoamine oxidase inhibitors: reappraisal of dietary considerations. *J Clin Psychopharmacology 3:* 249-52, 1983.
28. Wurtman RJ. Neurochemical changes following high dose aspartame with dietary carbohydrates (letter). *N Engl J Med 309:* 429-30, 1983.
29. Ferguson JM. Interaction of aspartame and carbohydrates in an eating-disordered patient. *Am J Psychiatry 142:* 271, 1985.
30. Schwartz RH, Peary P. Abuse of isobutyl nitrite inhalation (Rush) by adolescents. *Clin Ped 25:* 308-10, 1986.
31. Dalessio DJ. Carbon monoxide (CO) and headache. *Headache 22:* 89, 1982.
32. Talley JD, Crawley IS. Transdermal nitrate, penile erection and spousal headache. *Ann Intern Med 103:* 804, 1985.
33. Reeves JT, Moore LG, McCullough RE, et al. Headache at high altitude is not related to internal carotid arterial blood velocity. *J Applied Physiol 59:* 909-15, 1985.
34. Meehan RT, Zavala DC. The pathophysiology of acute high-altitude illness. *Amer J Med 73:* 395-403, 1982.
35. Wright JE, Vogel JA, Sampson JB, et al. Effects of travel across time zones (jet-lag) on exercise capacity and performance. *Aviat Space Environ Med 54:* 132-7, 1983.
36. Wilkinson M, Woodrow J. Migraine and weather. *Headache 19:* 375-8, 1979.
37. Cull RE. Barometric pressure and other factors in migraine. *Headache 21:* 102-4, 1981.
38. Dalessio DJ, ed. *Wolff's Headache And Other Head Pain.* pp 256-86. New York, Oxford University Press, 1980.
39. Check W. And as for migraine. *Medical News. JAMA 250(6):* 708, 1983.
40. Egger J, Wilson J, Carter CM, et al. Is migraine food allergy? A double-blind controlled trial of oligoantiallergenic diet treatment. *Lancet 2(8355):* 865-8, 1983.
41. Medina J, Diamond S. The role of diet in migraine. *Headache 18(1):* 31-4, 1978.
42. Komaroff AL. The "chronic mononucleosis syndromes". *Hospital Practice (off) 22(5a):* 71-5, 1987.
43. Goldenberg DL. Fibromyalgia syndrome. An emerging but controversial condition. *JAMA 257:* 2782-7, 1987.
44. Yunus M, Masi AT, Calabro JJ, et al. Primary fibromyalgia (fibrositis): Clinical study of 50 patients with matched normal controls. *Semin Arthritis Rheum II:* ISI-72, 1981.
45. Buchwald D, Goldenberg DL, Sullivan JL, et al. The "chronic, active Epstein-Barr virus infection: syndrome and primary fibromyalgia. "*Arthritis Rheum Oct 30(10):* 1132-6, 1987.

13

Analgesic Rebound Headache

Alan M. Rapoport and Randall E. Weeks

Analgesic rebound headache (ARH) is an often unrecognized clinical syndrome in which the frequent and excessive use of analgesics (aspirin, acetaminophen, etc.) by chronic headache sufferers perpetuates and worsens head pain rather than relieves it. Such consumption also interferes with the therapeutic efficacy of standard, usually effective, pharmacological and nonpharmacological treatment regimens, thus preventing expected improvement. ARH is a clinically important phenomenon that is often ignored by clinicians and researchers. This chapter will describe the clinical entity of ARH, review the relevant (though somewhat sparse) literature, summarize our three major clinical studies, discuss possible mechanisms of pain and research issues, and offer suggestions for treatment.

ARH: The Clinical Entity

Limited amounts of analgesics may offer some relief initially from tension-type headache, but patients with frequent or daily headache seem to habituate to the therapeutic actions of such agents. This begins a cycle of increased intake to achieve similar relief. At some point, increased consumption not only fails to provide pain reduction, but seems to perpetuate and intensify headache. This paradoxical effects of analgesics is called ARH.

Many abortive headache agents can be extremely helpful to the occasional headache sufferer when used properly. The following medications help intermittent headaches:
- Aspirin and combination medicines containing aspirin.
- Acetaminophen and combination medicines containing acetaminophen.
- Non-steroidal anti-inflammatory compounds.
- Vaso-active substances such as isometheptene mucate (Midrin).
- Ergotamine tartrate (Cafergot and Wigraine).
- Dihydroergotamine (D.H.E. 45).
- Butalbital containing compounds (Fiorinal, Fiorinal with codeine, Fioricet, and Esgic).
- Narcotics.
- Steroids.
- Anti-emetics (Phenergan and Reglan).
- Sedative-hypnotics.

When guidlines are followed, these medicines can be effective in the treatment of the occasional headache sufferer. However, the abuse of these medications may lead to dependency and/or analgesic rebound headache or ergotamine rebound headache. As physicians do not usually set limits with patients, they can inadvertently help the patient get into trouble by continuing to prescribe analgesics. Some patients get themselves into trouble by taking too many off-the-shelf medicines. Nasal sprays, antihistamines and sinus medications are also abused by headache sufferers.

Fiorinal (butalbital, aspirin and caffeine) or Fiorinal #3 (with codeine) are excellent medications to treat an acute tension-type headache or a migraine early in the course. But using these medications more than 3 times a day for more than 3 days a week on a regular basis can lead to analgesic rebound headache.

Cafergot (ergotamine tartrate with caffeine) is one of the best medications available to stop a developing migraine in its tracks. But using it more than 1-2 days per week can lead to ergotamine rebound headaches and increase the headache frequency.

The term "rebound" refers to the worsening of the headache as the analgesic effect wears off (usually after three to four hours), and an apparent withdrawal phenomenon whereby the patient experiences an escalation of pain after discontinuation of the medication. The Analgesic Washout Period (AWP) is the length of time required for reregulation of the nociceptive system and the renewed potential for pain relief.

Our group at The New England Center for Headache (NECH), including Dr. Fred Sheftell and Dr. Steve Baskin, has studied 2,500 patients with ARH. The following clinical trends have emerged.

Most patients with ARH are in their 30s or 40s and have a history of mild subacute, or chronic tension-type headache for many years. They experience pain two to four times a week before abusing analgesics. Many also have a history of intermittent migraine.

Headaches last from six to 24 hours and are described as mild, dull, nonthrobbing, steady, bilateral, fronto-occipital, or diffuse discomfort. They are not usually associated with visual complaints or autonomic symptoms (nausea, vomiting, diarrhea, sweating, pupillary changes, stuffed nostrils, etc.). There are no focal symptoms such as weakness, paresthesias, or speech problems. Frequency of pain and/or pain duration slowly increases and patients gradually begin to use off-the-shelf or prescription analgesics in larger amounts. Over time, the headaches may develop the characteristics of migraine and the syndrome becomes a mixture of several headache types. Patients also have sleep disturbances such as difficulty falling asleep and early morning awakening, depression, trouble concentrating, irritability, restlessness and tremor. There is often a family history of depression, substance abuse and headache.

Some patients use only one analgesic, but a significant percentage may use two or more. The most common preparation used is aspirin or acetaminophen in combination with a barbiturate; but off-the-shelf medications are also abused and may create the "rebound" effect. It is not clear whether ibuprophen can cause the rebound effect. Narcotics can be and are difficult to deal with as they can cause more significant degrees of dependency and withdrawal.

Patients note only temporary, partial relief and begin to take medication three to four times per day, often as soon as relief wears off. Some start to take medication in anticipation of a severe headache to ensure that their level of activity will not be compromised by pain.

A typical pattern of increased consumption is one in which analgesics, which were taken two times per day in small quantities in the early course of the headache pattern, begin to be taken regularly, habitually, and in excessive amounts. Patients frequently awaken in the morning with a headache and take medication before getting out of bed. They continue to take medication every three to four hours until bedtime, with total consumption ranging from five to 20 tablets per day. They may take up to five tablets at one time. There is little relief and the headache appears to worsen in spite of increased amounts of medication.

ARH: Relevant Research

Kudrow studied the paradoxical effect of frequent analgesic use in 200 daily headache sufferers [1]. One hundred patients were given amitriptyline HCl (Elavil, Endep) and 100 were not. The two groups were further divided into two equal subgroups (n = 50). One subgroup discontinued analgesics while the other did not. At the end of four weeks, the amitriptyline-treated group had a mean improvement of 30% in the subgroup using analgesics compared with 72% improvement in the analgesic-free subgroup. In the non-amitriptyline group, the corresponding figures were 18% and 43% respectively. These data support and underscore the need to have patients discontinue analgesics to maximize the likelihood of therapeutic benefit from amitriptyline or similar medication. Even in the absence of other treatment, a significant number of patients improve by discontinuing analgesics.

Isler studied 235 migraine patients who were consuming analgesics at a rate of 30 or more tablets per month (many of whom were also taking ergotamine) [2]. He found that they had twice as many headache days per month as those who took fewer than 30 tablets per month. It was found that the slow withdrawal of analgesics and ergotamine while maintaining appropriate prophylactic treatment (mostly beta-blocking agents combined with tricyclic antidepressants) improved chronic headache and decreased the frequency of headache days. He concluded that chronicity of headache was a direct consequence of abuse of medication designed for immediate effect. Restriction of the use of such drugs to once a week or less was recommended. A limitation of the study was that it combined analgesic abusers with ergotamine abusers and studied only migraine patients without addressing issues of tension-type headache.

Dichgans and colleagues studied the effects of abrupt withdrawal of mixed analgesics in 52 patients with chronic headache [3]. The patients developed withdrawal symptoms but improved markedly for long periods of time.

Mathew studied 200 patients who consumed excess quantities of symptomatic medication but continued to suffer from almost daily headaches [4]. He included patients taking pain and sleeping medications, ergotamines, nasal sprays, and antihistamines. All groups studied showed initial withdrawal reactions. All patients taken off symptomatic medication improved. Those placed on appropriate prophylactic medication improved the most.

Wilkinson studied non-headache patients who took large amounts of analgesics for other conditions (i.e. arthritis) and found that they do not develop analgesic rebound headache [5].

ARH: Clinical Studies at NECH

Our initial study examined personality variables in patients with ARH [6]. Twenty patients with daily headaches who consumed a minimum of 20 analgesic tablets per week were included in this study. Most used either aspirin, acetaminophen, or a compound containing aspirin, caffeine, and butalbital (Fiorinal). At the end of the four-month study period, the patients were divided into three groups. The pure analgesic rebound group were those who experienced at least a 50% decrease in daily, mild-to moderate headaches by simply discontinuing their analgesics. The chronic tension-type headache/depressive group experienced similar headache reduction but only after discontinuing analgesics and being placed on a tricyclic antidepressant, either amitriptyline or doxepin. The treatment failure group did not reach the criterion of

50% reduction on frequency of pain despite discontinuing analgesics and being given trials of antidepressants.

Minnesota Multiphasic Personality Inventory (MMPI) data from the three groups revealed that the pure rebound patients had elevated scale 1 (hypochondriasis) configurations with lower scale 2 (depression) and scale 3 (hysteria) scores. This suggested "somatic concerns" in apparently well-adjusted people who were anxious about their symptoms. The tension-type/depressive patients demonstrated a subclinical "conversion V" (a relatively high scale 1 and 3 and low scale 2). This suggested individuals with an awareness of physical symptoms with little apparent concern about them. "Masked depression" would be likely in a psychologically defensive individual. The treatment failure group had relatively lower scale 1 and 2 elevation with higher scale 3 scores. Such profiles suggested possible histrionic tendencies indicating that they might be individuals who would have exaggerated dependency needs and difficulty dealing with the expression of anger.

A later study examined 70 patients who had daily headaches and were consuming 14 or more analgesic tablets per week [7]. We recorded their headache indices over a four-month period after discontinuation of all analgesics to assess the percent of improvement. A number of patients were not given any other treatment and simply observed. Depending on the clinical picture, some patients were treated with 2 mg of cyproheptadine HCl (Periactin) and 50 mg of vitamin B_6 (pyridoxine). Others were treated with 10-30 mg of amitriptyline at night.

For the study, a significant decrease in headache was defined as a 67% reduction in the frequency of daily, mild-to-moderate headaches. Treatment results at one month showed four patients improved using no medication. Twenty-four patients improved on cyproheptadine and vitamin B_6 and 18 patients improved on amitriptyline. In all, 46 of 70 patients (65.7%) had improved at the end of one month. At the end of the second month, three more patients on cyproheptadine and vitamin B_6 improved as did eight more patients on amitriptyline. Thus, 11 more patients in the sample improved in the second month. A total of 57 of 70 patients (81.4% of the total sample) had significantly improved at the end of two months.

Our third study on ARH was an attempt to ascertain the length of time that the analgesic detoxification process takes [8]. Such data were important since the presence of analgesics appeared to compromise otherwise effective headache treatment and, therefore, may cause a delay in symptom reduction due to the detoxification process. Such information was believed to be important in terms of an awareness of an adequate length of treatment trial before a drug regimen should be considered "ineffective".

Ninety patients took part in this study of the Analgesic Washout Period. Inclusion criteria included daily, mild-to-severe generalized headache in patients taking a minimum of 14 analgesic tablets per week. Once again, significant improvement was defined as greater than 67% reduction in the frequency of headache.

The results indicated that 30% of the patients were significantly improved during the first month, 37% during the second month, 13% during the third month, and 2% during the fourth month. Some patients were asked only to discontinue analgesics, while others were treated, in addition, with cyproheptadine and vitamin B_6 or with small doses of amitriptyline, depending on the clinical picture.

The data suggest that the Analgesic Washout Period may be as long as 12 weeks for some patients, but is almost always 8 weeks. To evaluate fully any headache treatment modality, a trial utilizing that modality, 12 weeks after cessation of analgesics, is necessary when treating patients who have analgesic rebound as part of their clinical picture.

Discussion

The pain from chronic tension-type headache was thought at one time to be peripheral in nature (viz, secondary to contracted muscles and painful nerves in the head and neck). There is an emerging body of data that suggest it may be a central nervous system disorder. The analgesics may be more centrally active than the peripheral role they play in inhibiting prostaglandins. In fact, aspirin and acetaminophen work centrally to relieve pain and lower body temperature while toxic doses may cause central side effects.

Our research and studies from the biofeedback literature have shown that patients with chronic tension-type headache may or may not have high levels of muscle tension. Depression has been shown to be a factor in the pain experience in either a primary or secondary way. Hence, tension-type headache may include several different entities some more related to peripheral factors (scalp muscle contraction) while others more directly related to central brain mechanisms.

If the pain of chronic tension-type headache is central in origin and associated with tolerance, habituation, and rebound pain, then it may be secondary to suppression of a central antinociceptive system. The system most likely affected is the ascending and descending serotonergic system controlling sleep, dull pain, migraine and feelings of well being. Amitriptyline affects the system by preventing a reuptake of serotonin into nerve terminals and, thereby, increasing its concentration and prolonging its effects.

It is known that aspirin works centrally to increase serotonin levels. It used to be thought that the rate-limiting step in the availability of cerebral serotonin was the concentration of the enzyme 5-tryptophan hydroxylase. It is now known that the availability of tryptophan in the brain is the limiting factor of the level of cerebral serotonin.

Tryptophan is the only amino acid bound to protein. Salicylates break that bond and increase the availability of free tryptophan and hence serotonin in the brain. Studies show that one to two hours after administration of tryptophan, there is an increase in brain serotonin concentration. But, there is a paradoxical effect with increased head pain. The mechanism is not well understood. Probably, there is a down regulation of serotonin receptors with a reduction in the number of serotonin receptors sites in the brain or some other receptor dysfunction or blockade. This reduces the effectiveness of the increased amount of serotonin; the result is increased pain.

Peripheral pain impulses enter the spinal cord at the dorsal horn and travel along the neospinothalamic tract. It begins in the dorsal horn, crosses to the other side of the cord, and ascends in the lateral spinothalamic tract to the thalamus. This tract carries acute pain signals of sharp, stabbing nature.

The paleospinothalamic tract begins in the cord, is not arranged somatotopically, and carries chronic pain impulses that are less localized and carry more dull and burning pain sensations. This tract terminates in different areas of the brain, including the reticular formation, the hypothalamus, the thalamic nuclei, and the limbic system—the seat of emotions and the basic functions of sex, eating, drinking, the autonomic nervous system, and temperature regulation. The most important neurotransmitter in this system is the indoleamine serotonin (5-HT or 5 hydroxytryptamine).

There are descending and ascending 5-HT pathways that induce analgesia. Raphe spinal serotonergic nuclei in the medulla contain the cell bodies of descending pathways involved in pain control.

Ascending 5-HT pathways also play an important role in the regulation of pain sensitivity. Several reports concluded that reducing brain 5-HT by chemicals or lesions in the median forebrain bundle resulted in increased sensitivity to painful stimuli. Giving 5 hydroxytryptophan (5-HTP), the precursor of 5-HT, reversed the lesions and also the increased pain sensitivity.

Serotonin also blocks pain due to its relationship with the opiate receptor system. It is believed that serotonin increases the effectiveness of enkephalin-mediated analgesia, which can be blocked by serotonin antagonists such as LSD-25. Augmenting serotonin by giving 5-HTP or by blocking presynaptic uptake of serotonin with tricyclic anti-depressants such as amitriptyline, raises pain thresholds in conjunction with the enkephalin system.

The reason patients with ARH continue to take large amounts of medication in spite of the fact that it appears to be ineffective and may, in fact, be making them worse, is because they feel that they have to take something for their headache. Dr. Isler believes that analgesic combinations for immediate effect have psychotropic properties [9]. They are mildly euphoric, sedating, and habit forming. Relief of headache per se appears to cause euphoria even in the absence of euphoric drugs. Time estimation as well as general stimulus intensity estimation appear to be impaired in headache patients [10]. Previous time lapses of equal duration are generally underestimated [11]. This would seem a valid reason for taking the same drug earlier, in higher doses, and in increasing frequency.

While we feel that ARH is an important clinical consideration, it can also be a confounding variable with respect to evaluation of various headache treatment protocols. If one is studying a preventive medication for combination headache (migraine plus tension-type headache), it is common to say that if a patient used fewer analgesic tablets in the month after taking a preventative drug, the prophylaxis is effective. In our experience, however, reducing analgesic intake in and of itself, may be responsible for this reduction in head pain. Hence, studies that use analgesic intake as an outcome measure may create confusion regarding the true agents of change (i.e., is the change due to a new therapy or due to stopping the pain medication?). Adequate control groups are often difficult to obtain since allowing patients to continue abusing analgesics has been shown to inhibit relief. Ethically, such research is difficult.

Suggestions for Treatment

Our strong belief is that the patient must be withdrawn from all analgesics. In our experience, this is best done over a three-to-five-day period (but could be done abruptly) as long as there are no barbiturates, ergots or narcotics involved. This can sometimes be done on an outpatient basis. It may be necessary to hospitalize the patient if he has to be withdrawn from narcotics, tranquilizers, sedatives, ergots, or barbiturates, or if he has a medical condition that requires close monitoring such as cardiac disease or hypertension. It is certainly safer, more comfortable and ultimately more beneficial to the long term improvement of the chronic headache sufferer to hospitalize these patients in a specialized, inter-disciplinary headache treatment unit.

If no other medication is given, the patient will usually go through a withdrawal period accompanied by increased pain. We recommend treating the patient with either cyproheptadine 4 mg t.i.d. plus vitamin B_6 50-100 mg per day or Midrin (isometheptene mucate, dichloralphenazone, and acetaminophen), one capsule t.i.d. for one week. Other medications can be given as necessary: promethazine HCl (Phenergan) 25 mg t.i.d. or p.r.n. for nausea, alprazolam (Xanax) 0.5 mg t.i.d. or p.r.n. for sedation, etc. Dexamethasone (Decadron, Hexadrol) can also be used intramuscularly or orally in doses ranging from 4-12 mg/day for 1-3 days. We also use intravenous steroid preparations in our hospitalized patients. Dr. Raskin has described the use of intravenous D.H.E. 45 (dihydroergotamine) given as 1 mg administered intravenously every eight hours in the hospital [12]. This medication is preceded by an anti-emetic, usually metoclopramide HCl (Reglan) by mouth or intravenously. This regimen seems to help patients with all rebound phenomena whether from analgesics or ergotamine.

Attention to cognitive/psychological factors is important as patients may feel more helpless without their usual ritual of medication consumption. Cognitive/behavioral work as well as relaxation therapy (biofeedback training) are important components during the withdrawal phase [13].

The widespread use of analgesics for headache, and the lack of understanding of the concept of analgesic rebound in both the patient and treating physician leads to the ubiquitous problem of analgesic rebound headache today. The physician who is unaware of this concept will have much more difficulty treating his patient effectively. As Dr. Kudrow has shown, even treating the patient with proper preventive medications is not very effective when analgesics continue to be taken in large quantities. So, purely from the treatment point of view, it is vital to understand the concept of analgesic rebound. From the diagnostic point of view, the lack of understanding by neurologists and headache specialists of the concept of analgesic rebound adds to the problem of lack of reliability in headache diagnosis.

References

1. Kudrow L: Paradoxical effects of frequent analgesic use. *Adv Neurol, 33:* 335-341, 1982.
2. Isler H: Migraine treatment as a cause of chronic migraine, in Rose, FC (ed) *Advances in Migraine Research and Therapy.* New York, Raven Press, pp. 159-164, 1982.
3. Dichgans J, Diener, HC, Gerber WD et al: Analgetika-induzierter Dauerkopfschmerz. *Dtsch Med Wochnschr, 109:* 369-373, 1984.
4. Mathew N, Kurman R, Perez F. Drug induced refractory headache—clinical features and management. *Headache 30(10):* 634-638, 1990.
5. Lance F, Parkes C, Wilkinson M. Does analgesic abuse cause headaches de novo? *Headache 28(1):* 61-62, 1988.
6. Rapoport AM, Sheftell FD, Weeks RE et al: Analgesic rebound headache. Proceedings of the Twelfth Meeting of the Scandinavian Migraine Society 37-38, 1983
7. Rapoport AM, Weeks RE, Sheftell FD et al: Analgesic rebound headache: theoretical and practical implications. *Cephalagia, 5,(suppl 3):* 448-449, 1985.
8. Rapoport AM, Weeks RE, Sheftell FD et al: The "analgesic washout period": a critical variable in the evaluation of headache treatment efficacy. *Neurology, 36(suppl 2):* 100-101, 1986.
9. Isler H: Headaches combined with overuse of analgesics, in Carroll JD, Pfaffenrath V, Sjaastad O. (eds): *Migraine and Betablockade.* Uddevalla Bohuslaningns Boktryckeri AB, pp 180-183, 1985
10. Isler H, Solomon S: Impaired time perception in patients with chronic headache. *Headache, 24:* 160, 1984.
11. Ornstein R: *On The Experience Of Time* . New York,. Penguin, 1975.
12. Raskin NH: Repetitive intravenous dihydroergotamine as therapy for intractable migraine. *Neurology 36:* 995-997, 1986.
13. Rapoport AM: Analgesic Rebound Headache. *Headache 28:* 10, 662-665, 1988.

14

Ergotamine Dependency as a Cause for Refractory Recurring Migraine

Joel R. Saper

Ergotamine tartrate (ET) is considered the drug of choice for the treatment of severe acute attacks of migraine, with effectiveness estimated to range from 90% when used parenterally to 80% with rectal administration and 50% when given orally [1]. ET has a smooth muscle-stimulating effect producing vasoconstriction, an effect on medullary tissues causing a sympatholytic reaction, and a peripheral alpha-adrenergic blocking action [2]. Although traditionally considered to be related to vasoconstriction, ET's specific influence on migraine is not clearly understood. Earlier reports by Dalessio as well as more recent works have raised the possibility that the mechanism by which ergot derivatives affect migraine may be by both central as well as peripheral effects [1,3-7].

Common side effects of ET include nausea, vomiting, muscle achiness, diarrhea, and difficulty in swallowing. Ergotism is a progressive disorder characterized by severe vasoconstriction and resultant ischemia to major organ systems [1,4,8-13]. Serious reactions to ergotamine tartrate have occurred at modest treatment levels or when the drug is administered in the presence of contraindications, such as hypertension, peripheral vascular disease, and ischemic heart diseases [14]. Several years ago we drew attention to a phenomenon that had only been occasionally noted in the medical literature, but reflected the existence of a state of ergotamine dependency and its clinical consequences [5,15-17]. Previously referred to as ergot headache or rebound headache, the primary feature of this condition is a self-sustaining, rhythmic headache/medication cycle characterized by daily or almost daily migraine headaches and the irresistible and predictable use of ET as the only means of alleviating the headache attacks [18-21]. If left untreated, this condition may serve as the forerunner of frank ergotism, though this appears relatively infrequently.

The Argument for a Dependency Syndrome

To satisfy the criteria for physical addiction, the following conditions must be met: a predictable and irresistible pattern of usage, the development of tolerance (escalating usage without the presence of obvious adverse consequences), and a state of abstinence or withdrawal upon discontinuance [5].

These criteria seem to have been met as indicated by many reported cases; all well described cases reflect a predictable headache/medication cycle occurring on a daily or almost daily basis [5,15-22]. Consistently reliable effectiveness of ET is clearly demonstrated and is characteristically the only means of headache relief. But, despite daily and weekly dosages that frequently exceed safety limitations, patients demonstrate few serious consequences (tolerance) [5]. Upon discontinuance of the drug, a predictable and definable protracted and severely debilitating headache episode occurs, accompanied by autonomic disturbances and other somatic and mental complaints (abstinence). This prolonged attack usually occurs within 24 to 48 hours following withholding of the drug and may last 72 hours or longer once it begins [5,7]. In many cases, drugs considered useful for migraine had been employed without benefit, but demonstrated effectiveness following abstinence. In the cases described by Tfelt-Hansen, discontinuance of ET alone and without administration of prophylactic agents resulted in a marked reduction of headache frequency [22].

CLINICAL FEATURES

Table 14.1 summarizes the characteristic features of this syndrome. Headache of a migraine type occurs on a daily or almost daily basis. As the effects of the previous dose of ET diminish, the headache typically escalates until the next dose of ET is administered. Psychological dependence intensifies, and depression and sleep disturbance are frequently noted. Whether the latter symptoms are the direct result of the drug on central (brain) mechanisms or on other factors is undetermined. The headache is strikingly sensitive to ET, but will not generally respond to alternative symptomatic or preventive medications that would otherwise be expected to have an ameliorating effect.

Table 14.1 Criteria and clinical features of ergotamine dependency syndrome

History of intermittent, occasional migraine or mixed (combined) headache.
Insidious increase in the use of ET to more than two dosage days per week.
Parallel increased frequency of migraine, exceeding three days per week.
Irresistible and predictable use of ergotamine tartrate.
Predictable onset of headache, usually within 24 hours following last dosage.
Headache refractoriness to other appropriate treatments.
Increasing demands for greater amounts of ET.
Progressive depression, sleep disturbances, and loss of feeling of well being.
Symptoms of abstinence following discontinuance of ET.
Absence of other organic causes of daily headache.

DIAGNOSIS

Migraine, in its natural state, rarely occurs more than once or twice a week and often considerably less frequently [1,4,23-25]. Moreover, migraine is a variable disorder, the frequency of which changes from week to week and month to month. Daily or almost daily migraine is not considered typical and is outside the established criteria for migraine frequency.

Ergotamine tartrate is considered therapeutically specific to vascular headaches, such as migraine and cluster headache. Thus, a migraine-type headache occurring more than two or three times a week and selectively responsive to ET, while refractory to other symptomatic or preventive medications, should serve to alert to the possible presence of this disorder.

Patients will report an increasing frequency of headaches and will request larger supplies of ergotamine tartrate. Traditional restrictions and warning on the use of ET have been based upon the *total dosage per week,* not frequency of use. Thus, patient requests for more medicine may not seem particularly troublesome initially, since total weekly dose limits may not be exceeded in a patient taking, for example, 1 or 2 mg per day, five to seven days per week. Reported cases document that patients taking as little as one half to 1 mg three to four times per week may be affected by this syndrome, although most patients require greater doses and frequency [5,6].

From patient surveys, it appears that increasing usage resulted either from patient-determined preventive administration for expected but not yet present migraine attacks, or from attempts to treat nonmigrainous tension-type or daily chronic headache with ET. Patients also cite the advice of their physicians to take ET as early as possible in the course of a headache, thus prompting usage before the exact nature of the headache or its full manifestations become apparent. Patients confirm their use of ET at the first sign of any headache (many have nonmigrainous forms) or when experiencing some vague abnormal sense that they believe might represent a preheadache prodrome [26].

POSSIBLE MECHANISM OF THE SYNDROME

The exact order of events or mechanism of this phenomenon is unknown. The initial factor could be a natural increase in frequency, followed by the increasing use of ET and the subsequent development of dependency. Or, increasingly frequent use of ET initially might be followed by an ET-determined increase in frequency. It is likely that ET's central influences are critical. These include effect on the brainstem vasomotor centers, cortisol secretion, and neurotransmitter functions in the brainstem and hypothalamic regions [1,50,7,27,28]. ET affects serotonin and norepinephrine receptor function and has been shown to affect limbic hypothalamic pituitary adrenal axis regulation. Moreover, the depression and sleep disturbance accompanying this syndrome may reflect either natural components of the purported neurobiology of migraine or the central effects of ET.[26] Alteration of serotonin and norepinephrine function or receptor sensitivity along with the impact on the limbic hypothalamic pituitary adrenal axis could result in sleep and mood disturbances.

It is also possible that ET exerts its effect through chronobiological mechanisms. ET may capture the 5-hydroxytryptamine (serotonin) circadian rhythm, resulting in an alteration or disrupted phase relationship of the natural periodicity. Serotonin peaks during the day and falls during the night. Thus, the rhythmic pattern of ET dependency could imply a chronobiological disturbance in which ET becomes the synchronizer for an altered serotonin pattern.

Recently, Lance has shown that stimulation of the locus ceruleus in the pons results in the neurovascular changes recognized to occur during migraine [23]. The locus ceruleus is mediated by norepinephrine, and it is possible that the frequent or daily use of ET might alter the sensitivity of neurotransmitter functions in these areas, resulting in rebound or reflex hyperactivity following the discontinuance and/or reduction in blood drug levels after the last usage. The abstinence phenomenon (rebound) due to ET, thus, could be similar to the abstinence syndromes of opiate, nicotine, and alcohol, all of which are proposed to be initiated via the locus ceruleus [29-31].

Critical to the argument of dependency and the direct influence of ET on continuing migraine is the recognition that migraine is not customarily considered a daily headache process. ET is specific for vascular headaches. That patients report daily migrainous type headache, characteristically responsive only to ET, suggests a valid physiological relationship. Moreover, spontaneous improvement following discontinuance without treatment or with the use of prophylatic agents previously used, but ineffective in a particular patient, both support a direct physiological relationship [22]. Other pharmacotherapeutic variables, such as caffeine and barbiturates, which are common components of the ergot preparations, are not a contributing factor [6].

It is my opinion that many patients with this syndrome evolve from intermittent headache to a daily chronic nonmigrainous headache form. The increase in natural frequency as a result of this phenomenon prompts ET usage in an attempt to treat the daily nonmigrainous headache. The increased use of ET results in the development of dependency and the rebound headache. Upon discontinuance, a more natural frequency of migraine is reestablished, and the daily chronic nonmigrainous headache background once again appears.[26]

TREATMENT

The primary therapeutic intervention is discontinuance of ergotamine tartrate; once ET dependency is recognized, withholding of further administration of the drug, usually under controlled circumstances, is necessary. Patients must completely understand the reason for discontinuance and the withdrawal process and symptoms. Because patients' compliance is essential and because of the natural fear that they will be unprotected from intensifying headache, patients must be convinced that they will be well supported and managed during the period of this transition.

Hospitalization is frequently necessary when discontinuing ergotamine tartrate.[32] Intravenous fluids should be administered to maintain proper fluid and electrolyte balance if nausea and vomiting are severe. Symptomatic narcotic and phenothiazine administration and/or sedative treatments, usually via parenteral routes, are employed when necessary.

We are now employing a variation of the Raskin protocol for IV dihydroergotamine (DHE 45) therapy during the initial phases of ergotamine withdrawal.[33] An alternative IV preparation employs intravenous hydrocortisone therapy for three days during the period of acute ergotamine withdrawal. Clonidine may also help ease the withdrawal period. Patient compliance and willingness to undergo this detoxification process, which are essential elements in effective treatment, are greatly enhanced by a well trained team of supportive and experienced professionals, who, with appropriate drug and nondrug treatment protocols, assist patients during the acutely painful days of withdrawal.

The period of acute abstinence may last for two to four days following total ergot elimination, including IV DHE 45.[32] Gradually, over several days after the withdrawal, patients may notice a spontaneous and dramatic reduction in headache intensity. Although a natural improvement in headache frequency is generally forthcoming, many patients will require or prefer the security of some preventive pharmacotherapeutic intervention for at least a while.[22,32] The use of a beta blocker or calcium antagonist together with a tricyclic antidepressant is frequently effective. Symptomatic headache control can be achieved with isometheptene mucate, dichloral phenazone, and acetaminophen (Midrin), analgesics, or nonsteroidal anti-inflammatory agents (naproxen sodium, meclofenamate sodium, etc.).[34] The use of ET for acute headache may be allowed, but limitations must be carefully observed. Patients with a previous history of dependency should be restricted to no more than one usage day per week.

Syndrome Avoidance

It is clear from the experience of this author and others that ergotamine dependency can evolve when there is increasing ET usage that exceeds a frequency of more than two dosage days per week. Patients must be limited to this maximum frequency. Prophylactic agents must be used with appropriate intensity to maintain this control.

Careful monitoring of drug usage patterns and limited amounts of drug per nonrefillable prescription are strongly advised. Patients should be encouraged to call and report headache frequencies and migraine patterns that exceed these limits.

Summary

The frequent use of ET can result in a state of psychological and physiological dependency that appears to promote increasing usage of the drug and daily or almost daily headaches of a migraine type. Withholding of treatment or a delay in administration causes an intensifying headache and autonomic signs that reflect the abstinence syndrome and prompts continued administration of ET.

The onset of the condition is insidious and may result from either too frequent administration of the drug for nonmigraine forms of headache or from self-initiated prophylactic use. The actual mechanism may involve central disturbance of hypothalamic and brainstem function.

The recognition of this syndrome should result in withholding of further ET treatment and appropriate provisions for symptomatic relief during the period of withdrawal. The withdrawal itself is frequently characterized by severe migraine-type distress with autonomic accompaniments, usually occurring anywhere from 12 to 72 hours following discontinuance of the drug. The abstinence period may last several days before terminating spontaneously. Following withdrawal, the frequency of headaches generally diminishes or becomes more responsive to otherwise standard prophylactic regimens. This syndrome can be prevented by limiting the use of ergotamine tartrate to no more than two usage days per week.

References

1. Dalessio DJ. *Wolff's Headaches and Other Pain* 4th ed. New York, Oxford University Press, 1980.
2. Rall TW, Schleifer LS. Drugs effecting uterine motility, in Goodman LS, Gilman A (eds). *The Pharmacological Basis of Therapeutics* 6th ed. New York, Macmillan, 1980.
3. Dalessio DJ, Camp WA, Goodell H, et al: Studies on headache. *Arch Neuro 4:* 235-239, 1961.
4. Saper JR. *Headache Disorders: Current Concepts and Treatment Strategies.* Littleton, MA, Wright-PSG Publishers, 1983.
5. Saper JR, Jones JM. Ergotamine dependency. *Clin Neuropharmacol 9:* 244-256, 1986.
6. Saper JR. Ergotamine dependency: a review. *Headache 27:* 435-438. 1987.
7. Saper JR, Jones JM. Hypothalamic-pituitary-adrenal (HPA) disturbances in ergotamine "rebound" headache: clinical and mechanistic implications (abstract). *Headache 25:* 163-164, 1985.

8. Peters GA, Horton BT. Headache: with special reference to excessive use of ergotamine preparations and withdrawal effects. *Mayo Clin Proc 276:*153-161, 1951.
9. Senter HJ, Lieberman AN, Pinto R. Cerebral manifestations of ergotism: report of a case and review of the literature. *Stroke 7:*88-92, 1976.
10. Lucas RN, Falkowski W. Ergotamine and methysergide abuses in patients with migraine. *Br J Psychiatr 122:*199-203, 1973.
11. Merhoff BC, Porter JM. Ergot intoxication: historical review and description of unusual clinical manifestations. *Ann Surg 180:*773-779, 1974.
12. Goldfischer JD. Acute myocardial infarction secondary to ergot therapy: report of a case and review of literature. *N Engl J Med 262:*860-863, 1960.
13. Benedict CR, Robertson D. Angina pectoris and sudden death in the absence of atherosclerosis following ergotamine therapy for migraine. *Am J Med 67:*117-128, 1979.
14. Enge I, Silvertssen E. Ergotism due to therapeutic doses of ergotamine tartrate. *Am Heart J 70:*665-670, 1965.
15. Wolfson WQ, Graham JR. Development of tolerance to ergot alkaloids in a patient with unusually severe migraine. *N Engl J Med 241:*296-298, 1949.
16. Friedman AP, Brazil P, von Storch TJC. Ergotamine tolerance in patients with migraine. *JAMA 157:*881-884, 1955.
17. Horton BT, Peters GA. Clinical manifestations of excessive use of ergotamine preparations and manifestations of withdrawal effect: report of 52 cases. *Headache 2:*214-227, 1963.
18. Rowsell AR, Neylan C, Wilkinson M. Ergotamine induced headache in migraine patients. *Headache 13:*65-67, 1973.
19. Lippman CW. Characteristic headache resulting from prolonged use of ergot derivatives. *J. Nerv Ment Dis 121:*270-273, 1955.
20. Anderson PG. Ergotamine headache. *Headache 15:*118-121, 1975.
21. Ala-Hurula V, Myllylä V, Hokkanen E. Ergotamine abuse: results of ergotamine discontinuance with special reference to plasma concentrations. *Cephalagia 2:*189-195, 1982.
22. Tfelt-Hansen P, Krabbe AR. Ergotamine abuse. Do patients benefit from withdrawal? *Cephelagia 1:*29-32, 1981.
23. Lance JW. *Mechanisms in Management of Headache 4th ed.* Boston, Butterworth, 1982.
24. Diamond S, Dalessio DL. *The Practicing Physician's Approach to Headache 3rd ed.* Baltimore, Williams & Wilkins, 1982.
25. Raskin NH, Appenzeller O. *Headache.* Philadelphia, WB Saunders, 1980.
26. Saper JR. Changing perspectives on chronic headache. *Clin J Pain 2:*19-28, 1986.
27. Silbergeld EK, Hruska RE. Effects of ergot drugs on serotonergic function: behavior and neurochemistry. *Eur J Pharmacol 58:*1-10, 1979.
28. Fuxe K, Friedholm BB, Ogren S, et al. Ergot drugs and central monoaminergic mechanisms: a histochemical, biochemical, and behavioral analysis. *Fed Proc 37:*2181-2191, 1978.
29. Bakris GL, Cross PD, Hammarstein JE. The use of clonidine for management of opiate abstinence in a chronic pain patient. *Mayo Clin Proc 57:*657-660, 1982.
30. Glassman AH, Jackson WK. Cigarette craving, smoking withdrawal and clonidine. *Science 226:*864-866, 1984.
31. Gold MS, Pottach AC, Sweeny DR, et al. Opiate withdrawal using clonidine, a safe, effective, and rapid non-opiate treatment. *JAMA 243:*343-346, 1980.
32. Saper JR. Treatment of ergotamine dependency: techniques, outcome, and recidivism. *Headache (abstract) 27:*30, 1987.
33. Raskin NH. Repetitive intravenous dihydroergotamine as therapy for intractable migraine. *Neurology 36:*995-997, 1986.
34. Mathew NT Amelioration of ergotamine withdrawal symptoms with naproxen. *Headache 27:*130-133, 1987.

15

Treatment of Chronic Daily Headache

Joel R. Saper

Introduction

This chapter emphasizes the approach to and treatment of chronic recurring daily or almost daily headache. It also considers the phenomenon of "migraine transformation" in which episodic and typical primary headache conditions appear to evolve (transform) into chronic daily headache patterns.

In 1962, the Ad Hoc Committee on Classification of Headache offered what was to become the standard classification for head pain disorders for the next 20 years [1]. This report was based upon the premise of a clear distinction between migraine and tension-type headache (TH) and emphasized system-specific etiologies: vasculature in migraine, musculature in tension-type headache.

Despite its many citations and its traditional acceptance by researchers and clinicians alike, many authorities have been unable to reconcile the myriad of events and phenomena of migraine, tension-type headache, and cluster headache with the basic foundations of this classification [2-4,6]. During the past several years, the emphasis on peripheral phenomena (blood vessels and muscles) and separateness between migraine and tension headache disorders has been challenged and with this trend has come changing views in the treatment of these disorders.

Clinicians are now citing data that they believe support the view that migraine and tension-type headache are physiologically related entities, reflecting a varied symptomatic expression of central (brain) disturbances (transmitter or receptor function) within the upper brainstem, limbic, and/or hypothalamic regions [2,4]. Moreover, many headache authorities are now suggesting that tension-type headache may be less a disorder of muscle than a chronic disturbance of neural function with muscle factors playing a secondary role.

This "central hypothesis" gains its support from several observations. Among these are current understanding of brain mechanisms including the neurochemical and physiological events that are purported to occur during headache; symptom overlap between migraine and tension headache; general acknowledgement that the clinical phenomena, including pain, cannot be satisfactorily or entirely explained by disturbances of vascular or muscular structures; vascular flow studies that challenge traditional views linking pre-headache and headache symptoms of migraine with specific changes in blood flow; and therapeutic considerations that raise doubts as to the presumed mechanism of well-known therapeutic agents [2].

On this last point, drugs initially recognized to be useful for migraine or tension-type headache may be of value in both disorders. Moreover, a large number of agents found useful in the treatment of TH, migraine, or both conditions do not demonstrate a consistent system (vascular or muscular) specificity sufficient to explain their effectiveness. In fact, the wide ranging pharmacological actions of drugs found useful in chronic headache disorders appear to share an influence on the central brain mechanisms more than a specific vascular or muscular effect.

The perspectives on chronic headache are changing, and the villains of the past 100 years (blood vessels and muscles) are now coming to be seen as possible victims, affected by chronic, intermittent, or continuous disturbances of central phenomena. Currently, the International Headache Society (IHS) is undertaking the first major attempt to reclassify headaches since the Ad Hoc Committee Report of 1962. Ironically, controversy and disagreement already exist as to terminology and mechanism.

Daily Chronic Headache: Tension-Type Headaches or Combined Headaches

THE TRANSFORMATION CONCEPT

Tension-type headache is defined by the Ad hoc Committee as: "ache or sensation of tightness, pressure, or constriction, widely varied in intensity, frequency and duration; long-lasting, and commonly suboccipital, associated with sustained contraction of skeletal muscles — usually as part of the individual's reaction of life stress" [1]. Combined headaches (vascular and tension-type) are combinations of vascular headache of the migraine type and tension-type headache commonly which coexist in an attack.

Historically, physicians have used the term "tension headache" to characterize a daily or almost daily chronic headache disorder without vascular-type features and that are often but not necessarily associated with provocation by stress or emotional factors. Migraine and muscle contraction headaches were considered distinct entities [7].

So imprecise are the criteria for tension headache, and so casually has the diagnosis been applied, that to many the diagnosis is but a "wastebasket" entity. The diagnosis has been rendered to any headache disorder that ostensibly is not vascular (migraine, cluster) nor associated with identifiable structural disease, and that occurs when elements of stress, anxiety, or depression are evident.

The challenge to traditional views actually began with Dalessio's early observations (late 1950s) regarding the central actions of drugs used in migraine [5]. Raskin and Appenzeller, in their 1980 book *Headache*, described a "clinical continuum" they believed to be primary to the basic migraine/tension headache disposition [3]. Mathew described the transformation of intermittent migraine to "daily migraine" [9,10]. Saper expanded this concept further, demonstrating a pattern of transformation that involved large numbers (515) of daily chronic headache patients [6]. All patients had begun their headache course with intermittent typical migraine, but by 8 to 10 years following the onset, individuals were experiencing daily chronic headache indistinguishable from the historical description of tension headache. Other features of this transformation included a high incidence of depression, sleep disturbance, and analgesic over-usage. Family histories of these patients showed that over 90% of females and 84% of males had a close family relative with headache, and a higher than expected incidence of substance abuse, alcoholism, and depression. Daily analgesic use was present in 77% of patients and 26% demonstrated a neuroendocrine disturbance as reflected by abnormal cortisol suppression via the dexamethasone suppression test.

The European studies have similarly emphasized a centrally determined transformational process. They define common migraine as an "evolutive disease" characterized by progressive increase in the number of attacks, a gradual reduction of headache-free periods, and eventually reaching the state of "continuous migraine" with interparoxysmal headache (MIH). The interparoxysmal headache is acute migraine superimposed upon daily chronic background.

It is likely that common migraine and MIH as defined by the Europeans, and the transformational syndromes as intimated by Raskin and Appenzeller, and later specifically reported by Mathew and detailed by this author, are the same phenomena. The etiology is assigned to central biochemical dysnociception, due to disturbances of the monoamine system and/or endorphin disturbances, involving hypothalamic and brainstem mechanisms and hypothalamic chronobiological control.

A one-sided continuous headache is termed *hemicrania continua*. An episodic form has been described.

Treatment Considerations

NON-PHARMACOLOGICAL TREATMENT

Headache is a difficult illness to treat, and treatment efforts must include interventions beyond pharmacology alone. The treatment of headache actually begins the moment the patient enters the office. Historically, patients claim that the medical profession reacts differently to the complaint of headache and chronic pain than to other similar distressing illnesses. What is certain is that helping such a patient is enhanced by conveying a sincere interest in their distress, understanding the person with the complaint, and establishing worthwhile and frank communications [6].

A global recognition of the patient's life, emotional needs, and physiological vulnerabilities is essential. Likewise, the physician's ability to enlist trust, allay anxiety and fear, and encourage cooperation are similarly important. In the more complex cases particularly, the person, even more than the symptom, may require treatment and the traditional focus on symptoms must make way for an emphasis on the *individual* with the headache.

Although emotional factors are at times very important, emotional phenomena may have been overemphasized as an etiological basis for headache. Presumptions or premature emphasis on psychological elements early in the course of therapy is counterproductive and often clinically unfounded. Patients have come to feel defensive about these issues because they believe that many physicians harbor preconceived notions as to the relevance of emotional considerations in the etiology of chronic headache.

Preventative as well as symptomatic pharmacological treatment for chronic headache requires patience and resourcefulness. Therapy in all cases must be modeled to meet individual differences in general health, psychological makeup, headache pattern, and patient compliance.

DISCONTINUING DAILY ANALGESICS OR FREQUENT USE OF ERGOTAMINE TARTRATE

During the past several years, numerous reports have emphasized the importance of eliminating daily analgesics and/or frequent use of ergotamine tartrate as essential components to the treatment process [6,8,11]. Increasingly, it is clear that the daily use of analgesics and/or ergotamine tartrate imposes a refractoriness to treatment with other more effective agents.

The "rebound" phenomenon is defined as a clinical condition by which the daily or almost daily use of a symptomatic agent worsens headache severity and frequency. Personal experience suggests that this problem represents the single most important factor contributing to treatment refractoriness in longstanding headache patients. Several reports have documented the importance of this problem.

Recently, this author has delineated the condition of ergotamine dependency, by which the use of ergotamine tartrate three or more days per week involves the onset of a dependency state that leads to increasing tolerance and use, and a refractoriness to otherwise effective migraine prophylaxis [6,8]. Rapoport has detailed this phenomenon with analgesics [11].

Thus, an initial step in the treatment of patients with chronic recurring headache is detoxification and removal of offending agents from treatment regimens. This is often difficult since patients fear the elimination of analgesics or ergot before the establishment of an effective preventive treatment program, and thus resist the discontinuance of symptomatic drugs prior to efficacious prevention. But effective prevention is generally not possible *until* detoxification and removal of analgesics has occurred, thus providing a "catch 22" dilemma.

We have found that open communication and instruction on this point, the implementation of reasonable and flexible time tables, and use of comprehensive in-patient treatment setting are the key elements to successful transition from the overuse of abortive (symptomatic) agents to acceptable prophylaxis. Psychological as well as physiological dependency must be confronted, as must the practical considerations regarding the patient's need to remain functional.

OTHER NONDRUG TREATMENTS

Patients with chronic daily headache frequently require additional and adjunctive interventions that include biofeedback, stress management training, psychotherapy, family intervention, reduction of smoking, elimination of excessive caffeine, and a consideration of all aspects of their health.

It is this author's opinion that chronobiological principles should be considered in treatment programs. There is some evidence that headaches may in part reflect factors related to chronobiological dyssynchrony. Patients appear to fare much better when expected external stimuli, such as sleep times, diet schedules, exercise, daily activities, and even stress, can be kept on schedule. Regulation of these factors can be important in establishing headache control, since interruption of expected patterns appears to provoke headache.

While pharmacotherapy still represents the most important single treatment mode, reduction of analgesics and ergotamine tartrate, and the implementation of these adjunctive and perhaps primary treatments, may serve a critical role in determining whether the pharmacotherapeutic interventions will work.

Preventive Pharmacological Treatment

The preventive management of this disorder must be aggressive and innovative.

THE BETA BLOCKERS

The most important group of drugs for the prevention of migraine are the beta blockers. They are also important in chronic daily headache and their administration is similar to that in migraine prophylaxis. Nadolol (Corgard) and propranolol HCl (Inderal) appear to have the greatest value, but the exact mechanism by which these prevent headache is not understood.

Individual dose determination is required. Corgard is often begun at 20 mg once or twice a day and increased to the point of tolerance, often to a range of 120 mg to 160 mg/day. The traditional short-acting form of Inderal is used in a range of 20 mg to 40 mg three to four times per day, whereas the long-acting form (Inderal LA) is best employed in a twice-per-day regimen, beginning at 80 mg once or twice per day and increasing to 160 mg twice a day as tolerated. Other beta blockers may also be effective.

ANTIDEPRESSANTS

The tricyclic antidepressants (TCAs), particularly amitriptyline HCl (Elavil, Endep), nortriptyline HCl (Pamelor), and doxepin (Adapin, Sinequan) can be of dramatic value in daily chronic headache. In addition to addressing pain, these agents frequently ameliorate the sleep disturbance that is common, and frequently assist even at low dosages in the alleviation of depression. Amitriptyline is administered in a dosage of 25 mg to 150 mg/day, often in a single bedtime dose. Nortriptyline dosages range from 25 mg to 75 mg/day.

The monoamine oxidase inhibitors (MAOIs), particularly phenelzine sulfate (Nardil), can be dramatic in the prevention of migraine as well as daily chronic headache, especially in the presence of elements of endogenous depression. The traditional taboo over the use of MAOIs and the simultaneous administration of tricyclic antidepressants has diminished [12]. Combined MAOI and amitriptyline treatment regimens are used extensively for refractory depression and are now used increasingly in the treatment of headache.

When tricyclic antidepressants and MAOI agents are administered simultaneously, both drugs should be started at the same time, gradually increasing dosages to tolerance [12]. One regimen is amitriptyline 25 mg to 50 mg at night given concurrently with Nardil 15 mg two to four times a day. Imipramine HCl (Tofranil) or related drugs should not be used with MAOIs.

CALCIUM CHANNEL BLOCKERS

While the calcium channel blockers may well have a place in the treatment of daily chronic headache, at this point they do not enjoy the success of the above described agents. Nevertheless, the use of verapamil HCl (Calan, Isoptin), diltiazem HCl (Cardizem), and nifedipine (Adalat, Procardia) deserve consideration, although the latter drugs can produce headaches in up to 30% of patients.

SEROTONIN ANTAGONISTS

Methysergide maleate (Sansert), the oldest of the migraine prophylactic agents, is marred by a history of adverse consequences. Nevertheless, methysergide, when used selectively and for defined periods, is an effective preventive agent and can be safely combined with tricyclic antidepressants. It is presumed that a central mechanistic influence may in part, if not mostly, explain therapeutic efficacy; it may also act as an extra-cerebral vasoconstrictor. The usual dosage of methysergide is 2 mg three or four times per day.

NONSTEROIDAL ANTI-INFLAMMATORY AGENTS

The nonsteroidal anti-inflammatory drugs (NSAIDs) are used for both the symptomatic and preventive treatment of headache. Naproxen sodium (Anaprox) has been successfully established as an effective preventive agent. The dosage of naproxen sodium for prophylactic therapy is one or two 275 mg tablets twice a day. Other drugs such as meclofenamate sodium (Meclomen) may be useful at dosages of 100 mg to 200 mg two or three times a day. The chronic use of NSAIDs without interruption is discouraged. "Pulsed," intermittent use helps to avoid the GI, renal, and other consequences of uninterrupted treatment.

ALPHA-ADRENERGIC BLOCKING AGENTS

Clonidine HCl (Catapres) possesses alpha-adrenergic blocking properties and has not achieved the same therapeutic success as tricyclic antidepressants and beta blockers. Nevertheless, this agent is useful in many patients, particularly those who are withdrawing from analgesic or benzodiazepine medications.

OTHER AGENTS

Benzodiazepines, though historically unpopular because of the addiction potential, may be helpful in some patients. Short-term, well-controlled treatment trials are occasionally advisable. Phenothiazine therapy may also have a place.

Conclusions

Currently, no universally effective solution to this complicated health problem exists. It is clear that most of the pharmacological agents used do provide an indirect influence on the mechanisms of headache. However, no therapy, despite its importance, can be relied upon to universally benefit or satisfy the treatment goals. Indeed, from patient to patient with headache, effective treatment requires individual consideration and treatment planning.

Many patients with chronic daily headache will benefit from the programs described, including the comprehensive and multidisciplinary approaches now available at specialty centers and inpatient units. Headache is a disabling condition and medical science has not, until recently, begun to address it in a manner consistent with its widespread impact. But, despite the limitations in our current understanding as well as the historical prejudice directed towards patients with this condition, current understanding and treatment approaches can provide hope and relief for most patients who suffer from this disorder.

Unfortunately, not all patients can be satisfactorily helped. For some it is because their condition exceeds current knowledge; for others, the need to be sick or the fear of well-being can defeat even the most committed effort. Nonetheless, persistence, patience, and compassion will bring recognizable and satisfying relief for most who suffer from recurring headaches. Although the chronic headache patient is prone to isolation and despair, the awareness that a knowledgeable professional cares, understands, and is committed to help is extraordinarily important and sustaining.

Finally, while the use of multiple medication regimens is generally to be discouraged, this, like other aspects of therapy for difficult-to-treat illness, must be considered in perspective. Physicians commonly employ multiple treatment regimens for control of Parkinson's disease and epilepsy. Likewise, numerous concurrent therapies are used in the control of hypertension, ischemic heart disease, congestive heart failure, and multisystem disease. That such efforts are occasionally appropriate in the treatment of some refractory headache patients seems similarly justifiable. Attitudes that these efforts are excessive or inappropriate for this disabling disorder may be more a reflection of bias than a fair appraisal of current pathogenetic theories or treatment needs.

References

1. Ad Hoc Committee on Classification of Headache. *Arch Neurol 6*: 173-176, 1963.
2. Saper JR. Changing perspectives on chronic headache. *Clin J Pain 2*: 19-28, 1986.
3. Raskin NH, Appenzeller O. *Headache*. Philadelphia, WB Saunders Company, 1980.
4. Lance JW. *Mechanism and Management of Headache*, ed 4. London, Butterworth Scientific, 1982.
5. Dalessio DJ, Camp WA, Goodell H, et al. Studies on headache: The mode of action of UML-491 and its relevance to the nature of vascular headache of the migraine type. *Arch Neurol 4*: 235, 1961.
6. Saper JR. *Headache Disorders; Current Concepts and Treatment Strategies*. Massachusetts, Wricht PSG, Littleton, 1983.
7. Dalessio DJ (ed). *Wolff's Headache*. New York, Oxford University Press, 1980.
8. Saper JR, Jones JM. Ergotamine tartrate dependency: Features and possible mechanisms. *Clin Neuropharm 9(3)*: 244-256, 1986.
9. Mathew NT, Stubits E, Nigam M. Transformation of migraine into daily headache: Analysis of factors. *Headache 22*: 66-68, 1982.
10. Mathew NT. Prophylaxis of migraine and mixed headache: A randomized control study. *Headache 21*: 105-109, 1981.

11. Rapoport AM, Weeks RE, Sheftell FD, et al. The "analgesic washout period:" A critical variable in the evaluation of headache treatment efficacy (abstr). *Neurology 36 (suppl)*: 100-101, 1986.
12. Saper JR. Combined MAOI-tricyclic antidepressant treatment: Diminishing of a taboo? *Topics in Pain Management 2(5)*: 17-19, 1986.

16

Headaches in Children

Marcia Wilkinson

Children, like adults, often suffer from headaches. Most of these will be relatively minor, but in a certain proportion they may have serious implications. In a study done by Bille of 8,992 school children, 59% reported incidences of headache [1]. The headaches were infrequent in the majority, only 10% having fairly frequent headaches. Other studies include those of Sillanpää, who found that in a group of 2,915 children aged 14 years, 28% had a headache at least once a month; and Waters, who found that 27% of girls aged ten to 16 years had severe headaches at least once a month [2,3]. Any headache occurring in a child must be carefully assessed.

History

When a child presents with headache, a careful history must be taken with particular attention as to whether the child looks ill and if the headache is a new symptom or one in a series of attacks. Obtaining a good history depends on finding out from the child and his parents the exact nature of the symptoms. This means that there must be close cooperation and understanding among the doctor, patient, and parents, and this is best done in an informal way. My own practice is to see the child alone on the initial visit and ask him to tell me about his headaches. A simple question like this is usually enough to start the child talking, and much can be learned about the severity and number of attacks and the precipitating factors.

Recently, a child came complaining of headaches and when asked what brought them on, she said, "They always seem to be bad when my parents are having a row." This answer immediately suggested that the headaches were probably of the tension type rather than migrainous in nature. Subsequent interviews with the parents confirmed that there was considerable parental friction, the mother being of Irish descent and the father a rather unsuccessful Indian businessman. The child's most recent severe headache, which lasted for a week, had occurred on a visit to India when there had been considerable parental dissent.

It is important that the child be seen alone since pain is an individual affair and nobody but the sufferer can know the extent of it. If the parents are present, it is not uncommon for the mother to answer the questions rather than the child. If the child is seen on his own, he can be talked to as an individual, and not merely part of the family group. However, it is equally important to see the parents when the patient is present and also when he is not there. In some cases it is found that the child is manipulating his parents and in others the child plays a relatively passive role. For these reasons, I believe it is important that the doctor be the first in the treatment group to see the patient and that he should conduct the interviews himself.

Recently, much emphasis has been put on alternative methods of obtaining a history, either by getting the child and/or his parents to fill out a form that can then be analyzed by a computer or to get a third party to take the history. In the first case, it is difficult to construct a program that is acceptable and includes every possible question; and in the second, it is far more difficult to get the child's confidence if he has already talked to someone else, possibly about things that are upsetting to him. Any history must include details of the family history and past illnesses and should not be limited to questions about the headache. The disadvantage of this approach is that it is time-consuming; but if a complete history is taken at the first interview, many diagnostic errors and unnecessary investigations can be avoided. It should also be remembered that, although headache may be the presenting symptom, the underlying pathology may be elsewhere. After the history has been taken, a full examination must be done and, if indicated, special investigations including magnetic resonance imaging (MRI) and computed tomography (CT) scans.

Headaches of Recent Onset

ACUTE INFECTIONS

Some kind of infection is probably the most common cause of headache in children. Headache may accompany any type of fever, and it is very common for an attack of flu to start with headache. Other common childhood complaints such as exanthemata or gastrointestinal disorders may start in this way, and occasionally headache may be the presenting feature in disorders such as brucellosis.

INTRACRANIAL INFECTIONS

The main intracranial infections are meningitis and encephalitis. In meningitis, the infection may occur as a direct result of a skull fracture or a penetrating wound, or spread from the mastoid or other infected site. Ear infections are common in children and are often the cause of headache and fever. Children presenting with these symptoms should have an examination of the ears.

Tuberculous meningitis is now less common than it used to be, but it still occurs particularly among the immigrant population. The onset is insidious and there is almost always a prodromal phase of ill health. Headache, lassitude, anorexia, and weight loss are symptoms of meningitis; cervical rigidity and Kernig's sign only occur after a period of two to three weeks. If a child presents with these symptoms a lumbar puncture should be done to rule out tuberculous meningitis.

ENCEPHALITIS

There are several viral infections that may cause headache. These include the various types of epidemic encephalitis, inclusion body encephalitis, and encephalitis due to herpes simplex. Other viral infections that may present as headache are poliomyelitis and mumps. In all these disorders, special investigations are necessary to establish the diagnosis, beginning with lumbar puncture and serologic testing.

TRAUMA

Transient headache following an injury to the head is relatively common among children. If there is evidence of injury, the diagnosis is simple. In younger children, the injury may not be remembered and the child may present with headache as the only symptom. In this case, the child should be carefully examined for evidence of bruising. The possibility of nonaccidental injury must be considered as well as other evidence of child abuse. In very young children, even minor head injuries may cause intracranial hemorrhage and evidence of raised intracranial pressure should be looked for. Post traumatic headache associated with altered level of alertness and/or neurologic signs should be thoroughly investigated. Epidural and subdural hematomas are not common in children but should be considered when head trauma is followed by a decreased level of consciousness or focal neurological signs.

CHRONIC OR RECURRENT HEADACHES

The majority of children who present with chronic or recurrent headaches probably suffer from migraine or tension-type headaches. Less common causes are sinusitis or ocular muscle imbalance. A small percentage of children presenting with headache may have a serious neurological disorder including cerebral tumors, benign intracranial hypertension, and hydrocephalus. All of these disorders require investigation by a specialist. Adolescents being treated for acne with tetracycline and vitamin A should be investigated for benign intracranial hypertension.

CEREBRAL TUMORS

Among children under ten years, the incidence of headache due to a cerebral tumor is relatively low, approximately five per 100,000. However, as headache is the most common presenting symptom of tumors, especially in posterior fossa lesions, the possibility of headache due to a tumor must always be considered. In young children, the headache is usually accompanied by restlessness, vomiting, crying, and general irritability. The headache tends to occur every day and is sometimes made worse by coughing, sneezing, or straining.

Migraine

Migraine has been defined as a familial disorder characterized by recurrent attacks of headache widely variable in intensity, frequency, and duration. Attacks are usually unilateral and are associated with anorexia, nausea, and vomiting. In some cases they are preceded by or associated with neurological and mood disturbance [4].

A useful definition of migraine in children, similar to that used by the World Federation of Neurology, is that migraine is a paroxysmal headache lasting from three to 24 hours with total freedom from headaches between the attacks. The attack must be accompanied by visual or gastrointestinal disturbances, and the visual disturbances usually occur before the attack and last between 15 minutes and 45 minutes. Photophobia may also occur. The gastrointestinal disturbances include anorexia, nausea, vomiting, and diarrhea. If only gastrointestinal symptoms are present, the patient must have vomited in at least some of the attacks. Premonitory symptoms may occur before the attack, and after the headache is over, there is a recovery phase. In classical migraine (migraine with aura), there is an aura; this is usually visual, but there may also be paresthesia, motor disturbances, speech disturbances, hyperacuasis, or mood changes.

PREVALENCE

Migraine is a common disorder and occurs in about 13% of the adult population. It is essentially a disease of the young, 20% of all migraine sufferers having had their first attack before the age of ten and 60% before the age of 20. Hockaday found that 62% of her patients had developed migraine by the age of seven and 86% by the age of ten. A similar early onset was found by Congdon and Forsythe [5,6]. The incidence is higher among boys (about 60%), but after the onset of puberty, there is a female preponderance (about 75%).

FAMILY HISTORY

Most clinicians know of families where there is a strong history of migraine, but the epidemiological evidence in favor of it being a familial disorder is controversial. One difficulty is that most of the evidence for these studies has been obtained from questionnaires and there is difficulty in making an exact conclusion from this material. Another difficulty is that migraine is a common disorder (at least 10% of the population) and if the extended family—aunts, uncles, and grandparents—are included, epidemiological studies become very difficult.

PRECIPITATING FACTORS

There are many factors that may bring on migraine in children. These include stress, hunger, exercise, travel, lights, and unpleasant smells—similar precipitating factors to those found in adults.

STRESS

Any form of stress may bring on a migraine attack. The stress in children is usually either at home or at school, and if a child complains of migraine it is important to find out the cause.

Excitement is another form of stress that may precipitate an attack. A social event such as a party of an exciting day out or going to the cinema or theater, may cause an attack. One child had a bad migraine attack after an outing with his grandmother. She had taken him around London shopping, given him a lunch of fish and chips and ice cream and taken him to a cinema. On the way home, he complained of a severe headache and was sick.

Migrainous children may not be subjected to more stress and anxiety than the rest of the population but in some way they appear to be more susceptible to stress. However, at times of real anxiety, children usually remain free of headaches; it is rare for a migraine student to be unable to take an examination because of a headache.

Maratos and Wilkinson studied 45 children who were referred to a migraine clinic [7]. They found that one in six children suffered from more than one type of migraine and that there was a wide variation in the age of onset, with some of the children having had their first attack at the age of two. The frequency and duration of the attacks varied widely among the children but remained consistent for each child. An emotional upset was reported as the precipitating factor in 86%. In this series, a significantly higher proportion of migrainous children than controls showed signs of a neurotic disorder, mainly anxiety or depression, and had a higher prevalence of a neurotic disorder in the previous years. This increased prevalence was found to be associated with a disturbed parental relationship.

Hunger

Migraine sufferers may develop an attack if they miss a meal or eat insufficient amounts of food. Many children go to school without eating breakfast and sometimes have only a snack at midday, eating their main meal when they get home from school. These children can often be helped by being encouraged to eat breakfast and taking a packed lunch.

Diet

Diet is now thought to play an important part in about 10% of migraine sufferers, and the foods most commonly implicated are chocolate, cheese, and citrus fruits. Many studies have been done to find out the mechanism of dietary migraine. There is uncertainty as to whether the attacks are due to a reaction to a particular substance in foods or whether allergy to certain foods provokes migraine. Hannington thought that the provocative factor was probably an amine — either tyramine or phenylethylamine [8]. Recently, interest has centered on the possibility that migraine is a food allergy. In a double-blind controlled trial of oligoantigenic diet treatment, workers at the Hospital for Sick Children, Great Ormand Street, in London found that the majority of the 40 children with severe frequent migraine who completed the trial improved on this diet and relapsed on double-blind food challenges [9]. They also found that a wide range of associated symptoms and signs were also diminished by the restricted diets. However, although 28% of the 68 children tested had high serum IgE levels, IgE antibodies did not identify the foods thought to be causing the symptoms and the group treated was unusual in that there was a high incidence of personal and familial atopy.

In another study of adults, food allergy was thought to be the cause of the attacks [10]. In this trial, patients were put on diets avoiding certain foods. After each five-day period of excluding certain foods, challenges were carried out and the provoking food identified. These patients were then given either sodium chromoglycate or placebo in a double-blind manner with the foods previously identified as provocants. It was found that sodium chromoglycate exerted a protective effect that could prevent a hypersensitivity reaction as well as the symptoms of migraine. Challenging with the relevant food also led to the presence of immune complexes containing IgE. These were absent when the patient was pretreated with sodium chromoglycate but present when placebo was given.

Environmental Factors

Exposure to glare, flickering light, noise, heat, smells, cold, or changes in the weather have all been know to induce migraine. In order to induce an attack, these stimuli usually need to be either severe or prolonged, or more than one such stimulus may be necessary.

Many children find that a visit to the seaside will bring on an attack. Such an outing means an early start, a journey by car or train that may take several hours, exposure to sun, and the glare from the sun. This combined with an unsuitable diet — often ice cream, fish and chips, and cola — and fatigue may precipitate an attack.

Some children are particularly sensitive to smells, and substances such as paint and gas have been implicated. Other substances such as glue may cause headache, but the headaches resulting from glue sniffing should not be confused with migraine.

PHYSICAL EXERTION

Excessive physical effort may bring on a migraine, particularly if the child has missed breakfast or lunch. Running, football, or weight lifting have all been reported as the cause of migraine, and any child who is likely to get headaches should eat before and after exercise. Sometimes glucose tablets taken before or during exercise have been found to be helpful.

PREMONITORY SYMPTOMS

Premonitory symptoms are present in some children. The day before the attack the child may be listless, complain of heaviness in the head, yawn, feel sleepy, or crave a particular food or foods. The craving for food, if present, is usually a desire for sweet things or other carbohydrates. Sometimes the child may look pale, complain of abdominal discomfort, or be constipated.

HEADACHE

Headache is the essential feature of the attack in the majority of children. The headache tends to be unilateral and may begin on one side and remain there or become generalized. One characteristic of the headache is that although one side is primarily affected, some attacks may start on the other side. The pain is usually throbbing, in the temple or behind the eye, and when it is severe, the child wishes to sleep and not be disturbed. After a period of sleep, he wakes up feeling better, often requesting food.

NAUSEA, VOMITING, AND DIARRHEA

About 95% of children with migraine complain of nausea and vomiting; diarrhea occurs in about 10% [11]. The feeling of nausea may precede the headache by some hours but vomiting does not usually occur until the headache is at its worst. During the attack, the child often complains of feeling cold and may complain of abdominal discomfort. Much has been written about "abdominal migraine" or cyclical vomiting, and some regard recurrent attacks of abdominal pain in children as a migraine equivalent. While it is true that children with migraine do get recurrent attacks of headache associated with abdominal pain, it is extremely rare for the abdominal pain to recur without any headache. Lance comments, "abdominal symptoms are common in migraine but it is doubtful whether such an entity as abdominal migraine exists," and Hockaday considers that "the links between cyclical vomiting, the periodic syndrome, abdominal migraine and recurrent abdominal pain syndrome are not established" [12,13]. One difficulty is that many of the disorders considered are ill-defined and not easily distinguishable and therefore difficult to study in an epidemiological sense.

MIGRAINE EQUIVALENT

Terms such as "migraine variant" or "migraine equivalent" have been used to describe more unusual forms of migraine. Bruyn describes a "migraine variant" as "any form of dysfunction intimately tied to the migraine attack in a migraine sufferer," and the term "migraine equivalent" as "an episodic, transient dysfunction in a migraine patient which is not closely tied to the migraine attack and which may completely replace the attack or substitute for it" [14].

The other main types of clinical presentations in migraine are basilar migraine, hemiplegic migraine, and ophthalmoplegic migraine. These often occur without the severe headache, nausea, and vomiting of the common migraine (migraine without aura) attack so they are sometimes referred to as "migraine variants."

VERTEBRO-BASILAR MIGRAINE

This term was first used by Bickerstaff to describe patients, usually adolescent girls, who had attacks of visual disturbances, bilateral sensory changes, vertigo, dysarthria, dysphasia, diplopia, and sometimes loss of consciousness [15]. Hockaday reviewed a series of 132 children, 80 (61%) boys and 52 (39%) girls, the majority (82%) of whom were aged ten or under and suffered from vertebro-basilar migraine [16].

HEMIPLEGIC MIGRAINE

This is an unusual type of migraine in which weakness of one side occurs as part of the migraine attack. Either side of the body may be affected, sometimes alternating in successive episodes. The weakness usually clears up in 24 hours and the condition is sometimes familial. Before making this diagnosis, all other causes of intermittent hemiplegia must be eliminated by full neurological examination and investigations.

OPHTHALMOPLEGIC MIGRAINE

This is a term that has been used to describe recurrent attacks of headache associated with weakness of muscles supplied by one or more oculomotor nerves. The third nerve is the one most commonly affected, and the weakness usually outlasts the migraine headache by days or weeks and may become permanent after repeated attacks. It often occurs in children in the ten to 14 years age group. Before diagnosing ophthalmoplegic migraine, it is important to rule out all causes of oculomotor nerve compression. A full neurological evaluation including CT and/or MRI scans should be done. An MRI scan shows the midbrain, pons, and medulla better than CT scan, and, where available, is the preferred test to rule out structural disease of the brain stem. Testing for diabetes, Lyme disease and inflammatory neuropathy should also be included.

TENSION-TYPE HEADACHE

Tension-type headache may occur in children and is usually associated with stress of some kind. There may be a difficult family situation which the child feels unable to deal with or there may be difficulties in school. Whatever the cause, it is important that the correct diagnosis be made since drugs that are useful in migraine may not be helpful in tension-type headache.

The headaches tend to occur when the child is stressed; a morning headache may develop just before the child goes to school. Once the time for leaving has passed, the child often improves and may even lie in bed listening to pop music. If the attack is a true migraine, he will often look pale, be sick, and want to lie down in a darkened room and go to sleep. Unlike tension-type headache in adults, which may last all day, tension-type headaches in children usually last for three to four hours or less and rarely for as long as 12 hours. However, the attacks may occur daily, unlike migraines, which do not occur more than twice a week. A typical tension-type headache is usually mild, bilateral in the frontal, occipital, or vertex areas, steady and non-throbbing, and feels like a tight band or pressure in the head.

Treatment of Headache in Children

The treatment of headache as a symptom of some underlying pathology depends on the treatment of that condition. When a diagnosis of migraine or tension-type headache is made, a simple analgesic should be given. It is only necessary to give prophylactic treatment to children if the headaches are severe and occur more than twice a month.

ANALGESICS

The analgesic of choice is acetaminophen and the dosage schedule is as follows: children up to one year, 60 mg to 120 mg; children aged one to five years, 120 mg to 250 mg; children six to 12 years, 250 mg to 500 mg. These dosages may be repeated every four to six hours up to a maximum of four doses in 24 hours. It is best given in a soluble form. The present recommendation in the United Kingdom is that aspirin should not be given to children under the age of 12 years unless specifically indicated for childhood rheumatic conditions.

This is because of the possibility of developing Reye's syndrome which is a rare but severe neurological disorder complicated by hepatic dysfunction and predominantly affecting children.

In a typical case of Reye's syndrome, a previously healthy child contracts a common viral infection which is apparently taking a normal course. There is a sudden onset of profuse, persistent, effortless vomiting accompanied, or soon followed by, alteration in the level of consciousness. Liver involvement is indicated by grossly elevated levels of serum aspartate and alanine transaminase, and the blood ammonia level is usually raised.

The etiology of Reye's syndrome is believed to be multifactorial resulting from an abnormal reaction to a viral infection which is modified by an exogenous toxin, in a genetically susceptible host. Aspirin is one of the toxins which has been implicated. Because of this danger, acetaminophen is the analgesic of choice. Acetaminophen is similar in efficacy to aspirin, but has no demonstrable anti-inflammatory activity and is less irritating to the stomach than aspirin. Parents should be warned against exceeding the recommended dosage since an overdose of acetaminophen is particularly dangerous and may cause hepatic damage which is sometimes not apparent for four to six days.

Metoclopramide HCl

Over 90% of migraine sufferers have gastrointestinal symptoms, the most common of which are nausea, vomiting, and diarrhea. Most children respond well to a small dose of metoclopramide HCl (Reglan) or domperidone which is not available in the United States. Metoclopramide stimulates gastric emptying and small intestinal transit and enhances the strength of esophageal sphincter contraction. However, metoclopramide and, occasionally, domperidone, can cause extrapyramidal reactions in which there may be facial and skeletal muscle spasms and oculogyric crises. These are more common in children and may occur soon after starting treatment and subside within 24 hours of stopping the drug. Because of this possible reaction, metoclopramide should not be given to those younger than five and only with caution to those under 12 years. Patients should be warned to look out for increased jerky movements and if these should occur, the drug should be stopped immediately.

For children between five and 12 years, the dosage is 5 mg stat, given in syrup (5 mg/5 mL) or tablet form. In exceptional cases it may be necessary to give the drug intramuscularly. Other antiemetics such as cyclizine lactate (Marezine) or prochlorperazine (Compazine) are probably less effective in migraine than metoclopramide or domperidone as they tend to depress rather than promote gastrointestinal activity.

Ergotamine Tartrate

It is rarely necessary to give ergotamine preparations to children and certainly not to the very young. If the migraine attacks cannot be controlled without it, ergotamine tartrate should be given as one quarter of a suppository (0.5 mg of ergotamine tartrate as Cafergot). This dose may be repeated once. The use of ergotamine should be limited to two days per week.

Most attacks can be controlled with antiemetics and analgesics, and it is helpful if the child lies down in a darkened room. Most children with migraine want to lie still and go to sleep; if a child chooses to listen to pop music he is probably not suffering from migraine. If the child is restless and anxious, a small dose of a sedative may be helpful.

PREVENTIVE TREATMENT

Prophylactic treatment is recommended when the attacks are frequent or severe enough to be disabling and, in my experience, most children do not require prophylactic therapy for migraine. One point that must be remembered is that migraine is essentially a benign recurring disability with no underlying structural pathology. It is therefore important that the treatment should not be more unpleasant or dangerous than the disease. For this reason, I would not use any of the ergot derivations, such as methysergide maleate (Sansert) for the prophylactic treatment of migraine in children.

Because of both clinical and ethical difficulties in carrying out double-blind trials in children, there is relatively little published material on the efficacy of prophylactic treatment in children. Probably either pizotifen, comparable to cyproheptadine but not available in the United States, or propranolol HCl (Inderal) are the drugs of choice. In the United States, cyproheptadine is the drug of choice. The actual dose is best calculated using age, body weight, or body surface area, or a combination of these factors. If body weight is used, the dose may be expressed in mg/kg and young children may require a higher dose per kilogram of body weight than adults because of their higher metabolic rates. Body-surface estimates are more accurate for calculation of pediatric doses than body weight because many physical phenomena are more closely related to body surface area. Cyproheptadine dosage is 2 mg to 16 mg/day, the majority of which is given at bedtime.

NON-DRUG TREATMENT

If a trigger factor can be identified as the cause of migraine, it may be possible to eliminate. For instance, if eating chocolate or cheese is known to bring on a headache, these should not be eaten. If there is any doubt whether a particular food is causing migraine, a careful record of the headaches should be taken. The suspect food should then be eliminated for a month. If there is no improvement, the food can be reintroduced and another eliminated. In my opinion, there is no such thing as a "migraine diet" and if a child is put on a diet that excludes everything that has been said to bring on migraine, he is likely to suffer from malnutrition. Restriction diets have been tried, but such treatment is very difficult and very expensive to maintain [9]. Other treatments such as acupuncture, biofeedback, autohypnosis, and psychotherapy have not been adequately evaluated for children, and some of these treatments are not suitable for children.*

References

1. Bille B. Migraine in school children. *Acta Paediatr Scand 51 (suppl)*: 136, 1962.
2. Sillanpää M. Prevalence of migraine and other headache in Finnish children starting school. *Headache 15*: 288-290, 1976.
3. Waters WE (ed). *The Epidemiology of Migraine*. Bracknell, Berkshire, England. Boehringer-Ingelheim, 1974.
4. Cochrane AL (ed). World Federation of Neurology. *Definition of Migraine. Background of Migraine*, p 181. London, Heinemann Medical Books, 1970.
5. Hockaday JM. Late outcome of childhood onset in migraine and factors affecting outcome. In: Greene R, (ed), *Current Concepts in Migraine Research*. New York, Raven Press, 1978.
6. Congdon PJ, Forsythe WJ. Migraine in childhood. *Dev Med Chil Neurol 21*: 209-216, 1979.
7. Maratos J, Wilkinson M. Migraine in children: A medical and psychiatric study. *Cephalalgia 2*: 179-187, 1982.
8. Hannington E. Preliminary report on tyramine headache. *Br Med J 2*: 550-551, 1967.
9. Egger J, Carter CM, Wilson J, et al. Is migraine food allergy? *Lancet 2*: 8865-868, 1980.
10. Munro J, Brostoff J, Carini C, et al. Food allergy in migraine. *Lancet 2*: 1-4, 1980.
11. Volans GN. Absorption of effervescent aspirin during migraine. *Br Med J 4*: 265-269, 1974.
12. Lance JW. *Mechanism and Management of Headache*, 3rd ed, p 141. London, Boston, Butterworth, 1978.
13. Hockaday JM. Headaches in children. In: Vinken PJ, Bruyn GW, Klawans HL, (eds), *Handbook of Clinical Neurology*, vol 48, pp 31-42. New York, Elsevier Publishing Co, 1985.
14. Bruyn GW.. Migraine equivalents. In: Vinken PJ, Bruyn GW, Klawans HL, (eds), *Handbook of Clinical Neurology*, vol 48, pp 155-171. New York, Elsevier Publishing Co, 1985.
15. Bickerstaff ER. Basilar artery migraine. *Lancet 1*: 15-17, 1961.
16. Hockaday JM. Basilar migraine in childhood. *Dev Med Child Neurol 21*: 455-463, 1979.

---

* Editor's note: In the United States biofeedback is often used with great success in most types of headaches in children.

17

Post-Traumatic Cephalalgia

Morris Levin and L. Jay Turkewitz

Post-traumatic cephalalgia is a topic of great importance not only for neurologists and other specialists in pain management, but for most primary care physicians as well. The incidence of reported head injury in the United States is approximately three million per year; the incidence of post-traumatic cephalalgia has been quoted to range between 12% and 80%. Obviously this syndrome represents very large numbers, which means major expenditures in health care as well as great disruption at the work place and in the home environment. Coonley-Hoganson and colleagues, looking at 275 head trauma patients seen at a hospital emergency room with injuries not severe enough to warrant hospitalization, found that 27% had not resumed normal activity after 48 hours and 13% still had not after one week [1].

The occurrence of persistent post-traumatic cephalalgia does not correlate with electroencephalographic (EEG) abnormalities, skull fractures, blood in the cerebrospinal fluid, loss of consciousness, or the occurrence or severity of post-traumatic amnesia. This is not surprising, given the varied potential mechanisms for the development of post-traumatic cephalalgia. Interestingly, many severely injured patients do not develop post-traumatic cephalalgia or non-cephalalgic post-traumatic syndrome. Interestingly, chronic discomfort after neurosurgical procedures is distinctly uncommon.

Table 17.1. Potential Mechanisms of Post-Traumatic Cephalalgia

Immediate extracranial
    Lacerations
    Abrasions
    Skull or cervical spine fractures
    Whiplash (apophyseal joint injury, musculoskeletal injury, C2 root injury)

Immediate intracranial
    Arterial dilation (nonmigrainous vascular headache)
    Traumatic subarachnoid hemorrhage
    Arterial occlusion

Delayed extracranial
    Muscle contraction headache
    Entrapment or neuroma of sensory nerves (neuralgia)
    Carotid dissection
    Dysautonomia

Delayed intracranial
    Subdural hematoma
    Epidural hematoma
    Cerebral contusion with edema
    Cerebrospinal fluid leak (low pressure headache)
    Hydrocephalus

Other
    Sinus pathology
    Orbital pathology
    Temporomandibular joint dysfunction
    Posttraumatic migraine
    Posttraumatic cluster headache

Combination

Mechanisms of Post-Traumatic Cephalalgia

Kelly classified post-traumatic cephalalgia as being either of immediate or delayed onset and as having an intracranial or extracranial basis [2]. This will be an outline for discussing some of the more common etiologies of post-traumatic cephalalgia (Table 17.1).

In the immediate extracranial group, scalp lacerations and abrasions, subgaleal hematomas, and subperiosteal hematomas are obvious causes of pain. The upper cervical spine is another area of importance, with pain arising from apophyseal joints, ligaments, vertebral bodies, disc displacements, or root irritations, particularly the C2 root. C2 root pain generally involves the postcervical regions with radiation of pain anteriorly to the occiput and occasionally to more anterior areas, as well. The pain can be unilateral or bilateral, often stinging or burning in character. Secondary muscle contraction with aching discomfort and splinting is common.

Immediate intracranial mechanisms of post-traumatic cephalalgia include arterial dilation with resultant nonmigrainous vascular cephalalgia. This pain is often described as a deep aching sensation, worse when coughing, sneezing, bending, etc., and it can be associated with nausea and vomiting. Post-traumatic subarachnoid hemorrhage, usually the result of venous tearing, gives rise to a generalized discomfort, also associated with nausea, vomiting, and signs of meningeal irritation. Traumatic arterial occlusive disease, either via a direct blow to the anterior neck or due to stretching of the cervical spine with vertebral occlusion, may produce cephalalgia periorbitally or occipitotemporally [3].

Delayed extracranial etiologies make up the vast majority of mechanisms that produce post-traumatic cephalalgia. The most common mechanism is so-called muscle contraction pain, often in association with some other pain mechanism. Recent work has suggested that tension-type headache may be under central/hypothalamic control, which is of particular interest when one examines other non-pain aspects of the post-traumatic syndrome [4].

Aching pain at the site of trauma, with or without overt scar formation, may reflect entrapment of a sensory nerve with characteristic neuralgic pain. Local inflammatory changes in superficial blood vessels may also produce pain at the site of trauma. Post-traumatic carotid dissection occurs rarely and is usually associated with neck pain overlying the carotid artery, along with frontotemporal cephalalgia, Horner's syndrome, and occasionally focal neurologic dysfunction on the basis of cerebral ischemia.

A syndrome of dysautonomia with cephalalgia was described by Vijayan and Dreyfus [5]. In five patients who suffered anterior cervical triangle region injury, there were symptoms of episodic throbbing, ipsilateral frontotemporal pain, pupillary dilation, increased sweating, photophobia, visual blurring, and nausea. Sympathetic hypofunction was described between attacks. These patients responded to beta blockers but not to ergotamines, consistent with the authors' hypothesis of sympathetic overactivity.

Headache after trauma that is delayed in onset, either by hours or by days, particularly if associated with focal neurologic dysfunction, should be of particular concern. Potential intracranial etiologies include subdural or epidural hematomas, the development of edema surrounding cerebral contusion, low pressure headache associated with a cerebrospinal fluid leak or, rarely, the development of hydrocephalus.

Damage to the sinuses, orbits, or temporomandibular joints can all occur as a result of trauma. Dysfunction of these structures should be ruled out in the evaluation of post-traumatic cephalalgia patients. Clear cases of migraine, either of the classical or common variety (migraine with and without aura), as well as cluster headaches, have been described following head trauma. The mechanisms by which head trauma might produce these "primary" headache disorders are unclear. Recent understanding of brainstem neurochemistry may provide the answer.

Clinical Presentations of Post-Traumatic Cephalalgia

Post-traumatic cephalalgia can begin within the first several hours of an injury, but may develop several weeks or months later. In the latter case, drawing cause-and-effect conclusions can be very difficult, particularly if there are potentials for secondary gain. Post-traumatic cephalalgia can be a self-limited condition or can persist for years. Hence, prognostication, a key task for the treatment team, is often difficult.

One common mode of presentation in post-traumatic cephalalgia consists of a diffuse, pancephalic aching sensation that may wax and wane throughout the day on a daily basis or exacerbate several times per week. The character of the pain is often described as pressure, tightness, or a band-like sensation around the head. Associated stabbing pains that may or may not be related to the area of scar or injury are described by some patients. Nausea, with or without vomiting, scalp tenderness, photophobia, and phonophobia are common accompaniments, all reminiscent of migraine. This pattern has been termed the "mixed form" of post traumatic cephalalgia.

Another typical pattern, the cervical form, involves aching discomfort in the neck with a pressure sensation or tightness from the occipital regions to the shoulders. This is suggestive of a muscle contraction syndrome or dysfunction in the cervical spine (i.e., apophyseal joint, ligament, vertebral body, or disc). Accompanying sharp, stinging pain in the second cervical root distribution with or without tenderness over the occipital nerve is quite frequent.

These two common modes of presentation are often superimposed upon one another and may often coexist with the other mechanisms of post-traumatic pain. The evaluation of post-traumatic cephalalgia patients must be thorough so as not to overlook treatable pathologies.

Noncephalic Symptoms following Head Trauma

Along with cephalalgia, many post head trauma patients exhibit a typical constellation of other symptoms that are often more disabling than the head pain. These include dizziness (vertiginous or nonvertiginous), depression, anxiety, memory disturbance, loss of consciousness, passivity, anger outbursts, sleep disturbance, and other behavioral changes. Recent reports have pointed to the presence of previous neuropsychiatric disturbances as predisposing to the development of this syndrome [6-8]. However, increasing evidence of disruption in the central nervous system following head trauma suggests that these noncephalalgic post-traumatic symptoms may have an organic basis, rather than representing a functional illness [9,10]. Anatomical changes in brain stem structures, abnormalities in evoked potentials and event-related potentials, and reproducible objective changes in perception of light and sound all support this idea. Suggestions that brain stem, limbic system, and subcortical areas might be foci of dysfunction in patients with post-traumatic cognitive difficulties will require further investigation.

Treating the Post-Traumatic Cephalalgia Patient

In addition to the difficulty posed by the numerous, often coexisting, mechanisms of pain in these patients, issues of litigation, compensation, and other forms of secondary gain can cloud diagnosis and management of post-traumatic cephalalgia. This type of patient therefore requires an objective, painstaking approach. The traumatic event should be thoroughly characterized, including which area of the head was struck, whether there was a loss of consciousness, how fast the patient was moving, whether there was a discharge (bloody or watery) from the nose or ears, and whether there was amnesia or incontinence. If, as in many cases, the patient is a vague or poor historian, eye witness reports or interviews with close family members can be valuable.

A general neurologic history must be obtained and should include history of preexisting cephalalgia, history of seizures in the patient or family, alcohol or other drug use, complaints of focal weakness, sensory change, gait difficulties, and bowel or bladder dysfunction. A complete and thorough history of the pain, its location, duration, quality, and exacerbating or relieving factors, should be obtained. A history of any previous injuries and the patient's prior work status are also important.

The physical exam should emphasize the head and neck, looking for carotid, orbital, or cranial bruits; asymmetry in carotid pulses; tenderness over the scalp, especially in areas of scarring; tenderness over sinuses; and trigger points in the face or neck. Cervical spasm and range of motion should be assessed. The temporomandibular joint areas should be examined carefully for pain, tenderness, and clicks. Finally, a full neurologic exam should be performed. If the head trauma has been recent, the patient's neck should not be rotated or flexed until cervical spine x-rays have been reviewed. In acute head trauma, it is important to check for drainage from the nose and ears, as well as for ecchymosis periorbitally or retroauricularly (Battle's sign), both of which are signs of basilar skull fractures.

Depending on clinical suspicion, diagnostic radiographic testing might include cervical spine films with flexion and extension views, skull films, sinus films, orbital views, and temporomandibular joint views. A computed tomography (CT) scan (at the time of unjury) and magnetic resonance imaging (MRI) of the head (at a later point in time) should probably be obtained in all cases with significant trauma. Although EEG abnormalities have been described acutely in post-traumatic cephalalgia, these abnormalities are frequently minimal, nonspecific, and they do not aid in diagnosis [11]. An EEG should be reserved for patients whose symptoms are of an episodic nature consistent with seizure activity (i.e., absence, paroxysmal behavior changes, syncope, episodic dizziness, or paroxysmal cephalalgia).

Neuropsychometric testing, including the Minnesota Multiphasic Personality Inventory (MMPI), the Wechsler Adult Intelligence Scale (WAIS), the

Wechsler Memory Scale, etc., can be helpful in evaluating cognitive disturbances in post-traumatic cephalalgia patients. Unfortunately, these tests can be inadequate, due to subjective variations related to patient performance and examiner interpretation. Recent reports of abnormal cognitive event-related potentials in post head trauma patients raise hopes that this modality may provide an objective neuropsychological parameter of dysfunction in these patients [12]. MRI, with its ability to detect small subtle lesions in the brain stem, as well as in cerebral hemispheres, may be of increasing help in elucidating mechanisms of cognitive impairment in patients with post-traumatic syndromes.

Treatment

Once diagnoses such as seizures, chronic subdural hematoma, hydrocephalus, and other structural lesions have been excluded, post-traumatic cephalalgia patients should be clearly informed as to the presumably organic but non-life-threatening nature of their illness. A clear understanding of deficits and likely mechanisms on the part of patients has, in our experience, been a positive predictive factor for good outcome. A positive outlook on the part of the treatment team is also important. A multidisciplinary approach seems to be essential, including, when appropriate, the services of physicians, psychologists, physical therapists, specially trained nurses, and social workers. Family members or caretakers must be included in interviews, especially when cognitive dysfunction accompanies post-traumatic cephalalgia.

Regulating sleeping and eating patterns, as well as structuring daily activities, is often helpful for patients. Regular exercise at least twice weekly is also consistently helpful. Psychiatric and/or psychological consultation can help to uncover emotional factors in a patient's pain syndrome, and can also help to address psychological disturbances ensuing from the traumatic injury or from the resulting pain. Formal ongoing psychotherapy can be valuable when indicated.

Cephalalgia of the tension-type can often be successfully treated prophylactically with a tricyclic antidepressant. Sedating tricyclics such as amitriptyline (Elavil, Endep), are most appropriately given in a single bedtime dose. The initial dose of amitriptyline is 10 mg, which should be increased slowly to 50 mg, with a maximum of 200 mg daily. More activating tricyclics, such as amoxapine (Asendin) or protriptyline (Vivactil) can be given in divided doses throughout the day. A starting dose of amoxapine is 25 mg b.i.d. with a maximum daily dose of 200 mg/day. Serious tricyclic antidepressant toxicities are rare and include cardiac arrhythmias, seizures, and urinary retention. Behavioral disturbances and even frank hallucinations have been observed, particularly in older individuals. More common side effects include morning grogginess, dry mouth, increased appetite, weight gain, and constipation.

The use of beta blockers, such as propranolol HCl (Inderal) or nadolol (Corgard), either alone or in combination with tricyclic antidepressants, can also be very effective prophylactically in post-traumatic cephalalgia, especially in those cases with vascular headache features. Nadolol should be started at 20 mg b.i.d., increasing as tolerated to a maximum dose of 120 mg b.i.d., monitoring blood pressure and pulse carefully. More recently, calcium channel blockers have been found to be useful in selected patients. Diltiazem (Cardizem), in a dose of 30 mg t.i.d., is a standard starting dose, with a daily maximum dosage of 180 mg in divided doses. Verapamil (Calan, Isoptin) is also used. For patients in whom cephalalgia is very typical of migraine, methysergide maleate (Sansert) can be used if other agents are ineffective. Cyproheptadine (Periactin) has been described as being particularly useful in children [13].

For patients with lancinating or burning pain suggestive of neuralgia, anticonvulsant medications, such as carbamazepine (Tegretol), phenytoin (Dilantin), and divalproate sodium (Depakote), can be effective. Baclofen (Lioresal) and clonazepam (Klonopin) have also been used with good results. Recently we have found mexiletine (Mexitil), an oral lidocaine analogue, to be useful in selected patients with neuralgic features.

Monoamine oxidase inhibitors, lithium, and phenothiazines all have been effective in occasional patients with intractable post-traumatic cephalalgia. Methylphenidate (Ritalin) has been useful in several post-trauma patients who have had intractable headache, as well as excessive daytime somnolence. Benzodiazepines can be of use in some post-traumatic cephalalgia patients, especially those in whom an anxiety disorder coexists with pain. However, due to the potential for physiological dependency and drowsiness, they should be avoided except under extraordinary circumstances.

For symptomatic relief of pain, nonsteroidal anti-inflammatory medications, such as ibuprofen (Advil, Motrin) or naproxen (Naprosyn), are fairly effective, although gastrointestinal irritation can limit their use. Agents with muscle relaxant properties can help symptomatically, especially in patients with clear muscle spasm. We have found methocarbamol (Robaxin) helpful. Occasionally severe exacerbations of pain require the use of narcotic analgesic medications, either orally or intramuscularly, but obviously this must be kept to a minimum because of potential risk of substance abuse.

Patients with focal musculoskeletal/mechanical discomfort may benefit from physical therapy modalities (massage, hot packs, hydrotherapy, ultrasound, etc.). Cervical mechanical factors may be alleviated, on occasion, with the use of soft cervical collars or specially designed pillows. Transcutaneous nerve stimulation has been helpful in a number of patients with localized pain syndromes. Other forms of local stimulation, such as "evaporative" creams, heating pads, and ice packs, have been effective as well. The addition of salicylates or anesthetics to topical creams is of questionable benefit.

In patients with tender areas subcutaneous trigger point injections can be dramatically effective, either for the relief of acute pain or as a series of injections for chronic pain. Sites often involved include cervical paraspinal areas, occipitocervical junction areas, and supraorbital and infraorbital regions. Often, exquisitely sensitive nodules can be palpated, possibly representing neuroma formation, which respond well to local injection. We have used short- and long-acting anesthetics with or without steroid preparations. Selective neurectomies, such as greater occipital neurectomy, can be of great help in cases where local nerve blocks have helped only transiently, but these patients must be selected very carefully as chronic somatoform issues can be exacerbated by these techniques.

Biofeedback can be a very useful therapeutic technique in post-traumatic cephalalgia, especially when muscle relaxation and stress reduction are prime goals. Both skin temperature and scalp muscle activity monitoring should be used. Relaxation techniques, self-hypnosis, and other meditative techniques are also helpful in some post-traumatic cephalalgia patients.

Conclusions

The potential mechanisms of post-traumatic cephalalgia are varied, and the pathophysiology of an individual's pain often represent a combination of factors. Cognitive dysfunction and psychological factors, such as anxiety and depression, can confound diagnosis and interfere with treatment. However, we believe that most patients have organic disease and, with appropriate aggressive therapy, they can be restored to productive and enjoyable living.

References

1. Coonley-Hoganson R, et al. Sequelae associated with head injuries in patients who are not hospitalized: A follow-up survey. *Neurosurg 14(3)*: 315-317, 1984.
2. Kelly RE. Post-traumatic headache. *Handbook of Clinical Neurology 4 48*: 383-389, 1985.
3. Zimmerman AW, et al. Traumatic vertebral basilar occlusive disease in childhood. *Neurology 18(2)*: 185-188, 1978.
4. Schoenen J, Jamart B, et al. Exteroceptive suppression of temporalis muscle activity in chronic headache. *Neurology 37*: 1834-1836, 1988.
5. Vijayan N, Dreyfus PM. Post-traumatic dysautonomic cephalalgia: Clinical observations and treatment. *Neurol 32*: 649-52, 1975.
6. Keshavan MS. Post-traumatic psychiatric disturbances: Patterns and predictors of outcome. *Br J Psychiat 138*: 157-160, 1981.
7. DeMol J. Personality disorders in head-injured adults. *Schweiz Arch Neurol Neurochir Psychiatr 129(1)*: 37-45, 1981.
8. Servadei F, et al. Epidemiology and sequelae of head injury in San Marino Republic. *Neurosurg Sci 29(4)*: 297-303, 1985.
9. Waddell PA. Sensitivity of light and sound following minor head injury. *Acta Neurol Scand 69(5)*: 270-276, 1984.
10. Hasimoto I. Hyperexcitable state of brainstem in children with post-traumatic vomiting as evidenced by brainstem auditory evoked potentials. *Neurol Res 6(1-2)*: 81-84, 1984.

11. Jacome DE. EEG features in post-traumatic syndrome. *Clin Electroencephalogr 15(44)*: 214-221, 1984.
12. Saper JR, Turkewitz LJ, et al. Abnormal P-300 in post concussion syndrome (abst). American Academy of Neurology, 40th meeting. *Neurology 38 (suppl 1):* 355, 1988.
13. Lanzi G, et al. Late post-traumatic headache in the pediatric age. *Cephalalgia 5(4)*: 211-215, 1985.

Copyright © 1993 PMA Publishing Corp.
Headache: A Clinician's Guide to Diagnosis, Pathophysiology, and Treatment Strategies
Edited by Alan M. Rapoport, M.D. and Fred D. Sheftell, M.D.

18

Drug-Induced Headache

Amos D. Korczyn

While most headaches are of the vascular or tension-type variety, the list of possible etiologies is almost endless. Among those causes, iatrogenic headaches are frequently overlooked. Most common among the iatrogenic headaches are those caused by drugs and these may be particularly problematic since they may present as exacerbations of pre-existing head pain. It is therefore important to recognize these diverse clinical entities.

This chapter will review the more common drug-induced headaches as well as some more unusual presentations. In addition to the clinical importance of recognition of headache induced by drugs, chemically induced headache may also be helpful in the elucidation of the pathophysiological mechanisms of headache in general and may even indicate novel approaches to headache therapy.

Vasodilator Headache

Even before nitroglycerin was used as a drug, workers in the explosives industry exposed to glyceryl trinitrate were known to develop headache [1]. Recognition of this syndrome was probably instrumental in understanding the relationship between vasodilation and the headache phase of migraine. With the growing number of drugs known to cause vasodilation or actually used for this purpose, several are reported to induce headache in some, but not all,

Table 18.1. Drugs Inducing Headaches

Vasodilator drugs
    Nitrates and nitrites [20]
    Histamine [7]
    Dipyridamole (Persantine) [21]

Vasoconstrictor drugs causing withdrawal headache
    Caffeine [22]
    Ergotamine

Drugs causing hypertension
    Monoamine oxidase inhibitors:
        Phenelzine sulfate (Nardil)
    Antihypertensives causing hypertension upon withdrawal:
        Clonidine HCl (Catapres) and Propranolol HCl (Inderal)
    Sympathomimetics:
        Amphetamine
        Methamphetamine [23]
        Phenylpropanolamine [24]

Drugs causing intracranial bleeding
    Anticoagulants
    Drugs acutely elevating blood pressure

Drugs causing benign intracranial hypertension
    Antibiotics (particularly tetracyclines) [24]
    Nalidixic acid (Negram) [25]
    Vitamin A [26]
    Corticosteroids [27]
    Thyroxine [28]
    Lithium [29]
    Phenytoin sodium (Dilantin) [30]

Drugs worsening pre-existing headache
    Estrogen administered cyclically
    Progesterone
    Danazol
    Alcohol
    Analgesics
    Ergotamines

patients (Table 18.1). What differentiates the people who will develop headache from those who will not is not yet known.

The headache induced by vasodilator drugs is frequently of a dull aching quality and often accompanied by a flushed face. However, it may also be throbbing in nature and occur either occipitally or bitemporally. These characteristics may be similar to those of a migraine attack, and the suggestion was made that migraineurs are particularly susceptible to vasodilator headache [22]. A direct examination of this problem is still lacking. Schnitker and Schnitker [2] have reported that administration of nitroglycerin is so specific that it can be used as an absolute test to confirm the diagnosis of migraine. In their series of 250 patients, there were apparently no false negatives. They have not reported the nitroglycerin effect in other types of headaches or in normal subjects. However, in one study, administration of therapeutic doses of nitroglycerin precipitated headache in 69% of patients with coronary artery disease, and, since this is higher than the frequency of migraine, non-migraineurs must also be susceptible [3].

The pathophysiology of nitroglycerin headaches is probably related to induction of vasodilation. Firstly, the time course of the disorder, extending for 20 minutes in most cases, is similar to the biological half-life of nitroglycerin. It is thus likely that the headache results from a direct effect of nitroglycerin itself, rather than from an effect of nitroglycerin triggering a migraine attack. Another relevant observation is that doses of nitroglycerin insufficient to cause headache by themselves will do so if a small dose of alcohol, a known vasodilator, is subsequently consumed [1]. Nitroglycerin causes an abrupt rise of intracranial pressure probably due to the vasodilatory effects on capacitance vessels [4].

An interesting aspect of nitroglycerin headache is the rapid development of tolerance to this phenomenon. First demonstrated among industrial workers, it probably occurs in the clinical setting too. The degree to which tolerance occurs in patients using other vasodilators is still unclear.

The headache induced by nitroglycerin is reportedly aborted by the vasoconstrictor ergotamine in 40% of patients [5]. However, this study was not controlled and the 40% figure is not much higher than the expected placebo response. Interestingly, propranolol HCl (Inderal), whose mechanism of action in migraine is unclear, is useless in the prophylaxis of nitroglycerin headache [3].

Histamine, which has been used for decades to induce gastric acid secretion, is a potent vasodilator. It has been known for many years that systemic injection of histamine can induce headache that is frequently pulsating in nature [6]. Of course, histamine injection leads to vasodilation and a drop in blood pressure. Interestingly, headache does not start immediately after the injection of histamine but only when the blood pressure is restored. Presumably, intracranial blood vessels are still dilated and relaxed, and the elevation of blood pressure towards its normal value leads to their passive stretching, thus causing pain [6]. Recently, it has been shown that patients with chronic headache are much more susceptible to develop histamine headache than are people without a history of headache [7]. Moreover, the type of pain produced differs in patients with tension-type headache and in those with migraine, being predominantly pressing in the former and pulsating in the latter. While there was considerable overlap between the groups, the differential susceptibility was clear. The explanation, however, is not straightforward. Either patients with specific types of chronic headache have different pharmacological responses to histamine, or histamine triggers off the type of headache to which these patients are predisposed. Obviously, these two possibilities have different implications as to the understanding of the pathogenesis of endogenous headache. It may even be that the mere existence of chronic headache of any type may induce a state in which histamine may trigger an attack.

Hypertension and Headache

The complex relationship between hypertension and headache has been reviewed [8]. As a general rule, mild-to-moderate hypertension is unlikely to cause headache, although this symptom is rather common in more severe cases and is part of the syndrome of malignant hypertension.

The pathogenesis of headache in malignant hypertension involves an increase of intracranial pressure (ICP). Abrupt elevation of the blood pressure may cause headache even if it does not reach the excessive levels of malignant hypertension, particularly if the rate of blood pressure elevation is high and if compensatory mechanisms cannot counterbalance the changes. Elevated ICP in hypertension may be due to either increase of intravascular blood volume when the autoregulation capacity is exceeded or to intraparenchymatous or subarachnoid hemorrhage.

Several drugs can induce severe elevation of blood pressure (Table 18.1). Also, withdrawal of antihypertensives could cause a rapid rise, particularly with abrupt withdrawal of clonidine HCl (Catapres) and beta adrenergic blockers. Clinically, the headache relating to hypertensive response to drugs is of an acute onset and the investigation should include monitoring of cardiovascular parameters. However, further neurological examinations, including brain computed tomography (CT) and spinal tap, should be considered for the demonstration (or exclusion) of intracranial bleeding.

Paradoxically, several antihypertensive drugs were reported to induce headache. The list includes most of the commonly used agents, such as diazoxide (Hyperstat IV, Proglycem), reserpine (vide infra), methyldopa (Aldomet), prazosin HCl (Minipress), hydralazine HCl (Apresoline), and beta adrenergic blockers [9]. The mechanism has not been investigated but may be related to the vasodilatory effects of these drugs. The headache induced by propranolol HCl (Inderal) and metoprolol tartrate (Lopressor) is particularly troublesome, since these drugs are commonly used to prevent headache. Kuritzky and colleagues have shown that almost one third of migraineurs report exacerbation of headache by propranolol [10].

Intracranial Hypertension

The characteristic features of intracranial hypertension include headache that is posterior in location, occurring in the early morning hours, and frequently waking the patient from sleep. It may be accompanied by nausea and vomiting. However, many patients with elevated ICP do not develop headache (particularly if the pressure rises slowly) or have headache that is different from the classical description. This is particularly true if the cause of elevated ICP is a focal mass lesion, which itself causes displacement of pain-sensitive structures.

Drug-induced elevation of ICP has four major causes: benign intracranial hypertension (BIH), sagittal vein thrombosis, intracranial bleeding, and enhancement of tumor growth.

BENIGN INTRACRANIAL HYPERTENSION

Several drugs have been implicated in the production of this syndrome (see Table 18.1). Although it develops insidiously, symptoms may be abrupt in appearance. These often include headache, diplopia, and blurred vision, presumably depending upon the rate of rise of ICP. The diagnosis and treatment of BIH are discussed elsewhere [11].

SINUS VEIN THROMBOSIS

Thrombosis of major intracranial sinuses will elevate ICP since fluid egress from the cranial cavity is impaired. Several drugs known to promote coagulation and thrombosis have been implicated, particularly estrogens and glucocorticoids. The process is more rapid in its evolution than BIH and therefore its clinical manifestations, including headache, are more abrupt in onset.

INTRACRANIAL BLEEDING

Bleeding into the epidural, subdural, or subarachnoid spaces, or into the brain parenchyma itself may increase the content and pressure in the cranial cavity and thus cause stretching of pain-sensitive structures. Bleeding can result from the use of drugs causing elevation of blood pressure, in which case, bleeding will be into the brain itself or into its subarachnoid space. Bleeding also may be due to the administration of anticoagulants, in which case it occurs usually in the subdural or epidural space, but could be in the parenchyma of the brain.

ENHANCEMENT OF INTRACRANIAL TUMOR GROWTH

Some drugs may increase the size of intracranial tumors (primary or metastatic) and thus cause headache. It has been suggested that dopamine blockers, e.g. sulpiride, may induce the proliferation of prolactinomas. Metastases were thought to respond unfavorably to dacarbazine (DTIC-DOME) at least transiently, and in the case of cerebral metastases such a reaction may elevate ICP. The clinical features commonly include headache [12].

Drug Interacting with Aminergic Mechanisms

One theory of the pathophysiology of migraine is that acute attacks relate to release of platelet 5-HT [13]. Drugs blocking 5-HT uptake similarly will reduce platelet 5-HT and may increase circulating plasma levels of this amine. However, tricyclic antidepressants in general are not known to induce headache but rather to relieve pain. Some are used in pain conditions, including tension-type headache. A significant exception to this statement is zimelidine, a new antidepressant (not yet approved for general use in the United States) with 5-HT uptake blocking capacity but without antimuscarinic effects, which has been reported to induce headache [14,15]. The pathogenesis is obscure.

Ranitidine (Zantac), a relatively specific H_2 histamine receptor blocker, has been reported to induce headache in as many as 3% of patients exposed to it. The headache may be of a migrainous type, or it may lack specific characteristics [16]. It is unlikely that the headache results directly from blockade of histamine receptors since this side effect has not been reported following the more commonly used H_2 receptor blocker cimetidine (Tagamet).

Fenfluramine HCl (Pondimin) is an amphetamine derivative that is used as a hunger suppressant. Unlike its parent drug, it lacks stimulant and sympathomimetic effects and, at least in animals, its actions are antagonized by 5-HT blockers. It was reported that fenfluramine can induce headache attacks in chronic headache sufferers [17]. It is known that many headache sufferers will have an attack when fasting. However, in this study, there was no control for suppression of eating. Certainly, the role of 5-HT in this situation is complicated, as evidenced by the ameliorating effects of methysergide maleate (Sansert) and pizotifen in migraine. (Pizotifen is widely used in Europe but is not yet available in the United States.)

Reserpine has induced headache attacks in migraineurs following intramuscular administration; however, more prolonged therapy with this drug reduced the frequency of migraine headaches [18,19].

Oral Contraceptives

Oral contraceptives have been repeatedly observed to induce or exacerbate migraine. A review of the voluminous literature on this topic suggests that women with preexisting migraine are particularly susceptible, although this was never demonstrated in a prospective study. The relationship is far from simple, however. Attempts to correlate the prevalence of headache with the dose of either the estrogen or progesterone of the preparations have been unsuccessful; indeed, even pure progesterone contraceptives were reported to induce migraine. (It is possible that this side effect may depend on endogenous estrogens.) The onset of headache may be delayed for several months after the drugs are first taken. In particular, it should be recalled that these effects occur most severely between treatment cycles. This suggests that, like menstrual migraine, contraceptive-induced migraine is related to falling beta estradiol levels. In a similar fashion, menopausal women who take replacement estrogen cyclically often develop headaches after the medication is stopped each month. If progesterone is given five to ten days per month, headache may develop during administration.

Discussion

The approach to the patient with headache should obviously include consideration of the issues discussed. There is no reason to assume that the listing of drugs in this chapter is exhaustive. The physician should always be on the lookout for medication side effects, including headache.

Several factors complicate the identification of drugs as precipitating causes of headache. First, headache is a common symptom that is often not evaluated by the physician. Therefore, it is likely that many patients with drug-induced headache will never mention the symptom unless it is severe or associated with unusual characteristics. Even if mentioned, it will be difficult for the physician to decide whether this symptom is drug-induced or due to other, much more frequent, causes of headache. In clinical trials headache is often reported to be due to the new drug tested, but eventual analysis shows it to be as common during placebo periods. A second problem relates to the difficulty of differentiating drug-induced headache from disease-related headache. Many diseases commonly cause headache, either as an integral part (e.g., in pyrexic individuals) or as a consequence of anxiety and depression. The problem is highlighted by the case of ergotamine-induced headache that took long to be recognized, since this drug is prescribed for people who have headache in the first place.

In general, establishment of headache as drug related requires its disappearance following withdrawal and reappearance upon rechallenge, although the decision as to whether the patient should be exposed again to the suspected drug should be made on an individual basis.

References

1. Ebright GE. The effects of nitroglycerin on those engaged in its manufacture. *JAMA 62*: 201-202, 1914.
2. Schnitker MT, Schnitker MA. A clinical test for migraine. *JAMA 135*: 89, 1947.
3. Horwitz LD, Herman MV, Gorlin R. Clinical response to nitroglycerin as a diagnostic test for coronary artery disease. *Am J Cardiol 29*: 149-153, 1972.
4. Dohi S, Matsumoto M, Takahashi T. The effect of nitroglycerin on cerebrospinal fluid pressure in awake and anesthetized humans. *Anesthesiology 54*: 511-514, 1981.
5. Schwartz AM. The cause of relief and prevention of headaches caused from contact with dynamite. *N Engl J Med 235*: 541-544, 1946.
6. Pickering GW. Observations on the mechanism of headache produced by histamine. *Clin Sci 1*: 77, 1933.
7. Krabbe AA, Olesen J. Headache provocation by continuous intravenous infusion of histamine: Clinical results and receptor mechanisms. *Pain 8*: 253-259, 1980.
8. Korczyn AD. Headache and hypertension. *Practical Cardiol 6*: 113-117, 1980.
9. Gilbert GJ. Neurological complications of cardiovascular medication. In: Silverstein A, (ed). *Neurological Complications of Therapy*, pp 35-36. New York, Futura, 1982.
10. Kuritzky A. Ziegler DK, Hassanein R, et al. Relation between plasma concentration of propranolol, beta blocking and migraine. In: Rose FC, (ed). *Migraine*, pp 250-255. Basel, Karger, 1985.
11. Weisberg LA. Benign intracranial hypertension. *Medicine 54*: 197-207, 1975.

12. Hafstrom L, Per-Ebbe J. Symptoms of occult brain metastases initiated by systemic dacarbazine (DTIC-DOME) therapy in melanoma patients. *Clin Oncol 6*: 343-348, 1980.
13. Dvilansky A, Rishpon S, Nathan I, et al. Release of platelet 5-hydroxytryptamine by serum taken from patients during and between migraine attacks. *Pain 2*: 315-319, 1976.
14. Sommerville JM, McLaren EH, Campbell LM, et al. Severe headache and disturbed liver function during treatment with zimelidine. *Br Med J 285*: 1009, 1982.
15. Clarke IM. Severe headache and disturbed liver function during treatment with zimelidine. *Br Med J 285*: 1425, 1982.
16. Epstein CM, Klopper J. Ranitidine headache. *Headache 225*: 392-393, 1985.
17. Sicuteri F. Dell-Bene E, Anselmi B. Fenfluramine headache. *Headache 16*: 185-188, 1976.
18. Curzon G, Barrie M, Wilkinson BM. Relationship between headache and amine changes after administration of reserpine to migrainous patients. *J Neurol Neurosurg Psychiat 32*: 555-561, 1969.
19. Nattero G, Lisino F, Brandi G. Reserpine for migraine prophylaxis. *Headache 15*: 279-281, 1976.
20. Raskin NH. Chemical headaches. *Ann Rev Med 32*: 63-71, 1981.
21. Hawkes CH. Dipyridamole in migraine. *Lancet 2*: 153, 1978.
22. Anonymous. Headaches and coffee. *Br Med J 2*: 284, 1977.
23. Yarnell PR, Speed W. Headache and hematoma. *Headache 17*: 69-70, 1977.
24. Chadwick D. Antibiotics and benign intracranial hypertension. *J Antimicrob Chemother 9*: 88-90, 1982.
25. Gedroyc W, Shorvon SD. Acute intracranial hypertension and nalidixic acid therapy. *Neurology 32*: 212-215, 1982.
26. Spector RH, Carlisle J. Pseudotumor cerebri caused by a synthetic vitamin A preparation. *Neurology 34*: 1509-1511, 1984.
27. Fardal RW. Pseudotumor cerebri following steroid injections. *Hawaii Med J 41*: 414, 1982.
28. Van Dop C, Conte FA, Koch TK, et al. Pseudotumor cerebri associated with initiation of levothyroxine therapy for juvenile hypothyroidism. *N Eng J Med 308*: 1076-1080, 1983.
29. Saul RF, Hamburger HA, Selhorst JB. Pseudotumor cerebri secondary to lithium carbonate. *JAMA 253*: 2869-2870, 1985.
30. Kalanie H. Niakan E, Harati Y, et al. Phenytoin-induced benign intracranial hypertension (letter). *Neurology 36*: 443, 1986.

19

Behavioral Medicine Approach to Headache

Randall E. Weeks

Headache treatment has become more complex as clinical research has confirmed the interplay of biological, physiological, psychological, and environmental factors in the development, escalation, and maintenance of headache. Comprehensive, multidisciplinary treatment programs have emerged that adequately address the diverse factors that have been shown to affect the clinical picture of headache sufferers. This chapter offers a description of such an integrated approach by describing the contribution made by the Behavioral Medicine program at the New England Institute for Behavioral Medicine to the overall treatment program at The New England Center For Headache. The thrust of the chapter is clinical in nature with references offered only where appropriate to direct the reader to sources for amplification and/or clarification of subject matter.

Overview

The field of behavioral medicine has received widespread recognition since 1976, with the term specifically defined at the Yale Conference on Behavioral Medicine in 1977. It was concluded, "Behavioral Medicine is the field concerned with the development of behavioral science knowledge and techniques relevant to the understanding of physical health and illness and the application of this knowledge and techniques to prevention, diagnosis, treatment, and rehabilitation..." [1]. The prevalence of headache in the general population (approximately 40 million Americans experience chronic headache), and the fact that over 90% of headache complaints are not the result of underlying structural deficits, have made the study and treatment of headache an important arena for behavioral medicine specialists. With increased awareness of the impact that environmental and psychological factors can play in headache as well as the development of viable non-drug treatments for headaches, more emphasis has been placed on the multidisciplinary team approach in headache treatment.

Over the years, specialty clinics have been established solely for the treatment of headache. Most offer treatment options beyond just medication. Depending on philosophy, orientation has ranged from treatments consisting of medication, elimination diets, and on-site biofeedback training, to approaches where behavioral medicine is practiced as part of a multidisciplinary team approach. Such practitioners are involved in assessment, treatment planning, and the treatment implementation. What follows is the description of a program that is compatible with the latter model.

Assessment

Throughout their training, practitioners are taught that effective treatment is possible only after a proper diagnosis is made. This, in turn, can occur only after an appropriate initial assessment of the patient's history and status. Such an evaluation should include minimally a complete medical and headache history, a complete neurological examination, investigational testing when appropriate (e.g., EEG, evoked potentials, CT or MRI scan of the brain), and a psychophysiological evaluation. As the first three components are somewhat commonplace (and described elsewhere in this text), they will not be reviewed here. What follows is a description of the psychophysiological evaluation.

This part of the initial evaluation is done typically by a behavioral specialist (usually a psychologist or psychiatrist) with an in-depth knowledge of headache pathogenesis and treatment. The meeting with the patient usually lasts 60 to 90 minutes and takes place after the initial headache history has been taken, usually by one of our staff nurses. The first part of the session is devoted to reviewing the headache history that has been taken previously. A significant number of patients will modify some of the information that was obtained in the initial history (apparently independent of the previous interviewer's skills). Through this review, the history can be clarified and, hopefully, made more valid.

A second goal of the session is to assess the extent to which psychological issues such as depression and/or anxiety may be a part of the headache picture. One approach is through behavioral assessment, e.g., noting markers for depression such as decreased energy, presence of initial, middle, and/or terminal insomnia, decreased libido, etc., and indices of anxiety such as rapid heart rate, bruxism, cervical tightness, etc. A second strategy is to elicit self-report data with respect to the patient's view about his/her mood state. It is important to assess whether any acknowledged affective problem might be primary or secondary to the pain experience. Perceptions regarding possible causes for headache (e.g., are headaches related to stress?) and perceptions of significant others regarding the patient's headaches are solicited. When appropriate, interviews with significant others take place.

Patients are required to have completed a battery of self-administered psychological tests prior to this interview. These typically include the Minnesota Multiphasic Personality Inventory, a depression inventory (e.g., Beck, Zung, or Lubin), and the Holmes Life Change Index. They offer a rather efficient assessment of overall personality status as well as an index of stress and adjustment issues. Interpretations of test results must take into account that chronic pain can affect performance on these scales and that issues of depression and/or anxiety can precede or be secondary to the pain [2]. Results are reviewed with the patient during this session.

Physiological data are gathered as the final part of the evaluation. Such an assessment may be structured in a variety of formats [3]. An adequate physiological profile would include either a structured assessment utilizing muscle scanning or multisite electromyographic (EMG) readings and photoplethysmographic measures of vascular lability [4]. With the latter assessment, data are gathered across conditions of Baseline ("sit comfortably"), Relaxation ("just relax in whatever way works best for you"), Stress (e.g., mental arithmetic, free association, headache imagery), and Recovery ("just relax again"). External stressors (e.g., cold pressor, noise) may also be added. Results are presented to the patient with respect to the absolute magnitude of the responses as well as relative changes across conditions.

Such data help to clarify the muscular and vascular involvement in the pain experience and assist in the confirmation of diagnosis. Though these data are believed to be indicative of hypothesized underlying physiological mechanisms, they do not always confirm the tentative diagnosis from the headache history. For example, patients with supposed muscular headaches do not always manifest high levels of muscular tension and/or a great deal of muscular reactivity. Similarly, migraine patients do not always demonstrate marked vascular lability during this assessment. Such inconsistency may be reflective of the complexity of the pain process (e.g., central versus peripheral mechanisms), the effects of immobilization (protective guarding) with respect to chronic pain, the effects that mood may have on physiological functioning, and limitations of the assessment itself (not sampling the appropriate physiological indices and their changes). The biofeedback literature offers a more complete analysis of these factors [5].

What is the value of these data? First, readings reflective of hypothesized underlying mechanisms (elevated or reactive EMG for patients with muscular headaches or vasospasm problems for migraine patients) allow the patient to understand current thinking regarding etiology of their pain and to raise questions regarding stress, life-style issues, etc. Biofeedback training would be an appropriate treatment consideration for such patients. Patients whose symptoms elicit a diagnosis of scalp muscle contraction headache (tension-type headache) but who have low EMG readings could be treated initially with antidepressants or referred to programs to increase muscular mobilization through exercise. Practically, however, some of these patients might be appropriate candidates for biofeedback and stress management training in order to develop better coping skills and a sense of self-competence. Involvement in a biofeedback program allows a forum in which affective issues can be assessed more fully and a psychotherapy referral made, if appropriate. Headache patients are somewhat resistant initially to any type of psychiatric interpretation of their pain. Often, they are only able to look at underlying psychological factors after developing a trusting relationship with the behavioral medicine specialist.

The data are also used in clinical research to understand better headache diagnoses with respect to physiological and emotional factors. Hopefully, studies of this type will help to clarify controversial issues in this area.

Results from the psychophysiological evaluation are summarized and reported back to the multidisciplinary team along with diagnostic impressions and treatment recommendations. When appropriate, the behavioral medicine specialist may attend (or lead) the summary conference during which the treatment program is presented to the patient.

Treatment

The purpose of the behavioral medicine program is to combine behavioral and medical treatments to provide a multifaceted, comprehensive treatment for headaches. The program's goals are: *Education* — teaching the patient current concepts regarding the causes and treatments of headaches; *Dietary and Behavioral Restriction* — altering certain life-style patterns that could cause headache; *Self-Regulation* — teaching the patient to control various physiological responses to abort and prevent headaches; *Cognitive Behavior Modification* — examining and changing certain actions, thoughts, attitudes, and expectations that could cause heightened levels of physiological arousal that might lead to headaches; and *Participation* — involving the patient as an active participant in the treatment program through education and acquisition of the skills mentioned previously. The program is built on the premise that it is important for the patient to take some responsibility for headache improvement rather than the professionals having total control and responsibility. It exists as a series of appointments following the initial evaluation. The absolute number of sessions is determined by the components required for effective treatment.

Education

This portion of the program includes a complete explanation of the pathophysiology of the different types of headaches. Genetic predispositions for headache, the physiology of stress, and the relationship between stress and headaches are other topics.

Information regarding different classes of headache medications, their therapeutic mechanisms of action, and potential side effects is presented. Rationale for the selection of abortive or prophylactic medications are explained.

Traditionally accepted myths regarding personality factors and headache are examined and exposed as unfounded. Questions about biofeedback are answered. The anticipated course of treatment is explained with respect to detoxification of medications and "time lags" before reaching therapeutic levels of daily medication.

Finally, patients are taught how to keep a headache calendar, which is brought to each treatment appointment. Such a calendar should include the intensity of the pain (mild, moderate-to-severe, incapacitating), the time of day the headache begins (morning, afternoon, evening, during sleep), the duration of the headache (minutes or hours), types and amounts of medication taken, degree or relief from the medication (no relief, slight relief, most pain gone, total relief), and any particular dietary or emotional factors that may have triggered the headache. If applicable, women should note their menstrual days. Though the calendar may sound complicated, formats have been established to record these data efficiently and easily.

Dietary and Behavioral Restrictions

When appropriate, patients are put on an elimination diet to limit foods that have been shown in the research literature to trigger headaches. The diet is reviewed and patients' questions are answered. Patients are advised that if they "slip" and eat one of the restricted foods, they should note this on the calendar. They are also requested to decrease their caffeine consumption, with an explanation as to why this is necessary.

Some medications need to be discontinued, and patients are given structure and/or support with regard to reduction schedules and discontinuation. Rationale for the elimination of frequent ergotamine and analgesic usage as it relates to rebound headaches is presented, with an explanation of the time period before the "washout effect" is complete. Patients need a great deal of support and education regarding these factors.

Sleep is also an important consideration in headache treatment. Patients are advised to get enough sleep but to avoid oversleeping. Changes is sleep patterns may precipitate headaches, so patients are advised to keep to their usual sleep patterns, even on weekends and vacations. Sleep problems (initial, middle, and/or terminal insomnia) are noted and treated either pharmacologically or behaviorally.

Self-Regulation

The first step in physiological self-regulation is to become more aware of body functioning. Subjective feelings of relaxation are no guarantee that the person has, in fact, changed inwardly. Only when patients can alter muscle tone and stabilize the vascular system are they regulating their physiology to help control headaches. The focus of the self-regulation program is to retrain the physiological system's responses to the environment in an attempt to compensate for biological predispositions that lead to headache.

Biofeedback facilitates the self-regulation process. Instrumentation provides immediate, objective information about the patient's physiological response systems that is "fed back" to the patient. The feedback may be visual, auditory, or both. This allows responses to be "shaped" in the most adaptive direction (e.g., decreased muscle tension and increased peripheral blood flow). Patients learn what must be done to achieve the desired responses and become aware of internal feelings that accurately reflect a relaxed system.

The biofeedback program is a series of skills acquisition steps that take place over several sessions. Each step must be mastered before moving to the next one. The steps of the program are as follows:

Step 1 – Body awareness/breathing exercises
Step 2 – Deep muscle exercise (progressive relaxation)
Step 3 – Passive relaxation/imagery exercises
Step 4 – Scalp and facial relaxation/shoulder and neck relaxation
Step 5 – Limb warmth/limb heaviness
Step 6 – Autogenic phrases/body scan

Audio cassettes are given to patients for each step. Patients are required to use these for home practice and are to fill out a debriefing log after each practice session. Data included are pre-tape and post-tape levels of tension and headache. In addition, body sensations of relaxation or difficulties in the relaxation process are noted. Patients are required to bring their debriefing logs to each biofeedback session in order to monitor progress and determine how often the patient is practicing. Home biofeedback monitors (e.g., thermal rings, portable EMG units) may be given to provide more specific data regarding progress in home practice.

Generalization strategies are discussed to encourage the patient to use the self-regulation strategies on an ongoing basis. Patients learn mini-exercises that are to be utilized throughout the day to heighten body awareness and reduce physiological arousal. Booster biofeedback sessions are held on an infrequent basis to ensure continued maintenance of acquired responses.

Cognitive Behavior Modification

This portion of the program is often referred to as the "stress management" aspect of treatment. Behavioral issues such as time management, over-scheduling, and the need for increased pleasurable activities are discussed. Indices of Type A Behavior are reviewed with attempts at modification [6].

A variety of cognitive styles have been shown to affect levels of stress. Maladaptive styles of thinking and irrational beliefs are believed to enhance and sustain high levels of arousal, anxiety, or depression [7,8]. Coping strategies are discussed to help dispute traditional styles of thinking that perpetuate stress [9].

An analysis of the patient's life is made to determine the degree of these maladaptive behavior patterns and thoughts as well as to discover particular areas of stress in the patient's life. Significant others may be interviewed at this point to provide additional input regarding the patient's status. Often, they present a different view of the patient's level of stress. All strategies are designed to promote more effective coping skills and facilitate acquisition of a more adaptive, pain-free life style.

References

1. Schwartz GE, Weiss AM. Yale conference on behavioral medicine: A proposed definition and statement of goals. *J Behav Med 1*: 3-14, 1978.
2. Weeks RE, Baskin S, Rapoport AM, et al. A comparison of MMPI personality data and frontalis electromyographic readings in migraine and combination headache patients. *Headache 23*: 75-82, 1983.
3. Boudewyns PA. Assessment of headache. In: Keefe FJ, Blumenthal JA. *Assessment Strategies in Behavioral Medicine*, pp 67-180. New York, Grune & Stratton, 1982.
4. Cram JR. *Clinical EMG: Muscle Scanning and Diagnostic Manual for Surface Recordings*. Seattle, Clinical Resources, 1986.
5. Schwartz MS. Headache: Selected issues and considerations in biofeedback evaluations and therapies. In: MS Schwartz & Assoc, (eds). *Biofeedback: A Practitioner's Guide*, pp 263-287. New York. Guilford Press, 1987.
6. Friedman M, Ulmer D. *Treating Type A Behavior and Your Heart*. New York, Knopf, 1984.
7. Beck AT. *Cognitive Therapy and the Emotional Disorders*. New York, International Universities Press, 1976.
8. Ellis A, Grieger R. *RET: Handbook of Rational-Emotive Therapy*. New York, Springer Publishing Co, 1977.
9. Meichenbaum D. *Cognitive Behavior Modification*. Morristown, NJ, General Learning Press, 1974.

20

Psychological Considerations in Evaluation and Treatment of Headache Disorders

Fred D. Sheftell

Introduction

Much remains to be learned about the nature, etiology, and pathophysiology of primary headache disorders. Research over the past ten years has continued to demonstrate the importance of physiological and neurochemical mechanisms in their pathogenesis. Central neurotransmitters such as biogenic amines (catecholamines and indolamines) and peptides (endorphins and enkephalins), which appear to play important roles in headache disorders, are also known to play central roles in determining mood and behavior. Theoretically, these mechanisms begin to provide a biological link between head pain and psychological symptomatology. We have seen that a large percentage of patients who present with chronic pain of any type, including headache, demonstrate symptoms of depression. Conversely, large percentage of patients with depression also present with complaints of pain of various types. The connections here may not just be on a psychodynamic level but may well be explained on a biological basis. While psychological factors alone may be a causative element in only the minority of primary headache disorders, they do play contributory roles to a varying extent in the majority of chronic headache disorders. Headache sufferers, for the most part, have been maligned by a society that gives them the message that their headache represents some type of psychological weakness and their physical symptoms are not to be taken seriously. Headache disorders tend to present on a broad continuum. On one end are disorders that are exclusively psychological in nature, such as delusional disorders of the somatic type, and on the other end of the continuum we see psychological difficulties and symptoms resulting *from* chronic headache problems. Our experience and observations at The New England Center for Headache have led us to the view that we may be dealing with a group of psychophysiological disorders. A physiological disorder does exist (migraine, tension-type headache, cluster headache, etc) where psychological factors play a role, though not necessarily etiological in its expression. It would appear that some individuals possess a genetic, neurochemical, or neurophysiological predisposition to these disorders. Their expression may then depend on a host of factors, including personality and environmental factors related to the individual's ability to adapt successfully to his environment. Like other psychophysiological models, high vulnerability may lead to marked symptomatology, and low vulnerability may require greater stress or maladaptive responses to give rise to symptomatology.

Historically, it was Adolph Meyer in the early part of the century who spoke of the term "psychobiology", viewing brain, body, and behavior as a continuum. He attempted to connect the relationship between external influences in a person's life to internal processes such as those described in C. Bernard's Inner Environment and Canon's Homeostasis. Other researchers, including Horsley Gant and Pavlov, contributed information that provided links among psychology, biology, learning, conditioning, and behavior. This work paralleled Hans Selye's theories of the effects of stress, self-regulation, and visceral conditioning. Franz Alexander and colleagues also looked at mechanisms that linked mind and body.

An understanding of primary headache disorders that incorporates psychophysiological principles might then view any stimulus threatening to the organism as capable of producing an arousal pattern that is probably genetically determined. For example, some people respond to various threatening stimuli with cardiovascular symptoms while others may respond with gastrointestinal complaints. Prolonged arousal patterns may then give rise to tissue breakdown and disease in genetically predisposed individuals. Again, those with high genetic vulnerability may respond to the normal stresses and strains inherent in daily living with a somatic disorder and may not, by definition, have deep seated psychological conflicts. Others who have lower degrees of organ vulnerability would require greater stress or maladaptive responses for symptomatology to appear.

In summary, our current understanding views primary headache disorders as those involving complex central and peripheral mechanisms that can be influenced by a number of factors not limited to, but including psychological factors. Psychological causation of primary headache disorders as a single factor exists in only the minority of patients seen. Nevertheless, psychological factors are important and often play contributory roles in these disorders.

Relationships Between Primary Headache Disorders and Psychological Factors

Much has been written about the migraine personality; the relationship among chronic tension-type headache, posttraumatic headache, and depression; the relationship among cluster headache, cyclical mood disorders, and certain personality features.

MIGRAINE

The migraine personality, as initially described by Wolff, is characterized as rigid, perfectionist, controlled, orderly, tense, meticulous, and ambitious. It has been stated that these patients are fearful of making mistakes, are overly conscientious, and in need of approval from their environment. Psychoanalytical studies by Freda Fromm-Reichmann and Selinski indicated that migraine patients come from family backgrounds that are demanding, insistent, and emphasize high standards of performance and attainment. Their observations further reveal that these families have rigid standards of behavior and tend to punish the expression of any strong feelings whether they are aggressive or expressive. This environment resulted in a child with diminished self esteem and feelings of inadequacy. These children tend to develop extremely high expectations of themselves and others that are difficult to live up to. As children, they tended to try and please and have a markedly exaggerated sense of responsibility. They are not able to express negative feelings towards loved ones and through defense mechanisms of repression, denial, and reaction formation can not admit to these feelings. These patients will often portray their families in an idealistic manner and denial is often seen. Ultimately, these patients tend to compensate for their feelings of inadequacy by working hard and performing incessantly in an effort to prove their worth. Their observations of migraine patients brought them to the conclusion that migraine is an expression of repressed hostility toward loved ones. They believed that migraine attacks would occur in lieu of and as an indirect expression of the patient's anger. The patient can then express denied dependency needs in the only manner acceptable to them via the expression of physical symptoms. The families of these patients are better able to accept the expression of illness rather than of rage or anger.

We often ask the migraine patients at our Center to describe a typical day. We usually hear about busy and demanding schedules replete with obligations and responsibilities to others and little or no time for themselves. At the same time, these patients often tend not to view their lives as being stressful. In fact, a study conducted in 1980 by Price and Blackwell showed that migraineurs tended to minimize the severity of the situation viewed by normal controls as stressful. If they were better able to respond verbally or behaviorally to such stimuli, perhaps their physiological responses would be less. Many migraine patients will describe long hours, few, if any, vacations, and no time for recreation and rest. Many will have little or no sense of their own limitations as human beings and do not see themselves as overextended. They may view the admission of limitations, inherent in the human condition, as a weakness or defeat. Wolff saw migraine as a sort of "biological reprimand" at times for this type of frenetic activity and behavior. Patients may state that this pace is impossible to change because of the reality of the demands placed on them by their environment. They have minimal insight in terms of extraordinarily high demands that they continue to place upon themselves.

Though this constellation of behavioral patterns and psychodynamics is indeed seen among migraine patients, they are certainly not seen consistently in all migraine patients. There are many migraineurs who are certainly not obsessive-compulsive and of course there are many without migraine who demonstrate this rigid obsessive style. Crisp's studies in the late 1970's did not demonstrate consistency in obsessive-compulsive characteristics in migraine patients and other studies did not show marked personality differences between migraine and non-migraine controls. Thus, no cause and effect can be scientifically proposed on the basis of psychodynamics, personality, and behavior alone. This is not to say that in patients predisposed to migraine that such an orientation and style cannot or does not provoke attacks.

Oliver Sachs, in his book on migraine, proposed a creative way of classifying migraine according to factors that involved its provocation. He speaks of circumstantial migraine, those attacks related to specific circumstances. These "circumstances" may range from physiological to emotional. Provoking elements may include weather, let-down periods, foods, hormones, and many others. He states, however, that violent emotions exceed all other acute circumstances in their capacity to provoke migraine reactions. Rage, fright and elation are cited specifically.

Considering these factors, it is useful in the course of an evaluation, including a psychological one, to gather information related to possible provocateurs of attacks, be they physiological or emotional. Information related to the patient's and family's behavior during these attacks may also be relevant. For example, this may help to shed light on possible contributory emotional factors and issues of secondary gain often denied consciously by migraine patients. Some patients, because of psychological factors, may tend to receive a good deal of secondary gain as a result of "sick" behavior. This behavior may be positively reinforced by frequent prescriptions for analgesics, emergency room visits, admissions to hospitals, and an excessively over-protective attitude from the spouse and family. When this leads to avoidance reactions such as missing work, quitting work, and avoiding responsibilities, psychological and medical intervention become crucial. This is seen only in the minority of patients with migraine headache.

TENSION-TYPE HEADACHES

Tension-type headache, particularly the chronic variety, is generally viewed as a separate category from migraine. There are those who view tension-type and vascular headaches on a continuum, with the lines, save in classical or complicated migraine, not so clearly drawn. There are a significant number of patients with episodic migraine whose headaches evolve over the years into a daily or near daily occurrence. This particular group of patients has been referred to, by Mathew, as evolutive migraine.

The most common type of presenting problem to headache centers are the mixed headache disorders. From a psychiatric point of view, the dynamics and behavioral patterns among tension-type headache patients and migraine patients tend to demonstrate many similarities. Some authors have reported less elevation of neurotic and other traits as indicated on the Minnesota Multiphasic Personality Inventory, in 'pure migraine" patients as compared to those with chronic tension-type headache or mixed headache disorders.

Many researchers, including Blumer, Diamond, Lance, Dalessio, Lesse, Ziegler, and Engel, have explored the relationship between chronic head pain and depression. For example, some view the responsiveness of these headache disorders to tricyclic antidepressants and MAO inhibitors as evidence that this disorder is a "masked" or somatic depression. Blumer found that these patients presenting with chronic head pain showed a super normal picture and denied interpersonal and emotional difficulties. Pain is the only difficulty they would admit to; denial and repression was prominent. Like migraineurs, these patients with chronic headaches tended to idealize family relationships and had difficulty expressing anger, rage, and dependence. They tended to reject psychiatric intervention, seen as a manifestation of denial. Studies by Rosenbaum demonstrated that it would be more the patient's fear of being viewed as having psychological and not physical problems that motivated them to deny psychological issues. Freidman, in his study of tension headache patients in 1954, found that emotional factors were contributory in all patients, though only 72% of patients agreed. Again, the most central problems were related to the attempt to control anger toward family members. His studies also reported conflicts surrounding dependency, secondary gain, and attention. Kolb's observations in 1963 were similar.

In summary, psychological investigations in the area of both migraine and tension-type headaches appear to reveal similar, if not identical psychodynamic issues. In these headache disorders, where psychological issues play a major contributory role, the dynamics alone do not enable us to separate the disorders. In fact, similar core dynamics of dependency, repressed hostility, rigidity, anxiety, perfectionism, and high expectations appear to be present in all of these disorders targeting end organs of the autonomic nervous system and inducing such disorders as ulcer, asthma, etc. These dynamics are also present in more clear-cut psychiatric disturbances such as phobias, depression, and panic attacks. There certainly is no one psychiatric diagnosis associated with any given headache disorder. Once more, we may be dealing with genetic substrates of organ vulnerability to account for the differences in disease presentation. Many of these behavioral patterns seen in patients with migraine and/or tension-type headaches are similar to those seen in Meyer Friedman's description and concept of the "Type A" personality. He described a type of behavior that leads to a stressful life style and affects biological systems adversely. Type A personalities tend to seek out hectic environments and overreact to insignificant events. They tend to be overtly insecure, have exceedingly high expectations of themselves, and have the need to succeed, win, and dominate. The demands that they have on their own performance can ultimately lead to self-destructive behavior affecting the health and quality of their life.

Weeks, in his overview examining psychological factors in migraine and tension-type headache, had two interpretations of the previously existing data. First, there was great variability in methodological rigor at the core of these studies. Results ranged from a researcher's impression of case studies and/or histories, to information obtained from questionnaires and self-report forms, to control studies utilizing psychometric testing. Hence, he felt no generalizations could be made. Secondly, it became apparent that the data were nearly equivocal in almost every personality dimension examined. He felt that this was related to the design differences and to the lack of specification in many of the studies as to criteria for headache diagnosis. The lack of controls and the small number of subjects in many of these studies may have accounted for some contradictory results.

Cluster Headache

Psychological contributory factors in episodic and chronic cluster headache have not been studied as extensively as those in migraine and tension-type headache. Most researchers have not seen psychological factors as contributing to the mechanisms of cluster headache. There do appear to be a number of personality and physical factors that cluster patients share. They tend to present as active, energetic, social, affable, and very much a "man's man." They tend to smoke heavily, enjoy alcohol and drink to excess at times, and enjoy "macho" activities. Interestingly, they tend to be highly dependent on their spouses. Indeed, it is this headache group, more than others, where the spouse makes the appointment for the consultation visit and takes copious notes during the discussion. Graham portrays the dynamics between the couple as a large roaring lion being pulled in a tiny wagon by a little mouse. He suggested that cluster patients have difficulty meeting their commitments and in the attempt to do so, they go into cluster. He described the cluster male as basically timid, with strong hysterical traits and dependency needs, and yet, a need to appear manly.

Friedman described a cluster group as ambitious, efficient, overly conscientious, perfectionist, and prone to compulsive behavior. Kudrow, in his studies, found that patients with cluster headache differ little from non-headache controls. These findings were obviously in opposition to those described above. Non-pharmacological techniques, in particular psychotherapy, have offered no promising results in cluster headache. We do see a preponderance of attacks during let down periods, such as sleep time, during naps, in the evening after returning home from the job and following exercise. We have seen a number of our patients begin a series of cluster headaches following a hectic or intense period of time. Finally, some have considered cluster periods to be a type of "autonomic variant" of bipolar disease secondary to their responsiveness to lithium carbonate treatment.

Implications for Evaluation

With these psychological and psycho-physiological factors in mind, a number of implications are suggested for evaluation and treatment. A variety of tests have been found to be useful in evaluating psychological and behavioral styles. The Minnesota Multiphasic Personality Inventory (MMPI) is used at a number of headache centers during the course of an evaluation. The MMPI must be viewed within the context of the patient's disorder and presenting symptoms. For example, some research has shown enormous variability in MMPI scores in patients with intermittent and discreet attacks of migraine who have significant pain free intervals. In fact, these scores appear to be no different from those that may be seen in the general population. There is more consistency in MMPI results when one begins to look at patients who have either chronic tension-type headache or mixed headache disorders when chronicity of the pain becomes an important factor. In fact, this may be why these patients tend to show more evidence of depression on the MMPI.

Other psychometric tests that have been used rather extensively in headache work are Beck's depression inventory and the Zung self-rating depression scale. There are a variety of other tests that measure anxiety, life changes, type A behavior, marital adjustment, etc. and may be useful, depending upon the clinical presentation. A clinical evaluation from a psychological viewpoint may help to understand better the role of pain in the patient's life. One would want to examine carefully levels of premorbid adjustment in terms of what the patient was like before the onset of head pain. Patients who demonstrate profound changes from premorbid functional levels are more likely to demonstrate psychological factors as an important contributor to the clinical picture than those with minimal or no changes.

Issues of secondary gain are assessed. Both nuclear and extended family history is evaluated, including the nature and quality of relationships with significant others. History of alcoholism, drug abuse, behavioral problems, or depression in a patient or family is assessed. Were physical symptoms an attention-getting form of behavior? Did the patient learn to communicate feelings via physical symptomatology? This portion of the overall evaluation does not necessarily have to be performed by a psychologist or psychiatrist. Certainly, the nonpsychiatrist physician can begin to get some sense of what, if any, psychological factors might be involved. Again, it should not be assumed that psychological factors are causative because the work up is negative.

Primary Headache Disorders And Their Relationship To Psychiatric Disorders

As stated, some patients with primary headache disorders may also present with virtually any psychiatric disorder. There are several psychiatric disorders listed in the DSM IIIR in which headache may be an accompanying symptom.

Probably the most common DSM IIIR psychiatric diagnosis seen among the headache population is that of Psychological Factors Affecting Physical Condition. In previous diagnostic manuals, these were classified as psychophysiological disorders. DSM IIIR states that this diagnosis may be made when psychologically meaningful environmental stimuli are temporally related to the initiation or exacerbation of a specific physical condition or disorder. The physical condition involves either demonstrable organic pathology or a known pathophysiological process. Finally, the condition does not meet the criteria for somatoform disorders. Certainly migraine headaches would fall under this category.

Other psychiatric diagnoses where psychological factors alone may play the predominant role include: (1) Somatoform disorders in which severe and prolonged pain is the predominant disturbance. There is no demonstrable organic pathology or pathophysiological mechanism identified after thorough evaluation. Pain is in excess of findings and psychosocial factors are thought to be etiologically involved. Pain allows the patient to avoid activities noxious to them and dependency needs are gratified. Hypochondriasis is the unrealistic and abnormal interpretation of normal physical sensations. This leads to a preoccupation with the fear of serious disease. Physical findings are absent and fears persist despite reassurance, causing impairment in function. (2) Major depression, either single episode or recurrent symptoms here include a depressed, sad, or hopeless mood that is prominent and persistent. Four of the following will be seen almost daily for at least two weeks: changes in appetite or weight, psychomotor agitation or retardation, loss of interest, anhedonia, decreased libido, loss of energy, fatigue, feelings of worthlessness, self reproach, excessive guilt and recurrent thoughts of death or suicide ideation or attempts.

(3) Dysthymic disorder — similar to a major depressive disorder but ongoing for two years and not as intense. (4) Adjustment disorder — this is defined as a maladaptive reaction to an identifiable stressor occurring within three months of the onset of the stressor. Maladaptive responses might be impairment in functioning. (5) Delusional disorder - somatic type. Here the predominant theme of the delusion is that the person has some physical defect, disorder, or disease. Headache patients presenting with delusional disorders will describe their head pain and its cause in a very bizarre fashion. (6) Malingering - this is defined as the conscious production and presentation of false or exaggerated symptoms in pursuit of a goal that is recognizable. This may need to be considered, particularly in cases of post head trauma syndrome or post traumatic headache especially where litigation is involved.

Finally, a non DSM IIIR term often used to describe certain headache patients with marked psychological impairment is conversion cephalgia. The term is derived from conversion hysteria and is characterized by constant, severe, nonthrobbing pain with no temporal pattern. Patients will state that their pain is always severe and incapacitating. They describe their pain with classical "La Belle Indifference" manifested by an indifferent affect. Tranquilizers and analgesics are often abused and the patient is dysfunctional in all areas of living.

Implications for Treatment

A review of these psychological aspects provides a number of implications for treatment. It would appear from our work as well as others that headache patients are generally resistant to the idea of psychotherapy. Psychoanalysts might view this as a manifestation of denial or emotional problems in somatically oriented or fixated patients. Some patients will view the physician's suggestions that the patient pursue psychotherapy as evidence that the doctor does not believe the patient's pain to be real. Indeed, psychotherapy is often suggested as a result of physician's sense of frustration at the patient's lack of response to treatment. Referral for psychotherapy should not be made simply on the basis of exclusion of organic etiology. Ziegler has stated that it's certainly not to be assumed that severe headaches that are intractable to certain treatments are evidence of deep seated psychiatric disturbance. Sometimes intractability may be simply a matter of the physician's limitations in regard to headache diagnosis and treatment. If there is evidence of emotional disturbance, contributing to, accompanying, or resulting from the headache disorder, the referral should be positioned as an adjunct to treatment and thereby not convey the message that a psychotherapy referral represents a discontinuation of medical treatment. The referral should not imply that the psychiatrist is the last and only hope of recovery.

There are a number of types of psychotherapy. Headache patients, as a rule, tend to be more accepting of behavioral treatments including biofeedback, cognitive-oriented psychotherapy, and supportive psychotherapy. The non-psychiatric physician should not underestimate his or her ability to provide a measure of supportive psychotherapy for headache. As Karasu has stated, the therapist's primary role may be along the lines of gradually assisting the patient in recognizing connections between life events and symptomatology. Supportive psychotherapy incorporates a number of techniques. Simple reassurance in terms of explanation and education of headache mechanisms when known can be very beneficial. Allowing the patient to verbalize sources of stress in his environment may be helpful as well. This can be followed by advice or suggestions of more constructive ways of dealing with the environment and reducing stressful factors. As stated before, many patients do not see how over-extended they are, and simply pointing this out may be useful.

We believe that a behavioral orientation is important in many of these patients as these approaches emphasize the responsibility of the individual in participating in remediation of his problems. It assists the patient in helping himself and shifts the locus of control from an external source to an internal one, thus involving the patient in sharing responsibility for his treatment. Techniques may be self-monitoring of symptoms and medication intake, logging of provocateurs of symptoms, stress management, and relaxation techniques. Family or conjoint therapy certainly may be useful when marital problems or family problems predominate or play an integral part in the symptoms, as may exist with children. Finally, group psychotherapy may be useful, particularly from a supportive point of view, in patients who have chronic intractable head pain.

Conclusion

If we embrace Adolph Meyer's concept of psychobiology, then headache represents a psychobiological disorder. Body, brain, and mind remain inseparable and intertwined. Primary headache disorders are indeed multi-determined. Important interplays among genetics, learning, and environment are involved. An open and flexible approach in evaluation that ideally could involve several disciplines appears to offer the most promising results. Psychological factors should be viewed as contributory but not necessarily central in these disorders.

Bibliography

Blumer D, Heilbrohnn M. The pain prone disorder: a clinical and psychological profile. *Psychosomatics* 22:395-402, 1981.

Blumer D, Heilbrohnn M Chronic muscle contraction headache and the pain-prone disorder. *Headache* 22:180-183, 1982.

Dalessio DJ. Some reflections on the etiologic role of depression in head pain. *Headache* 8:28-31, 1968.

Davis O, Weiss JMA. Malingering and associated syndromes, in: *American Handbook of Psychiatry*, pp. 270-287. New York, Basic Books, 1974.

Diagnostic and Statistical Manual of Mental Disorders, ed 3. The American Psychiatric Association, 1987.

Diamond S. Depressive headaches. *Headache 4:*255-259, 1969.

Engle A. Psychogenic pain and the pain prone patient. *Am J Med 26:*899-918, 1959.

Friedman AP (guest editor). *Medical Clinics of North America. Symposium on Headache and Related Pain Syndromes.* Philadelphia, WB Saunders, 1978.

Hendler N. *Diagnosis and Non Surgical Management of Chronic Pain.*, pp. 12-15, New York, Raven Press, 1981.

Kolbe LC. Introduction - psychiatry and the patient with chronic pain. *Psychiat Ann 14:*773-777, 1984.

Kudrow L. *Cluster Headache Mechanism and Management.* pp. 71-98, Oxford, Oxford University Press, 1980.

Lance JW, Curran DA. Treatment of chronic tension headache. *Lancet 1:*1236-1239, 1964.

Lesse S. The multivariant masks of depression. *Am J Psychiatry 124(suppl):* 35-40, 1968.

Rapoport AM. Analgesic rebound headache. *Headache 28:*10, 662-665, 1988.

Raskin NH. *Headache.* ed 2., p. 224, New York, Churchill Livingstone, 1988.

Rosenbaum JF Comments on "chronic pain as a variant of depressive disease: The pain-prone disorder." *J Nerv Ment Dis 170:*412-414.

Sachs O. *Migraine: Understanding a Common Disorder.* Berkeley and Los Angeles, University of California Press, 1985.

Weeks RW. *A Comparison of Psychological and Physiological Components of Migraine and Combination Headaches.* doctoral dissertation. North Texas State University, 1981.

21

Ongoing Treatment Considerations in the Management of Headache Patients

Frances M. Arrowsmith

The initial intake interview of a headache patient is the first step in the diagnosis and treatment of headaches. This process is crucial in differentiating between muscular, vascular, mixed, or other types of headache, and in educating the patient regarding his particular headache type.

The nursing goals at the assessment interview are to establish a therapeutic relationship that convinces the patient of the nurse's empathy, respect, and genuine desire to help; to provide the patient with an understanding of headaches, including their prevention and treatment; and to discuss the expectations of treatment and appropriate therapeutic methods.

The intake interview is derived from questions based on a PQRST model. "P" stands for provocation of the headache. What brings it on? What makes it worse? What does the person generally do for it? What palliates or relieves the pain? "Q" deals with the quality of the pain. Is it sharp, dull, throbbing, aching, pounding, intermittent, or constant? "R" is the region of the pain. Is it unilateral or bilateral? Can the person point to where it is located? Does the pain radiate to another area? "S" questions associated symptoms, i.e., nausea, vomiting, dizziness, or sensitivity to light during the headache. "T" assesses the temporal qualities of the headache. Does it occur suddenly? When did it start? How often does it occur? How long does it last? The answers to these questions help determine the types of headache that an individual has. Muscular or tension-

Table 21.1. Self-Diagnosis of Headache Pain

	Type I Muscular (Tension)	Type II Vascular (Migraine)
Quality	• Pressure, band effect around head • Constant	• Throbbing, pulsating
Region	• Bilateral, back of neck, forehead • Generalized	• Unilateral usually, but can be bilateral • Temple and/or orbit
Other Symptoms	• Decreased concentration, memory, and energy; interruption of sleep	• Nausea, vomiting, sensitivity to light and sound • Dizziness • Withdrawal to bed (hibernation)
Time Factors	• More frequent • Daily • Late afternoon • Gets worse as the day goes on • Wakening with headache	• Frequency: 1 to 4 attacks/month • Sudden onset • Related to pregnancy, menses, oral contraceptives, or hormone replacement

type headaches are usually constant, bilateral, and create a band-like pressure around the head with associated symptoms of decreased energy, concentration, and sleep. They are more frequent and often daily. Vascular headaches are usually throbbing, one-sided headaches that are accompanied by nausea, vomiting, and sensitivity to light (Table 21.1)

The documentation of headache pain is an important consideration in the ongoing treatment regimen. Since the majority of individuals have at least two types of headache and conceivably as many as four types, enlisting their aid in objective charting becomes the basis for diagnosing and managing the headaches. The use of a headache calendar serves to document details of the headaches (Figure 21.1). An explanation of the particular headache pain, which is then translated into a number value, helps to assure a commonality in understanding the intensity of the headaches experienced. At the New England Center for Headache, we use only three levels of pain to simplify the conversion of subjective head pain into an objective intensity understood by both the interviewer and the interviewee. These intensities are: number 1 – a mild, low-grade pain; number 2 – a moderate to severe pain in which the individual is still functioning; and number 3 – an incapacitating pain, either because the individual is unable to function or because of the excruciating nature of the pain.

The duration of the pain experienced is equally as important as the intensity of the headaches. The patient charts whether there is a particular time of day at which the headache starts or feels worse, as well as whether the pain is there from the time he gets up in the morning until the time he goes to sleep at night.

The baseline frequency is obtained at the initial intake history and subsequent improvement is noted and compared with initial values. Sometimes the initial frequency may be inaccurate since the patient is giving a "guesstimate" as to the

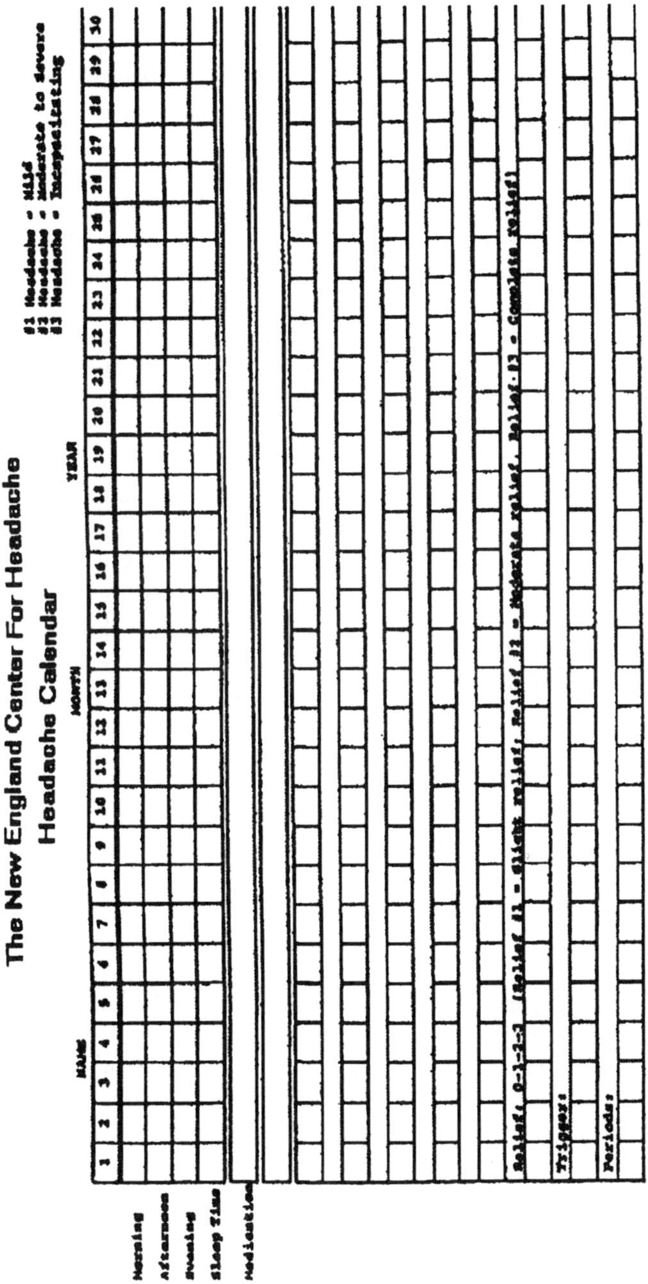

Figure 21.1 The New England Center for Headache Headache Calendar

particulars regarding headache frequency and intensity. Most individuals will underestimate rather than overestimate their headache frequency. This is important to consider when one is trying to determine the percentage of improvement between the initial evaluation and the first follow-up visit.

In addition to whether the frequency of headaches has improved, the intensity of the head pain and the duration of pain on a 24-hour basis is noted. It is important to see in a more objective manner whether there is improvement. It is not uncommon for individuals to say that they are the same and yet their objective charting reveals there has been a decrease in either the frequency, intensity, or duration of head pain. Likewise, patients may say they feel much better and yet their calendar reveals no appreciable improvement in any facet of their headaches. This latter group includes those individuals who were experiencing many side effects primarily due to the amounts of analgesics they were consuming.

The calendar becomes an educational tool that helps the patient assess possible causes of the headache, treatment efficacy, and feedback as to his improvement. Important information regarding possible "triggers" is built into the calendar. The individual can identify those situational factors that may have produced the headache. Some of these include stress, anger, anticipation, weekends, odors, and menses, to name only a few. These triggers are then recorded on the calendar as the precipitant of the particular headache. Patients can then begin to see their headache triggers and understand how they may have some control over the factors that may abort or reduce the frequency or intensity of the headache.

Another type of trigger is food. The individual is asked to restrict the intake of those foods that are known to be common offenders. These include chocolate, most alcohols, especially red wine, peanut butter, and foods that contain tyramine. This dietary restructuring is recommended during the first month so that identification of food triggers and control over them can be instituted early. If after the first month there has been some improvement in headache frequency in response to this measure, the individual is allowed to reintroduce the food groupings at the rate of one per week. Likewise, modifications in the quantity of caffeinated substances consumed is advised when it exceeds two cups of coffee, tea, or two caffeinated cola drinks per day. However, the caffeine restriction remains the same on an ongoing basis. (Figure 21.2)

If in fact the individual has noticed an improvement since following the diet, he is then encouraged to remain on a tyramine-restricted diet on an extended basis. Since skipped meals or fasting may be another triggering factor, it is strongly suggested that each individual adhere to eating three meals per day composed of the basic four food groups.

For women whose headaches occur perimenstrually, it is imperative that they avoid all dietary headache triggers during the days of the month that they are susceptible to headaches. Proper diet, sleep, and vitamin therapy are suggested

Figure 21.2. Helpful Hints for Headache Control

A variety of factors may act as triggers for headache. These vary from person to person. For example, hormonal factors may trigger migraine for some women but not for others. Diet, sleep patterns, over-exertion, stress, etc., affect some individuals.

The following should be helpful:
1. Do not skip meals. Eat nutritional meals at regular times.
2. Do not eat too much carbohydrate or high calorie foods at one sitting.
3. Get enough sleep, but *avoid oversleeping*. A change in patterns may precipitate headache. Keep to normal sleep patterns *even* on weekends. If necessary, arise at your normal *weekday* times and return to sleep.
4. Avoid overexertion and fatigue.
5. Avoid placing excessive demands on yourself. Schedule the necessary day to include *time for yourself*. Slow down and relax. Check for signs of tension — rapid and shallow breathing, wrinkled forehead, hunched shoulders, tight jaws, clenched fists, etc. Take slow, deep and even breaths, drop your shoulders, etc. This does not take much time and may be helpful.
6. *WATCH CAFFEINE INTAKE*. Excessive caffeine can trigger headache. One to two *cups* (not mugs) of caffeinated coffee is acceptable. None is preferable.
7. Avoid the following:

Chocolate	Onions	Herring
Canned figs	Pizza	Chicken livers
Nuts	Sour cream	Avocado
Peanut butter	Yogurt	Nutrasweet

    Ripened cheeses (cheddar, gruyere, brie, camembert, etc.) — Cheeses which are permissible are: American, cottage, cream, and Velveeta

    Vinegar — however, white vinegar is permissible

    Anything which is fermented, pickled, or marinated

    Hot fresh breads, raised coffeecakes, and doughnuts (due to activated yeast)

    Pods of broad beans (lima, navy, and pea pods)

    Monosodium glutamate — any foods containing large amounts (Chinese foods); meat tenderizers (Accent)

    Citrus fruits (Example: No more than one orange per day)

    Bananas (no more than 1/2 banana per day)

    Pork — Limit intake

    Tea, coffee, cola beverages (Avoid excessive amounts)

    Fermented sausage (bologna, salami, pepperoni, summer and hot dogs)

    Alcoholic beverages — *Avoid if possible*. Of all possible food triggers for migraine, alcohol is most frequently cited.
8. We recommend that you begin with a total elimination of the above for one month. If you observe a decrease in frequency or severity of headache, slowly re-introduce foods *one* at a time and observe the effect. If headache increases, eliminate that food and go on.

Please feel free to ask us any questions regarding information, medications, etc. Changing long-standing patterns is *not easy*, but successful treatment depends on it.

---

to control the cravings, irritability, and increase in headaches that become a part of the premenstrual syndrome.

The greatest amount of time is spent, both initially and on an ongoing basis, in educating the patient in the use of both preventive and abortive medications for their headaches. The first step is to learn the individual's perception of taking medication. Then, education begins with discussing the indications for use of the medication, mechanism of action, and potential side effects.

It is imperative that the caregiver recognize and work with the patient to deal with any resistance regarding medication. A thorough explanation about the medication is given, including indications for increasing the dose and the maximum dose allowed. This information should be written on the patient's headache calendars as well as on the prescriptions to insure compliance. Other important factors regarding compliance are an explanation as to how long it may take to derive benefit from the medication, an estimation of the length of time the medication will be used, and an explanation of side effects.

Some patients may be on a number of different medications. One may be prescribed on a daily basis as a preventative measure while another is prescribed to get through a rebound interval. Different medications may be used for moderate versus incapacitating headaches. Patients often experience information overload, especially when it concerns their medications. Written guidelines are given and telephone calls are encouraged to review any of the instructions that may be confusing. Not only does this help in clarifying the initial instructions but it also assists the individual in going through a difficult "rebound withdrawal" interval. Telephone communication is also important to continue the therapeutic relationship that was started during the initial interview.

Follow-up visits are scheduled according to need. Individuals with complicated medication issues should be seen two weeks after the initial evaluation. The usual follow-up visits can be at 4 week to 12 week intervals, depending on the complexity of the headache process and the distance the individual must travel. Multiple, frequent telephone calls indicate that the patient needs to come in sooner for individualized attention to address the problems encountered.

Figure 21.3a. Self-Care of Headaches

MUSCULAR HEADACHE TREATMENT
Preventive
Diet Therapy
1. Caffeine reduction.
2. Absence of daily analgesics (aspirin, acetaminophen, and prescription analgesics).
3. Well balanced diet, maintain ideal weight.

Environmental Factors
1. Sleep with a different size or shaped pillow.
2. Change body position throughout the day — practice range of motion and neck exercises.

Stress Reduction/Relaxation
1. Consciously control one's own life pace.
2. Maintain stable routines, habits, and life style.
3. Use situational groupings to talk problems over with others.
4. Practice time management techniques.
5. Learn and practice adaptive coping.
6. Learn assertiveness techniques.
7. Work tension off by physical exercise (jogging, swimming, bike riding) or meditative exercise (relaxation, biofeedback).

During Headache
Environment and Relaxation Techniques
1. Moist heat.
2. Massage.
3. Range of motion and neck exercises.
4. Relaxation techniques.
5. Withdrawal from stimuli.

Educating the patient to set realistic goals is an important basis of the treatment plan. Goals that are achievable are reinforcing and may alleviate some of the non-compliant behavior. The goals that need to be agreed upon for the first month include assessing symptoms and triggers to headache pain, distinguishing between muscular and vascular headaches, decreasing analgesic or prescribed medication abuse, and recognizing a headache of serious symptomatology that requires immediate self-referral. Goals to be achieved in the next three months include decreasing the frequency, intensity, and duration of headaches, and learning self-care techniques to meet these goals. This educational process may also include a program of stress management using biofeedback training as one modality. Other behavioral medicine techniques may be helpful. (Figure 21.3).

The attitude of professionals in caring for the headache sufferer is extremely important. Those who display empathy, respect, genuineness, concreteness, and gentle confrontation are facilitative to the individual. In the treatment of headaches, the professional must be caring; he or she must display a positive bias, that is, the belief that headache sufferers can be helped and that they possess the ability to tolerate the frustration of slow rewards or successes. Both the patient and the professional must set realistic goals. With chronic headaches, relapses are expected and are not met with discouragement or defeat.

Figure 21.3b. Self-Care of Headaches

VASCULAR HEADACHE TREATMENT
Preventive
Diet Therapy
1. Tyramine restricted diet: restrict strong cheeses, red wine, yogurt, alcohol, beer, pickled herring, fermented sausage, liver, bananas, avocados, figs, chocolate.
   Restrict nitrates, i.e.: hot dogs, salami, cured meats.
   Restrict MSG, i.e.: Chinese foods, Accent, meat tenderizers.
2. Restrict caffeine and alcohol
3. Increase foods high in vitamin B complex, especially B-6.
4. Eat three well balanced meals.
5. Absence of daily analgesics.
Environmental and Relaxation Factors
1. Keep normal routine and schedule. If sleeping later, get up at regular time and eat breakfast; then go back to bed.
2. Maintain normal regular exercise and sleep patterns.
3. Practice daily relaxation.
4. Eliminate fumes such as paint, chemicals, etc.
During Headache
Diet Therapy
1. Flat coke, saltines or toast for nausea.
2. Caffeine.
Environmental and Relaxation Techniques
1. Reduce environmental stimuli, i.e.: isolation, darkened room, decrease noise (hibernation).
2. Ice or heat; hot shower or ice to temples or sub-occipital region.
3. Fall asleep.
4. Massage.
5. Self-hypnosis, visual imagery.

The right amount of caring, nurturing, and "tough love" or confrontation are necessary in the treatment of this difficult and complex entity.

Copyright © 1993 PMA Publishing Corp.
Headache: A Clinician's Guide to Diagnosis, Pathophysiology, and Treatment Strategies
Edited by Alan M. Rapoport, M.D. and Fred D. Sheftell, M.D.

22

A Comprehensive Approach to Headache Treatment

Alan M. Rapoport and Fred D. Sheftell

This chapter summarizes and synthesizes our approach to the treatment of headache patients at the New England Center for Headache. An accurate diagnosis of headache type is an essential component of providing proper treatment. Though there are many workers in the field who see primary headache disorders existing on a continuum, we feel that accurate diagnosis of specific headache subtypes is important in selecting appropriate pharmacological and nonpharmacological treatment modalities. What follows is our standard approach to headache treatment. These treatments are usually effective in controlling headache in over 85% of the patients that we see.

Tension-Type Headache
(Muscle Contraction Headache)

ACUTE

Patients who have occasional or intermittent tension-type headache usually experience relief from over-the-counter analgesics. Other patients may require prescription medications that include combinations of salicylates, acetaminophen, short-acting barbiturates, and caffeine Fiorinal. In addition the combination drug containing isometheptene mucate, dichloralphenazone, and acetaminophen (Midrin) may be helpful. Nonsteroidal anti-inflammatory agents have also been successful. Patients who have occasional tension-type headaches may use these medications quite safely. In previous chapters, we emphasized the importance of not using these medications symptomatically on a frequent or daily basis, as this may create analgesic rebound headache.

Nonpharmacological alternatives are preferred by many patients and may include simple massage, relaxation, heat or ice, and exercise. The suboccipital ice pillow has been shown to be helpful. When patients can identify stressful situations that frequently produce the tension-type headache, appropriate avoidance or other adaptations may be made.

Chronic Tension-Type Headache
(Chronic Scalp Muscle Contraction Headache, Daily Dull Headache, Essential Headache, Chronic Daily Headache)

In chronic tension-type headache, the patient should avoid the use of daily symptomatic treatment. The first step in evaluating patients with daily headache is to document their analgesic intake and provide appropriate treatment to reduce and discontinue these analgesics. This can be done in a variety of ways. For patients using over-the-counter analgesics, medication may be discontinued abruptly without serious sequelae. However, for patients using medications containing barbiturates, narcotics, or ergotamines, a gradual tapering of the dosage is necessary to alleviate the symptoms of analgesic or ergotamine withdrawal. When our patients are told that they must decrease and discontinue analgesics, they are often frightened at the prospect. We start such patients on a gradually decreasing dosage of Midrin: t.i.d. for five days, b.i.d. for five days, and q.d. for five days. An alternative is the use of naproxen sodium (Anaprox) 275 mg in a similar fashion. This provides the patient with some degree of analgesia during the tapering process. Once this initial phase of discontinuing analgesics is completed, we have a more accurate picture of the underlying headache disorder, independent of the effect of daily analgesics. Patients are told to expect the withdrawal period to be difficult, and that they may experience some increased pain for up to three or four weeks. However, they are also told that by the end of this time period, most patients usually experience a reduction in daily pain even if no further treatment is given.

If daily headache persists for one to two months after the discontinuance of analgesics, the pharmacological treatment of choice would by tricyclic antidepressants, particularly amitriptyline HCl (Elavil, Endep). The nonpharmacological treatment of choice would be electromyographic biofeedback training. The same approach is used for patients with daily dull headaches in the absence of analgesic use.

Our usual starting dosage of amitriptyline is 10 mg one to two hours before bedtime. This is increased in 10-mg increments every five to seven nights as tolerated until the patient is at 30 to 50 mg. For patients with overt symptoms of biological depression, we may go to the usual antidepressant dosage of 100 mg or greater. We also look for evidence of anticholinergic side effects to evaluate our dosage. Usually patients begin to respond to the medication when the dosage level causes symptoms such as dry mouth. Other side effects frequently encountered are sedation, fatigue, increased appetite, constipation, and blurred vision. If sedation is a problem, we consider other tricyclics that are less sedating, such as nortriptyline HCl (Pamelor). Alternatives are doxepin HCl (Adapin, Sinequan), maprotiline HCl (Ludomil), and trazodone HCl (Desyrel). Generally, we have had greater success with the tricyclics that are more serotoninergic. Fluoxetine (Prozac) causes less weight gain but may not be as effective as amitriptyline in preventing headaches. Sertraline HCl (Zoloft) promotes weight loss and may be helpful in headache control.

When patients are refractory to tricyclics or cannot tolerate them, we consider the use of monoamine oxidase (MAO) inhibitors. Phenelzine sulfate (Nardil) has been used frequently in treating chronic headache disorders. Our starting dosage is 15 mg (one tablet) in the morning, increasing every five days up to two tablets in the morning and two tablets before 3:00 p.m. If patients receive this medication much later in the day, they may encounter sleep problems. Note that patients must stick to a strict diet.

When patients demonstrate a consistent, positive response to a given regimen (i.e., a 66% or greater reduction in frequency and intensity of headache) for four to six months, we begin to taper the medication slowly over a period of several months. During this time, patients continue to monitor their headache frequency, intensity, and duration. They may reach a critical dose below which they deteriorate. In these instances, we keep them on the lowest possible dose to provide reasonable control. We may try again for reduction in dosage in six months. Calendars monitoring frequency, intensity, and duration of headache and response to treatment are crucial to evaluate progress.

Vascular Headache

MIGRAINE WITHOUT AURA

The drug of choice to stop a migraine in its tracks is dihydroergotamine mesylate (D.H.E. 45) given intramuscularly or intravenously. The dose varies between 0.5 mg and 1 mg and is often preceded by an antiemetic. It is available in Europe as an oral preparation and a nasal spray. It has been tested as a nasal spray in the U.S. and it appears to be safe and effective. It should become available in 1993.

The most effective oral treatment for acute migraine is ergotamine. It is surprising how many patients with migraine have never been tried on ergotamine for the abortive treatment of their headache. Others have tried it once but could not tolerate it due to the nausea and vomiting sometimes associated with this medication. Therefore, we always prescribe an antiemetic prior to the use of ergotamine, particularly for the first several trials that a patient has with the drug. If the patient does not become unusually nauseated, the antiemetic can be omitted. Patients are told to begin their medication for the acute headache once they are relatively sure the headache will progress to a full migraine attack. We realize that all prescribing information for ergotamine states that patients should medicate immediately upon onset of their headache. Because most patients have mixed headache disorder and frequent headaches, this type of instruction usually leads to overuse of ergotamine and eventually to ergotamine rebound headache described in an earlier chapter.

If patients are nauseated at the onset of their attack, promethazine HCl (Phenergan), a 25 or 50 mg tablet, may provide relief. If vomiting is imminent, the patient is instructed to take Phenergan 50 mg by rectal suppository and wait 20 minutes before medicating with ergotamine. If this is too sedating or proves ineffective, there are alternative antiemetic agents. These include metoclopramide (Reglan) 10 mg tablet, trimethobenzamide HCl (Tigan) 250 mg capsule, 25 mg prochlorperazine (Compazine) suppository, and hydroxyzine HCl (Atarax, Vistaril) 50 mg tablet. If the antiemetic controls nausea, the ergotamine may be taken orally at a dosage of 2 mg initially and repeated in one hour if necessary. If the medication is not retained or not effective orally, the patient should switch to the suppository preparation, starting with 0.5 mg.. Other modes of ergotamine administration are sublingual and aerosol (recently discontinued).

We find that if 4 mg of ergotamine tartrate is not effective, then more ergotamine will not be effective and may cause side effects. Therefore, we limit the abortive use of ergotamine to 4 mg. In addition, patients are told to remain ergot-free for seven to ten days between doses; more frequent administration may, in fact, lead to an ergotamine rebound cycle with an increased frequency of "migraine." In certain special instances (e.g., menses), we do allow a patient to take ergotamines as frequently as two to three times in a given week, so long as that week is followed by ten days of ,o ergotamine usage.

There are various ergotamine preparations and routes of administration. It is sometimes necessary to try different preparations before giving up on the efficacy of ergotamine for migraine. If ergotamine is not effective, we prescribe ergonovine maleate (Ergotrate), an ergot derivative, 0.2 mg by mouth t.i.d. $5-HT_{1D}$ agonists may also prove useful when available, such as sumatriptan. Sumatriptan is available in several countries, including Canada, and will be marketed in the U.S. as Imitrex, probably in 1992. Experimental trials show it to work rapidly to improve a migraine and decrease nausea. Only minor side-effects are seen. The most effective dose is 6 mg subcutaneously; 100 mg by mouth is also helpful. It seems to work by inhibiting substance P release in the trigeminovascular system, thereby decreasing neurogenic inflammation in the dura mater. It is a vasoconstrictor. (See Chapter 1 and 3).

For those patients who are not responsive to ergotamine or who require frequent abortive medication, we have found some of the nonsteroidal anti-inflammatory agents to be useful. These include naproxen sodium (Anaprox) 275 mg, two tablets initially and repeated again in one hour, and meclofenamate sodium (Meclomen) 100 mg, two tablets initially and repeated in one hour if necessary. The use of the nonsteroidals, when effective, can be helpful in preventing ergotamine rebound and still leave patients with effective abortive medication. Midrin may be used in a similar way, two capsules initially and two capsules repeated in one hour if necessary. Butalbital containing medications such as Fiorinal and Fioricet, one tablet stat and again in an hour, may also be helpful.

When the above medications are not successful in alleviating a migraine attack at home, we have found the use of steroids to be beneficial, often preventing emergency room treatment. We prefer dexamethasone (Decadron, Hexadrol) 4 mg with a repeat of half a dose in one hour if necessary. In our experience, this will break 90% of prolonged migraine attacks at home. The frequency of steroid usage must be carefully controlled to two days per month or less.

For those patients whose migraine persists despite all abortive treatments, parenteral medications may be necessary. We have found the most beneficial combination to be 1 mg dihydroergotamine mesylate, 50 mg promethazine HCl, and 4 mg dexamethasone each administered intramuscularly in separate syringes. This is less sedating and is usually much more effective and faster acting than narcotics. D.H.E. 45 alone may also be effective.

PREVENTIVE TREATMENT

Preventive treatment is considered when migraine attacks occur three or more times per month or when there are four or more days during the month when the patient is incapacitated or debilitated as a result of migraine. Preventive medication may also be indicated when all abortive medications have been unsuccessful in treating the disorder. There are a variety of preventive medications available, as described in the earlier chapter on migraine. We prefer to start with either a beta blocker or calcium channel blocker. The calcium channel blocker of choice is verapamil HCl (Calan, Isoptin) given as an 80 mg dose on the first day, 80 mg b.i.d. on the second day, and 80 mg t.i.d. at eight-hour intervals on the third day. We sometimes start with 40 mg per day. If this is not effective within two to three weeks, the dosage can be increased up to a total daily dose of 480 mg. Side effects are not usually serious, the most common being constipation; atrial fibrillation has been reported. The other agent we use is diltiazem HCl (Cardizem). The usual starting dose is 30 mg/day increased up to 30 mg t.i.d. at eight-hour intervals. The maximum dose is 60 mg t.i.d. The most common side effects are fluid retention and constipation. The advantage of the calcium channel blockers is that there is less of an effect on mood, sedation, and energy than that experienced with the beta blockers. Nimodipine (Nimotop) and nifedipine (Procardia) have also been effective, but the latter occasionally worsens headache as it causes vasodilation.

Our beta blockers of choice are nadolol (Corgard) and propranolol HCl (Inderal). The usual starting dose of nadolol is 20 mg/day given as a single dose in the morning. Dosages are increased slowly up to an average dose of 80 mg to 120 mg/day. This can be increased if necessary. Propranolol HCl is usually taken several times during the day and, if effective, can be changed to the long-acting form Inderal LA. The usual starting dose is 30 mg/day, and it can be increased slowly to 240 mg/day if necessary. The most frequently encountered side effects are depression, fatigue, sedation, fluid retention, GI problems, decreased libido, and impotence. Therefore, one must be careful in evaluating migraineurs for treatment with beta blockers since existing depression may worsen with this medication. Proper patient education as to possible side effects improves compliance. Other beta blockers that may be effective include metoprolol tartrate (Lopressor) and atenolol (Tenormin). If a patient has chronic lung disease or asthma, it is important to use a selective beta$_1$ blocking agent, such as metoprolol, in low doses.

Tricyclic antidepressants have been reported to decrease migraine frequency. In our experience, however, they are not as effective as other drugs for prophylaxis of migraine.

Monoamine oxidase inhibitors have been used preventively with some benefit. We use phenelzine sulfate (Nardil), 15 mg in the morning, up to 4 tablets per day. Clonidine HCl (Catapres) has been tried at 0.1 mg/day gradually increasing to three doses per day, which may lower blood pressure and sometime cause drowsiness or irritability. A transdermal patch is easy to use.

Methysergide maleate (Sansert) is one of the oldest and best drugs for migraine prophylaxis but should be used cautiously because of the possible occurrence of retroperitoneal fibrosis as well as increased connective tissue growth around other organs. The starting dose is 2 mg per day and it is increased 2 mg daily up to three or four doses per day. If it is found to be effective, the patient must be tapered off the drug slowly for a minimum of one to two weeks every four to six months to prevent side effects. Periodic chest x-rays and intravenous pyelograms should be performed, along with tests of renal function. MRI can be a useful diagnostic test.

In children, cyproheptadine HCl (Periactin) can be very effective. Our usual starting dose is 2 mg at bedtime and this is increased gradually to a maximum of 16 mg/day. Interestingly, children tend to tolerate it better than adults and usually have no side effects. The most common side effects are increased appetite, weight gain, and drowsiness. Daily anti-inflammatory agents can be tried with caution.

Small doses of beta blockers and possible calcium channel blockers can be used in children if absolutely necessary. Childhood migraine may respond to anticonvulsants such as phenytoin (Dilantin), carbamazepine (Tegretol), and divalproex sodium (Depakote). These medications can also be effective in adult migraine and chronic daily headache. Depakote seems especially promising in resistant adult migraineurs.

MIGRAINE WITH AURA

The acute treatment of migraine with aura is similar to that of migraine without aura. Ergotamine taken during the aura can abort it; however, because of concern about worsening the probable vasoconstriction that occurs, we do not have patients use ergotamines initially during the aura. Patients are instructed to take their antiemetic drug as the symptoms of migraine with aura or complicated migraine begin, wait 20 minutes, and then medicate with the usual dosages of ergotamine described above. If the patient has used ergots successfully, we may tell him to use a small amount on one occasion during the aura. If there is either no effect on the aura or, in fact, a diminution of the aura using 1 mg of ergotamine, we allow the patient to take a full dose with subsequent headaches. In our experience, it is rare for a patient to have increased symptoms from taking ergotamine too early.

Preventive treatment in migraine with aura differs from migraine without aura only in that the calcium channel blockers seem to give greater and faster benefit than the beta blockers, and may be safer.

HORMONAL MIGRAINE

This term refers to those migraine attacks that occur with a fixed relationship in time to hormonal events. As a rule, menstrually related migraine is more refractory to standard treatment than nonmenstrually related migraine. In the same individual, there may be an effective response to ergotamine in nonmenstrually related headaches, and poor response to those that occur perimenstrually. These are the most difficult migraines to treat. The abortive measures described above for both migraine with aura and migraine without aura may be used in treating menstrual migraine. We have had some success with the use of preventive medication perimenstrually. If menses can be timed reasonably accurately, we start the regimen approximately four days before day one of menses. This regimen may include small dosages of cyproheptadine (2 to 4 mg) taken nightly four days before and through the end of menses. In addition to, or in lieu of, one may use naproxen sodium (Anaprox), 275 mg, three times a day a half hour after meals during the same time period. We have found that the use of these medications may either block the headache or help to enhance the response to ergotamines taken abortively during the attack. We have also tried using a beta blocker in conjunction with aspirin during the same time period.

Other medications that may be helpful are estrogen by skin patch (Estraderm), tamoxifen citrate (Nolvadex), a potent antiestrogenic agent, and danazol (Danocrine) which inhibits the output of gonadotropins from the pituitary gland. Other ancillary approaches may include the use of diuretics, depending on the degree of fluid retention, and the elimination of foods containing vasoactive chemicals during menses. We have seen many women who are not usually diet-sensitive except during menses.

Mixed Headache Disorders

The mixed headache disorder is the most common problem seen by headache specialists. The usual history is that of frequent or daily dull-to-moderate pain, with several days a month of very severe or incapacitating pain. Often these patients are not aware of having two distinct headache problems. It must be emphasized, however, that there are headache specialists who view common migraine and tension-type headache on a continuum and do not distinguish etiologically between the two. In evaluating the patient with mixed headache disorder, it is vital to get an accurate history of analgesic intake. Patients taking large amounts of over-the-counter or prescription analgesics must be withdrawn from these medications for either pharmacological or nonpharmacological treatment to be effective. During the early phase of treatment, we often use medications to provide for vasomotor stability, such as small dosages of cyproheptadine at bedtime (2 to 4 mg) in conjunction with decreasing doses of Midrin starting on a t.i.d. basis over a two-week period. This will help the patient to discontinue p.r.n. analgesic use. After the analgesic washout period has passed, daily headaches are usually much diminished in both frequency and intensity. (See Chapter 13).

Once the phase of analgesic rebound is over or we have determined that it is not an issue, we begin treatment of the underlying headache disorder. If daily, dull-to-moderate pain persists in combination with episodes of incapacitating or severe pain, we consider starting dosages of tricyclic antidepressants one hour before bedtime. We may start with small dosages of amitriptyline or doxepin, beginning at 10 mg and titrating upwards slowly to 50 mg if necessary. It is not necessary to use antidepressant doses of these medications (100 to 300 mg) to get a beneficial response. It may take one to four weeks to see any improvement. In our experience, the proprietary drug Elavil is superior to the generic form (amitriptyline) in terms of efficacy and lower incidence of side effects.

In mixed headache disorders, we find it beneficial to begin with tricyclic antidepressants, as they may lower the incidence not only of the daily dull headaches, but of migraine activity as well. If patients return in three weeks with a decreased frequency of daily headaches but an unchanged frequency of migraine (more than three per month or lack of effective abortive treatment), prophylactic medication specific for migraine might be added. A variety of nonpharmacological approaches may be useful as well, the most effective of which is biofeedback training.

Patients are monitored on a quarterly basis once they have begun to do well. When their calendars begin to show a consistent decrease in headache frequency, we begin a slow downwards titration of their medication. Some patients cannot get below a critical dose without return of their headaches.

Cluster Headache

Episodic cluster headache is the common form of cluster headache (90%) and often the easiest to treat.

EPISODIC CLUSTER HEADACHE

Oxygen therapy is effective in 82% of patients with episodic cluster headache in 70% of attacks [1]. The patient can rent an oxygen tank (D cylinder) and administer oxygen to himself through a loose-fitting mask over the nose and mouth in the sitting position at a rate of 7 liters of oxygen per minute for up to 20 minutes. If this does not break the attack, the patient takes 1 mg to 2 mg of ergotamine, usually sublingually but sometimes in tablet form. We usually prescribe Cafergot or Wigraine tablets. Ergotamine suppositories, usually Cafergot, are used when sublingual or oral preparations are ineffective. Patients sometimes respond even better when ergotamine is given preventively. For example, if patients have predictable attacks, such as after coming home from work or after falling asleep, one to two tablets of Cafergot are given approximately two hours before the expected headache. If the patient has trouble sleeping because of the caffeine content, a barbiturate can be added.

D.H.E. 45 is effective i.m. or i.v. to abort a cluster headache. A nasal spray has been tested and appears effective and safe. Daily use may be possible for a short period of time. It should be available by 1993. Sumatriptan (Imitrex), 6 mg subcutaneously, appears to be helpful in experimental studies.

PREVENTION

Preventive medication should be used when the attack frequency is high and the timing is unpredictable. For example, prophylaxis is indicated for an attack frequency of two or more per day that cannot be predicted and are debilitating and for which abortive measures are not adequate.

The short-term use of steroids can be extremely effective in decreasing the frequency of cluster attacks. It may also be useful in decreasing the duration of an attack period in episodic patients. We generally use a starting dose of 40 mg or 60 mg of prednisone, tapering off over a three to four week period. When steroids are effective, we see a dramatic response within 48 hours. Patients generally do extremely well during the initial phases of steroid therapy but may develop breakthrough attacks toward the end of the tapering cycle. If this occurs and the attack frequency is still high enough to warrant preventive therapy, other medications may be considered. Patients should be warned about the potential side effects of steroids, including aseptic necrosis.

CALCIUM CHANNEL BLOCKING DRUGS

There are a number of calcium channel blockers, most notably verapamil HCl, which can be used effectively in the prevention of both episodic and chronic cluster headache [2]. We usually start with an 80 mg dosage q.d. and increase by one tablet per day up to t.i.d. or q.i.d. The medication is tolerated extremely well and the most common side effect is constipation. There is a small percentage of patients who may not respond to 320 mg/day but may respond to 480 mg/day. Diltiazem HCl may be used as well. Nifedipine (Procardia) may exert too strong a vasodilating effect and therefore may worsen the cluster attack. Nimodipine (Nimotop) may be useful at a dose of 30 mg t.i.d.

ERGOTAMINES

Ergotamines may be used preventively for episodic or chronic cluster headache. We may have patients taking Cafergot on a b.i.d. basis, one tablet in the morning and one or two tablets at bedtime. The combination of calcium blockers and ergotamines seems to be quite effective in decreasing the frequency of cluster attacks. Cluster patients should not need more than 3 mg/day of ergotamine; they seem to handle ergotamine very differently from migraine patients. Interestingly, we have not noted much ergotamine rebound headache with cluster patients, compared with migraineurs. There may be some inherent physiological differences during cluster periods. It is rare to observe emesis as a side effect of ergotamine in cluster patients, although it is common in migraineurs.

LITHIUM CARBONATE

Lithium carbonate (Eskalith, Lithane, Lithobid) has been used most effectively in chronic cluster headache, but may be used in patients with episodic cluster headache who do not respond to the above regimens. Since the introduction of verapamil HCl for cluster headache, there is a tendency for clinicians to use lithium less frequently than in the past. Lithium may be added to verapamil and ergotamine in intractable cases. Usually dosages of 300 mg b.i.d. is adequate.

We have not found that therapeutic lithium blood levels correlate with an improvement in cluster patients. Certainly in patients with cyclical mood disorders or recurrent unipolar disorders, lithium levels in the appropriate ranges are required for effective treatment. There is debate as to whether this is necessary in cluster. Lithium levels should be taken during the use of the drug. We find that patients do well at levels between 0.4 and 0.6 mEq/l; toxicity often occurs at levels above 1.2 mEq/l. Patients should be educated as to the signs of lithium toxicity, especially tremor. Dehydration and the use of diuretics should be avoided with lithium therapy.

Methysergide Maleate

Methysergide maleate (Sansert) may be used in the treatment of cluster headache. However, our experience has been that it becomes less efficacious over a period of time. In other words, cluster patients who respond well during one cluster period may in fact not respond adequately in future periods. It certainly is not the drug of choice in this disorder. The dosage is usually 2 mg on a t.i.d. or q.i.d. basis. The dangers of prolonged methysergide therapy (i.e., six months or longer) are possible fibrotic changes around the ureters and kidneys (retroperitoneal fibrosis) and lungs, etc. We generally avoid the use of this medication in patients over age 40 because of its marked vasoconstrictive action. We also taper and stop the drug every three to four months for a one- to two-week period.

Nonsteroidal Anti-Inflammatory Drugs

Nonsteroidal anti-inflammatory drugs have been used in cluster headache, particularly indomethacin (Indocin). Dosages range from 25 mg t.i.d. to 50 mg q.i.d. Indocin may be useful in certain cases, but it is not the drug of choice.

Experimental treatment with intranasal capsaicin (Zostrix) (0.025 % cream) has been shown to be effective. So has bright light therapy.

Chronic Cluster Headache

The treatment of choice for chronic cluster headache is increasingly focused around the use of calcium channel blockers. Verapamil HCl is used in much the same way as described above. If verapamil alone is not effective, the next step would be the addition of ergotamine on a b.i.d. basis. If these two medications are not effective, lithium, 300 mg b.i.d., is added to the regimen. With the use of these medications, 75% to 90% of cluster patients should experience a greater than 50% decrease in headache frequency and intensity.

Preventive treatment in patients with chronic cluster can make them episodic patients. In other words, chronic patients may do very well on medication with rare and infrequent attacks for long periods of time. They may then experience a period during which their cluster activity picks up. Patients may be tapered off their preventive medication and given a brief course of steroids as described above. We feel comfortable with this use of short-term steroid therapy—up to three times a year. When chronic cluster patients go on vacation, they will often carry steroids in case of a breakthrough. As a rule, if chronic patients have enjoyed a remission for several months with no evidence of cluster headache, we may have them slowly decrease their medication. If during the tapering they find an increased headache activity, they are told to go back to the usual dose of preventive medication.

For patients who have not responded to the above regimens, we occasionally give intramuscular ACTH (H.P. Acthar Gel) in the dose of 80 units three times a week for four to six weeks. This may be effective without causing the typical side effects of steroid medication.

For those patients who persist in having one or two attacks a day, dihydroergotamine mesylate (D.H.E. 45), 1 mg intramuscularly one or two times a day, administered at home or at a doctor's office, can be an effective treatment. Dihydroergotamine nasal spray should also be helpful.

IN-PATIENT TREATMENT

When a patient with chronic cluster headache is unresponsive to any of the above treatments and cannot tolerate the frequency of attacks, we admit them to the in-patient treatment unit at the Greenwich Hospital. They may respond to special protocols including intravenous histamine desensitization or some combination of intravenous dihydroergotamine and steroids. Most pharmacological therapy that is effective in migraine headache is not effective in cluster headache (beta blockers, antihistamines, clonidine, etc.).

Some studies have shown the effectiveness of sphenopalatine block with either cocaine spray or 4% lidocaine. We have not found these to be frequently effective and are concerned about giving patients daily cocaine. We have also tried greater occipital nerve blocks using 160 mg of methylprednisolone acetate (Depo-Medrol) but have not usually found this to be helpful [3]. Other forms of therapy include chronobiological education such as having the patient go to sleep and awaken later than usual and stopping shift work. Bright light therapy is a new form of treatment that may be efficacious.

The literature cites many references to usually effective forms of surgery for cluster headache. Sine 1979 at the New England Center for Headache, we have rarely sent a patient for surgery. Even the effective forms of surgery may be somewhat short-lived. Patients sometimes will develop pain on the opposite side and there are possible complications from surgery.

When therapy resistance is encountered, the patient usually has either the chronic or subchronic form of cluster headache. Treatment has to be innovative, bridging the gap between an episodic and a chronic cluster patient. The newest form of treatment that has been tried for both episodic and chronic cluster headache patients is divalproex sodium. It was first tried by Kuritsky because of its GABAergic potential (it increases gamma amino butyric acid levels in the brain) [4]. It has been found to be effective in a moderate percentage of patients and has few side effects. Our typical regimen starts at 250 mg the first day, 250 mg b.i.d. the second day, and then 250 mg t.i.d. Most patients need 1,500 mg/day or less. The maximum dose is 60 mg/kg/day, but most patients use much less.

Chronic Paroxysmal Hemicrania

Chronic paroxysmal hemicrania is totally responsive to indomethacin in appropriate doses that range from 25 mg b.i.d. to 50 mg q.i.d. Episodic forms have been described.

Seizure Equivalent Headache

Seizure-equivalent headaches are an interesting type of headache that is somewhat controversial. By this term we mean patients who have headaches that are often difficult to characterize, usually sudden in onset, relatively brief, and associated with a paroxysmal and sharp electroencephalogram interictally. These patients usually are very responsive to standard doses of typical anticonvulsants such as phenytoin, carbamazepine, and divalproex sodium.

Post-traumatic Headache and Post-Head-Trauma Syndrome

Patients suffering from post-traumatic headache and post-head-trauma syndrome are among the most difficult to treat for a variety of reasons. First, we know that many patients with post-head-trauma syndrome are less likely to respond to treatment if litigation is still pending. The treatment of this disorder is pharmacologically similar to that described in mixed headache disorder and analgesic rebound. Additional help may be needed for the various cognitive deficits that one finds in this disorder. Neuropsychological testing is important and counseling will be necessary in order to restore a reasonable level of functioning. We believe that the occasional use of narcotics immediately following head trauma is permissible for a six week period.

Indomethacin Responsive Headaches

A small percentage of patients will present with syndromes that may be variants of migraine, probably prostaglandin mediated, that are exquisitely indomethacin responsive and are among the most gratifying headache disorders to treat. These disorders are:

BENIGN EXERTIONAL HEADACHE (COUGH HEADACHE)

These are characterized by sudden onset of head pain, usually orbito-frontal in location, brought on by exertion such as coughing, weight lifting, bending, sneezing, straining (e.g., valsalva maneuvers). These can occur frequently and episodes may last minutes to hours. One must rule out more serious organic causes of exertionally triggered head pain. Indomethacin at 25 mg t.i.d., 1/2 hour after meals will usually eliminate these attacks within 24 hours. If not, the dosage should be doubled. Patients may titrate the medication downward and monitor return of symptoms. These syndromes are self-limited and will eventually cease, eliminating the need for medication. Some patients are able to use indomethacin on an as-needed basis, e.g., 1 hour prior to exercise.

ICE PICK HEADACHE ("JABS AND JOLTS")

These present as spontaneous episodes of extremely sharp, electrical-like pain in various areas of the head which can be excruciating but short-lived (a few seconds to a few minutes). They may occur occasionally or they may occur frequently throughout the day (20 to 30 times). In the latter case, indomethacin treatment is indicated and, once again, the response is dramatic.

CHRONIC PAROXYSMAL HEMICRANIA

This entity is mentioned earlier. Its indomethacin responsivity is one of the major diagnostic criteria for the disorder. There is an episodic form.

HEMICRANIA CONTINUA

This is characterized by a continuous, unilateral, dull ache with superimposed ice-pick-like head pain often provoked by exertion plus focal, throbbing, intense pain several times daily, usually triggered by alcohol or exertion. Most of these patients are effectively treated with indomethacin. Aspirin, ergotamine, and tricyclic antidepressants can also be helpful. There is an episodic form.

References

1. Kudrow L. Response of cluster headache attacks to oxygen inhalation. *Headache 12*: 1-4, 1981.
2. Gabai IJ, Spierings ELH. Prophylactic treatment of cluster headache with verapamil. *Headache 29*: 167-168, 989.
3. Anthony M. Arrest of attacks of cluster headache by local steroid injection of the occipital nerve. In: Rose FC, (ed). *Migraine: Clinical and Research Advances*, pp 169-173. Basel, Karger, 1985.
4. Kuritsky A, Herring R. The treatment of cluster headaches with sodium valproate. A new approach. *Headache 27:* 301, 1987.

23

The Inpatient Headache Treatment Unit

Alan M. Rapoport and Randall E. Weeks

Despite the existence of quality outpatient headache treatment programs, there remains a subset of headache patients who are "treatment failures" and require hospitalization. These patients have the most favorable response to treatment programs in specially designed, multidisciplinary inpatient headache units. There are relatively few of these units in the United States and none in other countries. The New England Headache Treatment Program, which is a joint venture of the Greenwich Hospital in Greenwich, Connecticut and The New England Center for Headache in Stamford, Connecticut, set up such an inpatient unit for the purpose of treating these recalcitrant patients. The unit was opened in the summer of 1988 in Greenwich Hospital, and the following is a description of its program, staff, and physical environment.

Philosophy of Treatment

The treatment philosophy is based upon an interdisciplinary therapeutic milieu model that is typical of chronic pain programs [1]. Basically, this entails treatment from a variety of disciplines whose singular goal is to reduce the degree of pain and suffering of these individuals [2]. Patients are required to become active participants in their treatment as opposed to passive recipients of medical care. They are taught treatment strategies by the program team members, and assume a great degree of responsibility for their own improvement [3]. The interdisciplinary nature of this treatment allows an integration of a variety of therapeutic modalities without any one being established as the most important (i.e., this is not a medical unit or a psychiatric unit). This leads to a significant crossover of practice among disciplines, allowing a great deal of education and cross-fertilization of techniques and strategies in treating the headache patient. All-team conferences are held twice a week in which various disciplines meet to define goals for each patient, which are then incorporated into an overall comprehensive treatment program.

The unit is directed by a medical director and, administratively, all disciplines report to him. There is a program director who is responsible for the clinical functioning of the program and implementation of the therapeutic milieu. A nursing administrative coordinator is in charge of the nurses on the unit, interfaces with nursing administration, serves as liaison to the outpatient unit, and has administrative responsibilities (e.g., budget, marketing, nurse scheduling, etc.). These three individuals make up the executive committee of the headache unit whose functions are to make policy and report on operations through the medical director of the unit, a the senior vice president of the hospital.

The clinical team is made up of a staff of specially trained registered nurses, a medical social worker, a physical therapist, an occupational therapist, the hospital chaplain, a dietitian, and a pharmacist. The current medical director is a board-certified neurologist, the associate medical director a board certified psychiatrist, and both program directors are clinical psychologists.

The physical aspects of the unit are designed to be part of the therapeutic environment. Carpeting, wallpaper, drapes, furniture and upholstery were carefully selected to create a warm, comfortable atmosphere. Lighting on the unit was specially designed and is non fluorescent, recessed, and indirect to reduce glare and create a pleasant and comfortable environment. Special heating and cooling units were designed to function with a low noise level and a comfortable flow of air. Lighting and noise issues are important as many patients with head pain are photo- and sonophobic (their pain will increase or be initiated by exposure to bright light or loud noise). Smoking is not permitted.

The unit contains both small and large group rooms in which program meetings and groups take place. There is a dining area for patients and staff to eat together (patients are not allowed to eat in their rooms). There are rooms for biofeedback training and for physical therapy instruction and exercise which are always available. Nurses utilize the nursing office and a nursing area, which includes the drug preparation room, the lounge for nurses, and the nursing station itself, as well as a secretarial area for the unit secretary. There are consultation offices for the medical director, the program director and the social worker. Since patients are required to dress in street clothes, not pajamas, bath robes, or other "sick-role" clothing, there is a laundry area to allow them to wash their own clothes. The unit contains 15 patient beds. There are five single rooms designed along the more typical medical/surgical model. In addition, there are five rooms with two platform style beds that have more of a dormitory appearance. All patients are required to make their beds and straighten their rooms on a daily basis. A pain control room has anesthesiology equipment for special procedures.

Admission Criteria

Individuals selected for admission to the unit are patients who are dependent on analgesics, ergotamine, narcotics, tranquilizers, or barbiturate-containing medication; patients who have significant medical or psychosocial problems that make it unlikely they can benefit from outpatient treatment; patients who have become chronically incapacitated by their head pain and have not responded to usually effective outpatient treatment strategies; patients that may have a complex headache history and require a more comprehensive diagnostic workup; and patients with chronic or severe cluster headache who have not responded to out patient therapy. Patients are advised prior to admission that no narcotics are used on the unit and that they will be taken off all medications not considered appropriate. In addition, they are expected to take part in all of the activities of the program even when they are not feeling well. They are not allowed to smoke on the unit and are urged to decrease and stop their smoking habit.

The Program

The following are components of the program, their frequency of occurrence, and a brief description. Most patients require six to fourteen days of hospitalization. Rarely, a patient will leave earlier if they are doing well and, occasionally, a patient will stay longer if the detoxification has not gone as smoothly as predicted.

Orientation Groups (two times per week) The purpose of these meetings is to acquaint the new patient with unit functioning and to allow patients who have been on the unit for a period of time to offer their assistance in orienting the new patients along with the nursing staff.

Biogenics Group (four times per week) The purpose of these groups is to educate patients about physiological functioning in a group relaxation format. The goal is to get the patient to be an active participant in his/her treatment by learning various relaxation techniques and having a greater degree of body awareness. Coping skills and pain management issues are discussed.

Social Work Groups (four times per week) The purpose of these groups is to explore the impact of the patient's pain on the family unit. There may also be more structured tasks such as constructing genograms and ventilation exercise such as drawing pictures of their head pain.

Physical Therapy Groups (three times per week) The purpose of these groups is to demonstrate proper stretching and mobilization techniques, as well as to point out the role posture can play in a person's pain experience.

Occupational Therapy Groups (two times per week) The purpose is to help make patients aware of the importance of leisure activities, time management, and utilization of relaxation skills during the day. Behavior strategies to change chronic pain lifestyles are discussed.

Pharmacy Group (twice per week) The purpose of this educational group is to familiarize patients with different types of headache medication, the biochemical explanation as to their efficacy, and the rationale for proposed pharmacological intervention.

Nutrition Group (once per week) The purpose of this group is to examine how diet can trigger and/or contribute to one's headache experience.

Discharge Groups (two times per week) The purpose of these groups is to discuss hospital course and examine concerns patients might have about leaving the hospital. It is a time for formulating questions that the patient and significant other might choose to ask at the discharge meeting.

Chaplain's Group (one time per week) The purpose is to discuss spiritual and consciousness raising issues.

Other groups such as laughter therapy, music therapy, and different lectures are planned. Pharmacist consultations are available.

Headache Unit Evaluations

Prior to hospitalization, all patients have had a complete diagnostic evaluation at The New England Center for Headache in Stamford, Connecticut. This information has been relayed to the inpatient unit prior to each admission. When patients arrive at the unit, a nurse gives a brief tour of the facility and describes the first day's program. This is typically a series of diagnostic interviews done by the various Headache Team members.

The first evaluation is a structured interview conducted by a nursing member of the Headache Team. Questions are posed regarding headache history, current medications, allergies, etc. Once again, patients are welcomed to the unit, and any questions regarding unit functioning are answered.

The patient then has a neuropsychological consultation with a doctoral level medical psychologist. During this consultation, further history is obtained regarding the patient's headache problem as well as an examination of issues with respect to present level of functioning in social, family, vocational, and psychological realms. An assessment of cognitive functioning is made (including a mental status examination) as well as a determination of current physiological status. The psychologist formulates his impressions and makes recommendations for treatment course.

The patient and significant other are then interviewed by the medical social worker who gathers detailed information about family systems. The impact that chronic pain may have on families is discussed. Family members are required to be a part of a patient's treatment.

The patient next has an admitting history, physical and detailed neurological examination which allows the physician to formulate impressions and treatment strategies. This information is combined with input from the other evaluations, and a tentative treatment plan is made. There is then a discussion with the patient and nurse about the plan in terms of further work-up and medical treatment. This usually includes withdrawing the patient from certain medications and adding others, both orally and intravenously.

Other evaluations on the first day are performed by the physical therapist, occupational therapist, and nutritionist. The patient may also be seen by the pharmacist and hospital chaplain, if appropriate.

Input from all disciplines is given the following morning at an all-team conference. Their recommendations are incorporated into a set of goals and into a comprehensive treatment plan which serves to guide the treatment team and patient through the hospital course. The patient is invited into the conference at this point and the treatment plan is discussed and questions are answered.

The Medical Program

Patients are seen daily on rounds by the physician, psychologist, nurses and other treatment team members. Medical consultation and laboratory testing is requested as needed. When indicated, patients are seen for individual sessions of biofeedback training, psychotherapy, physical therapy, family therapy, and more in-depth nutritional counseling. Patients are also involved in a variety of leisure activities designed to keep them active and out of the typical "pain lifestyle".

Pharmacologically, most patients are treated with intravenous medications that may include the use of intermittent repetitive dihydroergotamine mesylate (D.H.E. 45) and dexamethasone. Limited symptomatic medications are permitted according to treatment protocols and, if effective, may be utilized on an as needed basis once the patient leaves the hospital. The patient is required to keep a headache calendar while on the unit at the hospital as well as after discharge. This allows for an accurate recording of the amount and severity of pain, as well as types, quantities and effectiveness of medications used. Women track the relationship of headache to menstrual cycle. Team members review the calendar with the patient daily.

At the time of discharge, the patient and significant other meet with the nurse, psychologist, and physician to discuss thoroughly what medications the patient will be taking post discharge, how to use them, and potential side effects. Maximum limits of symptomatic medication are discussed. In addition, it is clearly stated what medications should *not* be used. Information sheets about prescribed medications are given to the patient in addition to a sheet of discharge instructions and prescriptions.

The discussion also encompasses the dietary regimen, physical activity, exercize and date of return to work, the decision regarding timing of follow-up visits is made. In most cases, the first follow-up appointment is within two to three weeks post discharge to confirm that the patient is following the treatment protocol and improving. The patient and significant other are encouraged to ask any questions they might have.

Since the Greenwich Hospital inpatient headache treatment unit has opened, over 80% of the patients admitted to the program have done remarkably well in the short period of time they have spent in the hospital. These are patients who have failed previous attempts at outpatient therapy and, usually, have had headaches for more than half of their lives. The majority have been abusing medication (possibly dependent upon it) and have had severe headaches on a daily basis. Most have done better than they had anticipated, but need several weeks or months to reach their maximum benefit. A surprisingly large number of patients, 96%, indicate on exist interviews their feeling that the program was definitely beneficial for them and more helpful than they had expected. There is a small number of patients who do not do well during and after hospitalization and, to a great degree, these are patients with significant psychological or social problems who are looking for that "magic pill" to cure their headaches. Obviously, both groups are resistant to taking greater responsibility for their pain management and are difficult patients to motivate or educate within the program. Such findings are consistent with outcome data from the few other inpatient units in the country.

We strongly believe that inpatient treatment in a comprehensive hospital program such as The New England Headache Treatment Program is both essential and beneficial for a significant percentage of headache patients and, without it, many of these patients would continue to suffer needlessly.

References

1. Newman RI, Seres J. The interdiscliplinary pain center: an approach to the management of chronic pain, In Holtzman AD, Turk DC (eds). *Pain Management: A Handbook of Psychological Treatment Approaches.* pp. 71-85. New York, Pergamon Press, 1986.
2. Fordyce WE. Learning process in pain, In Sternbach RD (ed). *The Psychology of Pain, ed 2.* pp 49-66. New York, Raven Press, 1986.
3. Holtzman AD, Turk DC, Kearns RD Jr. The cognitive behavioral approach to the management of chronic pain, In Holtzman AD, Turk DC (eds). *Pain Management: A Handbook of Psychological Treatment Approaches.* pp. 31-50. New York, Pergamon Press, 1986.

Index

Abdominal migraine, 191-192
Abortive (symptomatic) treatment, 31, 32, 91-93, 179
Abscess, 47, 131-132
Abuse of medication, 160
Acebutolol HCl, 73
Acephalalgic migraine, 44
Acetaminophen, 92, 158, 159, 164, 171, 193, 194, 243
Acetazolamide, 151
Acetylcholine, 20
Acidosis, 87
Acoustic nerve assessment, 38
Acquired immune deficiency syndrome (AIDS), 52-53, 131, 133
Acromegaloid look, 29
ACTH, intramuscular (H.P. Acthar Gel), 254
Acupuncture, 195-196
Ad Hoc Committee on Classification of Headache, 175, 176
Adalat, 21, 180
Adapin, 180, 245
Addiction-proneness evaluation, 116
Adenopathy, 154
Adenosine triphosphate, 69
Adjustment disorder, 231
Admission criteria for inpatient unit, 259
Adrenal endocrinopathy, 134
Adrenaline, 64, 65
Advil, 203
Affect, assessment of, 36
Age
  factor in biofeedback training, 108-109
  headache and, 27, 83, 112, 185, 188-189
Agitation, 44
AIDS (acquired immune deficiency syndrome), 52-53, 131, 133
Air travel, 115
Alcohol, 30, 32, 95-96, 115, 116, 119, 122, 147, 149
  blood levels of, 54
  nitroglycerin and, 209
Alcoholism, 177
Aldomet, 210

Allergies, 2, 95, 152-154
Alpha-adrenergic blocking agents, 181
Alprazolam, 164
Alprenolol, 73
Altitude, 30, 96, 115, 151
Altitude hypoxia, 119
Amenorrhea, 53, 102, 145
Aminergic mechanisms, 211-212
Amitriptyline, 21, 74-75, 78, 91, 94, 103, 104, 105, 154, 159-160, 161, 162, 180, 202, 244-245, 250
Amnesia, 44, 197
Amobarbital, 74
Amoxapine, 104, 202
Amphetamines, 31
Amphotericin B, 143
Amyl nitrite, 70, 74, 85, 148
Amyloid angiopathy, 132
Amytal, 74
Analgesic detoxification process, 161
Analgesic rebound headache (ARH), 31, 157-165
  clinical studies, 160-162
  research, 159-160
  treatment, 164-165
Analgesic washout period (AWP), 158, 161-162
Analgesics, 30, 31, 92, 103, 108, 171
  discontinuing daily use of, 178-179, 244
  non-habituating, 103
  in treating children, 193-194
Anaprox, 154, 181, 247, 249
  in discontinuing analgesics, 244
Anatomical correlations to vascular head pain, 4-5
Anemia, 134
Aneurysm, 44, 124, 140
Aneurysmal subarachnoid hemorrhage (SAH), 45
Anger and headache, 122
Angina pectoris, 72
Angiography, cerebral, 51-52
Angioparalytic migraine, 64
Anhedonia, 230
Animal studies, 6-7
Ankle jerk, 41
Anorexia, 29, 83, 84, 102, 187
Anticonvulsants, 203
Antidepressants, 94, 103-104, 105, 180

263

See also Tricyclic antidepressants
Antiemetics, 92, 158, 249
Antihistaminic tricyclic antidepressants, 31
Antihypertensives, 210
Anti-inflammatory drugs, nonsteroidal, 7
Antimigraine drugs, 7-8, 93-94
Antiphospholipid antibodies, 49
Antiserotoninergics, 69, 75
Anxiety, 30, 188-189
Aphasia, 37
Appetite changes, 102
Apresoline, 149, 210
Aqueduct of Sylvius, 48, 133
Aqueductal stenosis, 133
Arachidonic acid metabolism, 21
Arachnoid cysts, 132-133
ARH, *See* Analgesic rebound headache
Arnold-Chiari malformation, 48, 49
Arterial blood gases, 53
Arterial dilation, 198
Arterial occlusive disease, traumatic, 199
Arteries sensitive to pain, 129-130
Arteriovenous anastomoses, 20, 66-67
Arteriovenous malformation (AVM), 44, 45, 46, 85, 124
Arteriovenous oxygen measurements, 66-67
Arteritis, 85, 135-136
Arthralgias, 154
Asendin, 104, 202
Aseptic necrosis, 252
Aspartame and carbohydrates, 150
Aspergillosis, 143
Aspirin, 7, 92, 105, 158, 159, 193-194
Assessment, of patient's history and status, 216-218
Asthma, 31, 248
Atarax, 246
Ataxia, 29, 132
Atenolol, 73, 94, 248
Athetoid movement, 40
Atmospheric pressure change, 143
Atony and dilation of stomach, 92
Attention, assessment of, 36
Aura, 2, 9, 10, 12, 74
Aura symptoms, 29-30, 83-85
Autogenic phrases for self-regulation, 220
Autohypnosis, 196
Autonomic dysfunction, 117
Autonomic symptoms, 90, 134
AVM (arteriovenous malformation), 44, 45, 46, 85, 124
Avoidance, in treatment of cluster headache, 122
AWP (analgesic washout period), 158, 161-162
Babinski reflex, 41
Baclofen, 203
Bacon, 96, 148
Ballistic movement, 40
BAEP (brain stem auditory evoked potential), 55
Bananas, 149
Barbiturates, 159, 243, 244
Barometric pressure, 96, 152

Basilar migraine, 44, 192
Battle's sign, 201
Beans, fava or broad, 149
Bear liver, 148
Beck Depression Scale, 57, 216, 229
Beef liver, 148
Beer, 122, 149
Behavior, 30, 115-116
Behavior modification, 146
Behavioral assessment, 32-33
Behavioral medicine
 defined, 215-216
 approach to headache, 215-221
Behavioral tests, 56-57
Behavioral therapy, 165
Behavioral treatment, 231
Benign exertional headache, 255-256
Benign intracranial hypertension (BIH), 52, 133, 211
Benzodiazepines, 181, 203
Beta adrenergic blockers, 210
Beta adrenoceptor blockers, 72-73, 94
Beta blockers, 31, 171, 180, 203, 247-248
 vs. calcium channel blockers, 249
Beta endorphin, 10
Beta estradiol levels, 212
Bethanechol chloride, 105
BIH (benign intracranial hypertension), 52, 133, 211
Bilateral pain in migraine, 28
Biochemical modulators of trigeminovascular system, 2
Biochemistry of migraine, 9-14
Biofeedback, 91, 93, 108-109, 141, 162, 179, 196, 204
 in behavioral treatment, 232
 in self-regulation process, 220
 training, 165, 217, 250, 261
Biogenic amines, 103
Biogenics groups in inpatient program, 259
Biological reprimand, migraine as, 226
Birth control pills, 30, 31, 95, 212
Blocadren, 73, 94
Blood, 47, 135, 197
Blood-brain barrier, 72
Blood dyscrasia, 132, 134, 135
Blood flow, 71, 76, 85-86
Blood gases, arterial, 53
Blood pressure, 36
Blood tests, 53-54
Blood vessels sensitive to pain, 129-130
Blurred vision, 105, 211
Body awareness, 220, 259
Bologna, 148
Bony erosion, 49
Bradykinin, 2, 69, 88
Brain
 cells, 75
 CT scan of, 47-48
 5-HT$_{1D}$ receptors in, 20

mapping, EEG, 52
Brain stem, 103
  auditory evoked potential (BAEP), 55
  neurotransmitter functions, 170
Brain tumor, 50, 130-133, 135
Breathing exercises, 220
Bregmatic headache, 140, 144
Bright light therapy, 253, 254
Broad beans, 149
Bromo-LSD, 69
Bromocriptine mesylate, 10, 11, 145
Brucellosis, 187
Bruits, 36, 136, 201
Butalbital, 108, 158, 247
Butorphanol, 93
C2 root pain, 198
Cafergot, 92, 158, 195, 251, 252
Caffeine, 32, 92, 145-146, 158, 243
  abuse, 146
  restriction, 179, 219, 238
Caffeine withdrawal headache, 146
Calan, 21, 76, 94, 124, 180, 203, 247
Calcitonin gene related peptide (CGRP), 5, 7, 13, 136
Calcium antagonist, 171
Calcium channel blockers, 180, 203, 247, 248, 252, 253
  vs. beta blockers, 249
Calcium entry blockers, 75-77, 94
Capsaicin, 5-6, 253
Carbamazepine, 203, 248, 255
Carbohydrates and aspartame, 150
Carbon dioxide (CO_2), 56, 70, 85
Carbon monoxide (CO), 53, 150
Carbonic anhydrase inhibitor, 151
Carboxyhemoglobin, 53, 150
Carcinomatosis, 134-135
Carcinomatous infiltration of meninges, 47
Carcinomatous meningitis, 52
Cardiac arrhythmias, 94, 105, 124
Cardiovascular disease, 31, 32, 123
Cardizem, 94, 180, 203, 247
Carisoprodol, 108
Carotid artery disease, 137
Carotid body dysfunction, 119-121
Carotid bruits, 36, 201
Carotid Doppler, 51
Carotid pulse asymmetry, 201
Catabolite accumulation, 74
Catapres, 105, 181, 210, 248
Catch 22 dilemma in detoxification, 179
Catecholamines, 11, 13, 54
Causative treatment, 95-96
Cavernous plexus, 4-5
Cavernous sinus thrombosis, 143
CEBV (chronic active Epstein-Barr virus) syndrome, 154
Central (brain) disturbances, 176
Central hypothesis, 176
Central involvement, 71-72

Central nervous system (CNS), 14, 19, 39, 40, 53, 88-90, 145, 149, 162
  central vs. peripheral effects, 162
Centrax, 107
Cephalalgia, post-traumatic, See Post-traumatic cephalalgia
Cerebellar hematoma, 132
Cerebellar tumor, 4
Cerebral A-V malformation, 51
Cerebral angiography, 51-52
Cerebral arteriogram, 45
Cerebral atrophy, focal, 48
Cerebral blood flow, 71, 85-86
Cerebral edema, 131, 133
Cerebral infarction, 46, 47
Cerebral ischemia, 199
Cerebral neoplasm, 133
Cerebral tumor, 46, 188
Cerebritis with fever, 131
Cerebrospinal fluid (CSF), 10, 197
  examination, 44, 50, 52-53
  leak, 52, 134, 199
  outflow obstruction, 131, 133
  rhinorrhea, spontaneous, 50
Cerebrovascular disease, 136-137
Cervical arthritis, 108
Cervical collars, 203
Cervical form of post traumatic cephalalgia, 200
Cervical rigidity, 187
Cervical spine problems, 31, 46, 49-50, 198
Cervical triangle region injury, 199
CGRP (calcitonin gene related peptide), 5, 7, 13, 136
Chaddock reflex, 41
Chaplains group in inpatient program, 260
Character of pain, 28
Cheek, 5
Cheese, 95-96, 148
Chicken livers, 149
Child abuse, 187
Children, headaches in, 185-196
  acute infections and, 186-187
  patient history, 185-186
  recent onset headaches, 186
  treatment, 193-196, 248
Chinese food, 96
Chinese restaurant syndrome, 147
Chlordiazepoxide, 105, 107
Chlorzoxazone, 108
Chocolate, 95-96, 149
Cholecystokinin-8, 5
Chronic active Epstein-Barr virus (CEBV) infection, 154
Chronic and subchronic cluster headache, 111, 124-125, 253-254
Chronic daily headache, 175-182, 244-245
Chronic headache in children, 187-188
Chronic hypomotility, 140
Chronic lung disease and beta blockers, 248
Chronic meningitis, 52, 134-135

Chronic mononucleosis, 139, 154
Chronic obstructive pulmonary disease, 53
Chronic pain impulses, 163
Chronic paroxysmal hemicrania (CPH), 116-117, 255, 256
Chronic recurrent headache, 46
Chronic scalp muscle contraction headache, 244-245
Chronic subdural hematoma, 132
Chronic tension-type headache, 28, 29, 78, 244-245
Chronic viral fatigue syndrome, 154
Chronic vs. acute headache, 102
Chronicity of headache, 160
Chronobiological disturbance, 170
Chronobiological dyssynchrony, 179
Chronobiological pacemakers, 119-121
Chronobiological principles in treatment, 179
Cigarette smoking, 32, 116, 150, 179
Cimetidine, 212
Cinnarizine, 76
Circle of Willis, 2, 4
Circumstantial migraine, 226
Citrus fruits, 95-96
Classic migraine, 10, 13, 83-84
Classification of headache, 111, 175-176
 Ad Hoc Committee on, 175, 176
Claviceps purpurea, 64
Clinical team in inpatient unit, 258
Clomipramine HCl, 74
Clonazepam, 203
Clonidine, 105, 171, 181, 210, 248
Cloudiness, 96
Cluster headache, 4-5, 13, 28, 29, 112-114
 classification, 111
 clinical features, 112-116
 cluster period, 112
 comprehensive treatment approach, 251-254
 diagnosis of, 111-119
 pathogenesis of, 119-121
 psychological considerations, 228-229
 thermography in, 57-58
 treatment of, 121-125
CNS (central nervous system), 14, 19, 39, 40, 53, 88-90, 145, 149, 162
CNV (contingent negative variation), 11
CO (carbon monoxide), 53, 150
CO_2 (carbon dioxide) reactivity, 56
Coagulation disorder, 85
Cocaine, 31
Codeine, 108, 158
Coffee, 31, 32
Cognitive behavior modification, 218, 221
Cognitive functioning assessment, 260
Cognitive-oriented psychotherapy, 232
Cognitive therapy, 165
Coital headache, 44, 45
Cold extremities, 29, 84, 94
Cold remedies, 149
Collagen diseases, 49, 85
Colloid cysts, 48, 132-133

Combination medications, 243-244
Combined headaches (vascular and tension type), 176
Common migraine, 13, 84
Communicating hydrocephalus, 133
Compazine, 194, 246
Complexion, ruddy, 29
Complicated migraine, 85
Comprehensive approach to treatment, 243-256
Computerized EEG topography (EEG brain mapping), 52
Computerized tomography (CT) scan, 44-48, 186, 201, 210, 216
 contrast enhanced, 45-46
 vs. MRI, 193
Conduction disorders of the heart, 94
Confusion, 44
Congestive heart failure, 94, 105
Conjunctival suffusion, 115, 116
Consciousness, impairment of, 31, 44, 197
 assessment of, 36
Constipation, 94, 105, 124
Contingent negative variation (CNV), 11
Continuous migraine with interparoxysmal headache (MIH), 177
Conversion cephalgia, 231
Coordination testing, 39-40
Coping skills in inpatient program, 259
Coping strategies, 32-33, 221
Corgard, 73, 94, 180, 203, 248
Corneal temperature, 117
Coronary atherosclerotic heart disease, 151
Corticosteroids, 7, 54
Cortisol secretion, 170
Cough and cold remedies, 106
Cough headache, 255-256
Counseling, 202
CPH (chronic paroxysmal hemicrania), 116-117, 255, 256
CPS (cycles per second)
 128: vibratory sensation test, 40
 256: hearing test, 38
Cracked tooth syndrome, 140
Cranial bruits, 201
Cranial nerves, 37-39, 47, 49, 129, 131
Cranial X-rays, 49-50
Cream, 149
CSF, See Cerebrospinal fluid
CT (computerized tomography) scan, 44-48, 186, 201, 210, 216
 contrast enhanced, 45-46
 vs. MRI, 193
Cured meat products, 96
Cycles per second (CPS)
 128: vibratory sensation test, 40
 256: hearing test, 38
Cyclical vomiting, 191-192
Cyclizine lactate, 194
Cyclobenzaprine HCl, 108

HEADACHE 267

Cyproheptadine, 21, 71, 72, 78, 161, 162, 164, 195, 203, 248, 249, 250
Cysts, arachnoid, 132-133
Dacarbazine (DTIC-DOME), 211
Daily chronic headache, 176-178
Daily dull headache, 244-245
Daily morning headache, 146
Danazol, 249
Danocrine, 249
Darvocet, 108
Darvon, 108
Daytime drowsiness, 94
Death wishes, 32, 102, 114, 230
Decadron, 164, 247
Decongestants, 31, 106
Deep muscle exercise, 220
Deep tendon tap technique, 41
Degenerative diseases, 140
Delusional disorder, 231
Demerol, 106
Dental bite appliances, 141
Dental disease, 31, 114, 140-141
Depakote, 203, 249
Depo-Medrol, 254
Depression, 30, 56, 94, 154, 159, 177
 assessment of, 32
 in children, 189-190
 family history of, 32
 inventory, 216
 major, 230
 scales, 57, 216, 229
 spreading, 71, 76, 85-87
Depressive disorder, 30, 102
Dermoids, 49
Desipramine, 104
Desyrel, 104, 245
Detoxification of habituated patient, 103, 109, 171, 179
Dexamethasone, 164, 247, 261
 suppression test, 54
D.H.E.45 (dihydroergotamine mesylate), 7, 13, 20, 67, 70, 93, 158, 164, 245, 247, 251, 254, 261
Diabetes mellitus, 53, 94, 139, 193
Diabetic ketoacidosis, 143
Diadochokinesis, 39
Diagnosis
 of brain tumor, 131
 differential, 116-119
 socially acceptable, 103
Diagnostic testing, 43-58
 blood tests, 53-54
 cerebral angiography, 51-52
 cerebrospinal fluid examination, 52-53
 cranial X-rays, 49-50
 CT scan of brain, 47-48
 electroencephalography, 52
 evoked potentials, 54-55
 indications for diagnostic work-up, 43-44
 magnetic resonance imaging, 48-49
 neuroimaging in headache, 46-47

 psychological and behavioral tests, 56-57
 radionuclide cisternography, 50-51
 temporal artery biopsy, 54
 thermography, 57-58
 timing and selection of tests, 44-46
 transcranial Doppler, 55-56
 urine tests, 54
Diamox, 151
Diaphoresis, 84
Diarrhea, 29, 83, 84, 191-192
Diazepam, 74, 107
Diazoxide, 210
Dichloralphenazone, 92, 164, 171, 243
Diet, 190, 262
Diet aids, 106, 149
Diet-related headache, 145
Dietary and behavioral restriction, 218, 219-220
Differential diagnosis, 116-119
Digitolingual paresthesias, 84
Dihydroergotamine mesylate (D.H.E.45), 7, 13, 20, 67, 70, 93, 158, 164, 245, 247, 251, 254, 261
Dilantin, 105, 119, 203, 248
Diltiazem, 94, 180, 203, 247, 252
Diplopia, 192, 211
Disability issues, 33
Discharge groups in inpatient program, 260
Disorientation, 44
Diuretics, 124, 250, 253
Divalproex sodium, 203, 249, 254, 255
Dizziness, 29, 106, 151
Domperidone, 194
Dopamine, 106
Dopamine—hydroxylase, 90
Dopamine blockers, 211
Dopamine-containing foods, 106
Dopaminergic stimulation, 10
Doppler, 51, 55-56
Dosage calculation for children, 195
Doxepin, 103-104, 160, 180, 245, 250
Drug abuse, 32, 116
Drug and alcohol levels in blood, 54
Drug-induced headache, 149-151, 207-213
Dry mouth, 94, 105
DSM IIIR disorders with headache, 230
DTIC-DOME (dacarbazine), 211
Dura mater, 1, 7, 88, 129
Duration of headache, 28-29, 114, 117
Dysarthria, 37, 192
Dysautonomia with cephalalgia, 199
Dysdiadochokinesia, 40
Dysphasia, 192
Dyspnea, 151
Dysthymic disorder, 231
Dystonic movement, 40
Ear, 141, 187
Early antigen antibody (EA-Ab), 154
Eating disorders, 150
EBV (Epstein-Barr virus), 139, 154
Ecchymosis, 201
Edema, 5, 131, 133

Education of patient, 218, 219, 239-241
EEG topography, computerized (EEG brain mapping), 52
Elavil, 21, 74-75, 91, 103, 104, 154, 159-160, 161, 180, 202, 244-245, 250
Electroencephalogram (EEG), 44, 46, 52, 197, 201, 216
Electromyographic biofeedback, 244
Emotional distress, 102
Encephalitis, 45, 52, 133, 187
Endep, 21, 74-75, 91, 103, 104, 154, 159-160, 161, 180, 202, 244-245
Endocrine disorders, 143-145
Endorphin function disturbance, 103
Energy loss, 32, 94
Enkephalin, 88, 163
Enkephalinase, 10, 13-14
Enkephalinergic interneurons, 71
Environmental factors, 151-152, 190-191
Epidermoids, 49
Epidural abscess, 132
Epidural blood patch, 53
Epidural hematoma, 132, 199
Epilepsy, 94
Epinephrine, 106
Episodic cluster headache, 111, 251
  in patients over 30, 124-125
  in patients under 30, 122-124
Episodic nature of migraine, 27
Epistaxis, 141
Epstein-Barr virus (EBV), 139, 154
Equanil, 107
Ergonovine maleate, 246
Ergot alkaloids, 7
Ergotamine, 1-2, 7, 31, 65-66, 68, 74, 87, 88, 125, 249
  cluster headache and, 251, 252, 253
  comprehensive treatment approach, 245-247
  dependency, 167-172
  detoxification, 171
  gradual discontinuance of, 244
  rebound pain, 31
Ergotamine dependency syndrome, 168, 170-171
Ergotamine tartrate (ET), 70, 92, 122-123, 124, 158, 167, 178-179
  in treating children, 194-195
Ergotamine trial, 31
Ergotin, 64
Ergotism, 167
Ergotrate, 246
Ergots and serotonin receptors, 20
Esgic, 108, 158
Eskalith, 123-124, 252
Essential headache, 244-245
Estraderm, 249
Estradiol, 95
Estrogen, 2, 95, 211, 212
Estrogen replacement therapy, 30, 31
ET, *See* Ergotamine tartrate
Ethmoid sinus pain, 142

Eutonyl, 107
Evaporative creams, 203
Evoked potentials, 11, 54-55, 216
Evolutive migraine, 227
Examination, general, 36
Exanthemata, 187
Excitement, 122, 189
Exercise, 202, 244
Exertion and headache in children, 191
Extracerebral lesion, 45
Extractum secalis cornuti aquosum, 64
Extremities, cold, 29, 84, 94
Extrinsic trauma, 140
Eyelid edema, 5
Eyes, 29, 30
Facial hyperalgesia, 115
Facial nerve assessment, 38
Facial pain, 114
Facial sweating, 5
Facial trigger zones, 119
False transmitter, 96
Family history, 32, 116, 177, 189, 230
Family intervention, 179
Family relationships, 32
Family therapy, 232, 261
Fast-wave coefficient (FWC) in VEP, 55
Fasting, 30
Fatigue, 29, 32, 94, 106, 150, 230
Fava beans, 149
Fenfluramine HCl, 212
Fermented sausages, 149
Fever, 45
Fibromyalgia, 139
Fibromyalgia syndrome, 154
Fibrous tissue formation, 94
Figs, 149
Finger flexor test, 41
Finger temperature, 93
Finger wiggle test, 40
Finger-to-nose testing, 39
Fioricet, 158, 247
Fiorinal, 108, 158, 243, 247
First occurrence of sudden onset headache, 44-46
5-HIAA (5-hydroxyindoleacetic acid), 70, 71, 93
5-HT, *See* 5-hydroxytryptamine
5-HTP (5-hydroxytryptophan), 163
Flash P1 and P2 components of VEP, 55
Flash VEP, 54-55
Flexeril, 108
Flow velocities, intracranial, 56
Fluid retention, 29, 124
Flunarizine, 76, 77, 94
Fluoxetine, 245
Follow-up to inpatient treatment, 262
Food additives, 96
Food allergy, 190
Food triggers, 95-96
Foot-tap test, 40
Foramen of Monro, 132
Foramina of Luschka and Magendie, 133

Forehead, 5, 93
Fortification spectra, 29, 84
Free fatty acid level, 11, 90
Frequency of headaches, 27-28, 114
Frigidity, 102
Frontal headache, 4
Frontotemporal cephalalgia, 199
Fructose, 147
Functional hypoglycemia, 144
Fungal disease, 142, 143
Fungal meningitis, 52
Fungizone, 143
FWC (fast-wave coefficient) in VEP, 55
Gait, 40, 44
Gait apraxia, 133
Galactorrhea, 53, 145
Galanin, 5
Gallium scan, 50
Gastrin levels, 14
Gastrointestinal disorders, 31, 83, 187, 188, 194
Gastrointestinal motility, 92
Gene related peptide, 5, 7, 13, 136
Geriatric patients, 27
Glaucoma, 94
Glioma, 131
Glossopharyngeal nerve testing, 38
Glucocorticoids, 211
Glucose tolerance tests, 144
Glutamate headaches, 147
Glycerol, 121
GR 43175, 20
Grand mal seizures, 149
Granuloma, 131
Granulomatous disease, 85
Group psychotherapy, 232
Growth disorders, 141
Guanethidine sulfate, 105
Guilt, 32, 230
H_2 histamine receptor blocker, 212
Habit history, 32, 116
Habituation, 31, 103
Hallucinations, 44
Ham, 96, 148
Hand tremor, 124
Hangover headache, 147
Hatband distribution, 102
Head banging during headache, 30
Head injury, 187
Headache
    Ad Hoc Committee on Classification of, 175, 176
    in children, 185-196
    due to pain sensitive structures within head, 129-137
    pathogenesis, 66-67
    treatment of, 91, 121-125, 175-182, 193-196, 218-219
Headache calendar, 219, 236-238, 261
Headache history, 25-33
    behavior during attack, 30
    behavioral assessment, 32-33
    coping style factors, 32-33
    directing diagnostic skills, 35
    family history, 32
    habit history, 32
    medical history, 31-32
    medication history, 30-31
    onset, 27
    pain characteristics, 27-30
    precipitating factors, 30
    prodromal symptoms, 29
    types of headache, 26-27
Heat therapy, 108, 244
Heating pads, 203
Heavy metals, 54, 134
Heel-to-knee test, 39-40
Hematoma, 47, 132
    cerebellar, 132
    epidural, 132, 199
    intracerebral, 132
    intracranial, 132
    subdural, 48, 50, 132, 199
    subgaleal, 198
    subperiosteal, 198
Hemicrania continua, 178, 256
Hemicrania sympathicoparalytica, 64
Hemicrania vasomotoria, 64
Hemiparesis, 29
Hemiparetic migraine, 44
Hemiplegic migraine, 85, 192
Hemodynamics, intracranial, 55-56
Hemorrhage, 44-45
    aneurysmal subarachnoid (SAH), 45
    intracranial, 45, 187
    intraparenchymatous, 210
    parenchymal, 136
    subarachnoid, 52, 132, 199, 210
Hepatitis, 123
Heredity, 91
Herpes zoster infection, 119
Hexadrol, 164, 247
5-HIAA (5-hydroxyindoleacetic acid), 70, 71, 93
Hibernation during headache, 30
Hiccupping, 134
Histamine, 2, 69, 96, 115, 119, 121, 209
H_2 histamine receptor blocker, 212
Histamine-containing agents, 31
Histamine desensitization, 254
Historical perspectives on migraine, 9-10
History
    assessment of, 216-218
    of child with headache, 185-186
    family, 32, 116, 177, 189, 230
    of habits, 32
    of headache, *See* Headache history
    medical, 31-32
    medication, 30-31
    neurologic, 32, 201
    occupational, 32-33
    psychiatric, 32, 102-103
    short, 46

Hoffman test, 41
Holmes Life Change Index, 216
Home biofeedback monitors, 220
Homonymous hemianopia, 85
Homovanillic acid (HVA) excretion, 11
Hormonal migraine, 249-250
Horner's syndrome, 51, 117, 121, 199
Hostility, repressed, 225
Hot dog headache, 148
Hot dogs, 96
Hot packs, 203
5-HT, See 5-hydroxytryptamine
5-HTP (5-hydroxytryptophan), 163
Hunger, 189, 190
HVA (homovanillic acid) excretion, 11
Hydralazine HCl, 149, 210
Hydrocephalus, 47, 133, 188, 199
Hydrocortisone therapy, 171
Hydrotherapy, 203
5-Hydroxytryptamine (5-HT), 11, 163, 170, 211-212
   5-HT$_1$ receptors, 7-8, 19, 20, 125
   5-HT$_{1C}$ receptors, 21
   5-HT$_{1D}$ agonists, 7-8, 66, 70, 246
   5-HT$_2$ receptors, 19, 21
   5-HT$_3$ receptors, 19
5-Hydroxyindoleacetic acid (5-HIAA), 70, 71, 93
5-Hydroxytryptophan (5-HTP), 163
Hydroxyzine HCl, 246
Hyperalgesia, 71
Hyperepinephrinemia, 144
Hyperparathyroidism, 49, 144
Hyperprolactinemia, 144-145
Hypersomnia, 32, 103
Hyperstat IV, 210
Hypertension, 31, 167, 133, 210
Hypertensive crises, 149
Hypertensive therapy, 31
Hyperventilation, 52
Hypervitaminosis, 134
Hypochondriasis, 56, 230
Hypoglossal nerve testing, 38-39
Hypoglycemia, 53, 144
Hypophyseal dysfunction, 53
Hypotension, 105-106, 124
Hypothalamic neurotransmitter functions, 170
Hypothalamus, 103, 119-121, 163
Hypotonicity, 39
Hypoxemia, 119
Hypoxia, 70, 75, 76, 90, 151
Hysteria, 56
Ibuprofen, 159, 203
Ice cream headache, 148
Ice packs, 203, 244
Ice pick headache (jabs and jolts), 256
ICP (intracranial pressure), 133-134, 187, 210
Idiopathic functional hypoglycemia, 144
IgE serum levels, 152, 153
IHS (International Headache Society), 176
Imagery exercises, 220

Imipramine, 74, 103, 104, 107, 180
Imitrex, 7, 69-70, 93, 125, 246, 251
Immunoelectrophoresis, 53
Immunological modulators of trigeminovascular system, 2
Impotence, 94, 102
Inattention, 44
Inderal, 72-73, 91, 107, 180, 195, 203, 209, 210, 248
Indium, 50
Indocin, 253
Indomethacin, 7, 117, 253, 255-256
Infarct, 46, 47, 136-137
Infection, 123, 186-187
   chronic active Epstein-Barr virus (CEBV), 154
   herpes zoster, 119
INH (isoniazid), 107
INMAs (isolated neurological migraine accompaniments), 77, 85
Inpatient headache treatment unit, 254, 257-262
Insomnia, 32, 94, 102, 103, 105
Insulin, excess, 144
Insulinoma, 53
Intake interview, 235
Intellect, evaluation of, 36
Intellectual functioning, 44
Intensity of headaches, 27-28, 114-115
Interdisciplinary organization of inpatient unit, 257-258
Interictal state, 10-11
International Headache Society (IHS), 176
Interparoxysmal headache, 177
Intracellular pH, 87
Intracerebral hematoma, 132
Intracranial abnormality, 124
Intracranial abscess, 131-132
Intracranial aneurysm, ruptured, 44
Intracranial bleeding, 211
Intracranial bruits, 36
Intracranial hematoma, 132
Intracranial hemorrhage, 45, 187
Intracranial hypertension, 133, 188, 210-211
Intracranial hypotension, 134
Intracranial infections, 187
Intracranial masses, 50
Intracranial pain-sensitive structures, 129-130
Intracranial pressure (ICP), 133-134, 187, 210
Intracranial tumor, 211
Intraocular pressure, 117
Intraparenchymatous hemorrhage, 210
Intravenous pyelograms, 248
Investigational testing, 216
Ionic modulators of trigeminovascular system, 2
Irritable bowel syndrome, 31
Ischemia, 48, 86, 199
Ischemic aura, 9
Ischemic heart disease, 140, 144, 167
Ischemic stroke, 45
Ismelin, 105
Isobutyl nitrite, 148

Isocarboxazid, 106, 107
Isolated neurological migraine accompaniments (INMAs), 77, 85
Isometheptene mucate, 68-69, 92, 158, 164, 171, 243
Isoniazid (INH), 107
Isoptin, 21, 76, 94, 124, 180, 203, 247
Isordil, 149
Isosorbide dinitrate, 149
Jabs and jolts headaches, 256
Jaw jerk, 41
Jet lag, 152
Judgment, assessment of, 36
Kernig's sign, 135, 187
Ketoconazole, 143
Klonopin, 203
Knee jerk, 41
Lacrimation, 5, 115, 116
Lacunar infarct, 137
Language assessment, 37
Late insomnia (early awakening), 102, 103
Laterality of pain, 28
Lateralizing sensory asymmetries, 40
Laughter therapy in inpatient program, 260
Lead poisoning, 54
Leão's spreading depression, 71, 76
Left ventricular failure, 124
Leonine appearance, 29
Lesions of brain, 47
LH (luteinizing hormone), 121
Libido, decreased, 230
Librium, 107
Lidocaine analogue, 203
Life changes, 33, 122
Life circumstances, 27
Light, sensitivity to, 29, 115, 200
Limb warmth and heaviness exercises, 220
Limbic hypothalamic pituitary adrenal axis regulation, 170
Limbic system, 163
Limbitrol, 105
Lioresal, 203
Liqueurs, 149
Lithane, 252
Lithium, 123-124, 203, 252, 253
Lithobid, 123-124, 252
Litigation issues, 33
Liver lovers' headache, 147-148
Location of pain, 28, 114-115
Location of Raeder's paratrigeminal neuralgia, 117
Locus ceruleus, 12, 13, 170
Lopressor, 73, 94, 210, 248
Loss of consciousness, 31, 197
Low-grade fever, 154
LSD, 11, 69, 163
Lubin depression inventory, 216
Ludomil, 104, 245
Lumbar puncture (LP), 134, 135
Luteinizing hormone (LH), 121
Lyme disease, 53, 193

Lymphocytes, 53
Lymphoma, 133
Lysergic acid, 69
Magnetic resonance imaging (MRI), 44, 46, 48-49, 186, 201, 202, 216, 248
  vs. CT, 193
Maladaptive behavior patterns, 221, 231
Malignant hypertension and headache, 210
Malingering, 231
MAOb (monoamine oxidase b), 10, 12
MAOIs (monoamine oxidase inhibitors), 103, 105-107, 148, 150, 180, 203, 245, 248
Maprotiline HCl, 104, 245
Marezine, 194
Marital relationships, 32
Marplan, 106, 107
Massage, 108, 203, 244
Masses, abnormal, 36
Masticatory muscle disorders, 140
MCAFV (middle cerebral artery blood flow velocity), 56
Mechanical modulators of trigeminovascular system, 2
Mechanism of migraine pain, 13-14
Meclofenamate sodium, 171, 181, 247
Meclomen, 181, 247
Medical history, 31-32
Medical program for inpatients, 261-262
Medication abuse, 160
Medication history, 30-31
Melatonin, 121
Memory testing, 37
Menarche, 30, 95
Meningeal irritation, 134-136, 150
Meningioma, 48, 131
Meningismus, 36
Meningitis, 44, 45, 47, 52, 134-135, 187
Menopause therapy, 95
Menses, 27
Menstrual hormonal changes, 95
Menstrual irregularity, 53
Mental status, 36-37, 260
Mentation, impaired, 133
Meperidine, 93, 106
Meprobamate, 107
Meprospan, 107
Mesitil, 203
Metanephrines, 54
Metastases, 49, 211
Metastatic carcinoma, 133
Metastatic disease, 32
Methocarbamol, 203
Methyldopa, 210
Methylphenidate, 203
Methylprednisolone acetate, 254
Methylxanthines, 145-146
Methysergide, 7, 21, 70-71, 72, 74, 78, 88
Methysergide maleate, 21, 69, 93-94, 123, 181, 195, 203, 212, 248, 253
Metoclopramide, 92, 164, 194, 246

Metoprolol tartrate, 73, 94, 210, 248
Mexiletine, 203
Microadenoma of pituitary, 145
Midbrain, 13
Middle cerebral artery blood flow velocity (MCAFV), 56
Midrin, 68-69, 92, 158, 164, 171, 243, 247
  in discontinuing analgesics, 244, 250
Migraine, 11-13, 87-90
  aura, 4, 77, 84-85, 249
  biochemistry of, 9-14
  as biological reprimand, 226
  in children, 188
  comprehensive treatment approach, 245-247, 249
  continuous, with interparoxysmal headache (MIH), 177
  diagnosis, pathogenesis, and treatment, 83-96
  equivalent, 192
  historical perspectives, 9-10
  interictal state, 10-11
  menstrual, 95
  ophthalmoplegic, 51
  pain mechanism, 13-14
  personality, 225-227
  post attack phase, 14
  serotonin receptor pharmacology in, 19-22
  thermography in, 57-58
  transformation, 175
  variant, 192
MIH (migraine with interparoxysmal headache), 177
Miltown, 107
Minipress, 210
Minnesota Multiphasic Personality Inventory (MMPI), 56, 116, 161, 201-202, 216, 227, 229
Miosis, 5, 29, 115, 116, 117
Miscellaneous headache types, 139-155
Mixed form of post traumatic cephalalgia, 200
Mixed headache, 109, 250-251
MMPI (Minnesota Multiphasic Personality Inventory), 56, 116, 161, 201-202, 216, 227, 229
Monoamine oxidase b (MAOb), 10, 12
Monoamine oxidase inhibitors (MAOIs), 103, 105-107, 148, 150, 180, 203, 245, 248
Monoaminergic function disturbance, 103
Mononucleosis syndrome, chronic, 139
Monosodium glutamate (MSG), 30, 96, 147
Mood, 32
Morning headache, 146
Motion sickness, 31
Motor systems evaluation, 39
Motrin, 203
MRI (magnetic resonance imaging), 44, 46, 48-49, 186, 201, 202, 216, 248
  MRI vs. CT, 193
MSG (monosodium glutamate), 30, 96, 147
Multidisciplinary team approach, 216
Multi-site electromyographic (EMG) readings, 216
Mumps, 187

Muscle contraction headache, *See* Tension-type headache
Muscle relaxants, 92, 141
Muscle scanning, 216
Muscle tonus, 36, 39
Muscle twitching, 105
Music therapy in inpatient program, 260
Myalgia, 124, 154
Myeloma, 49, 53
Myofascial pain dysfunction disorders, 140
Nadolol, 73, 94, 180, 203, 248
Naloxone HCl, 12-13
Nap, 29, 122
Naprosyn, 203
Naproxen, 154, 171, 181, 203, 244, 247, 249
Narcan, 12-13
Narcotic addiction, 124
Narcotics, 158, 244
Nardil, 106, 107, 180, 245, 248
Nasal discharge, 5, 141
Nasopharyngeal carcinoma, 49
Nausea, 29, 46, 83, 84, 106, 132, 150, 151, 191-192, 200
Neck and shoulder relaxation, 220
Neck examination, 36
Neck flexion, 117
Neck stiffness, 45
Neoplasms, 130-131, 133
Neural modulators of trigeminovascular system, 2
Neurectomies, 204
Neuro-otological work-up, 44
Neuroendocrine disturbance, 177
Neurogenic inflammation, 7
Neuroimaging, 46-47
Neurokinin, 6, 88
Neurokinin A, 5, 136
Neurological examination, 35-41, 201, 216
  coordination testing, 39-40
  cranial nerve function, 37-39
  deficiencies, 150
  general examination, 36
  history, 32, 201
  mental status, 36-37
  motor systems, 39
  reflexes, 41
  sensory systems, 40
  station and gate, 40
Neurological problems, 31
Neuronal mechanism, 90
Neuropathy, inflammatory, 193
Neuropeptide Y, 13, 136
Neuropeptides and trigeminal vascular system, 5-6
Neuropsychometric testing, 201-202
Neurosyphilis, 52
Neurotensin, 9-10
Neurotic characteristics, 116
Neurotransmitter defects, 103
Neurotransmitter functions, 170
Nicotinic acid, 74
Nifedipine, 21, 76, 94, 180, 247, 248, 252

Nimotop, 76, 94, 247, 252
Nitrates, 30, 31
Nitrites, 96, 148
Nitroglycerin, 69, 115, 119, 144, 149, 208-209
    transdermal, 150-151
Nizoral, 143
NMR spectroscopy, 87
Nolvadex, 249
Noncephalic symptoms following head trauma, 200
Non-pharmacological, 178-179, 195-196
Nonsteroidal anti-inflammatory drugs (NSAIDs), 7, 108, 141, 158, 171, 181, 203, 243-244, 246-247, 253
Nonvascular headaches, 57
Noradrenaline, 67-68, 90
Noradrenaline uptake, 75
Norepinephrine, 20, 103, 106
Norepinephrine receptor function, 170
Norflex, 108
Norgesic, 108
Norgesic Forte, 108
Norpramin, 104
Nortriptyline HCl, 104, 180, 245
NSAIDs (nonsteroidal anti-inflammatory drugs), 7, 108, 141, 158, 171, 181, 203, 243-244, 246-247, 253
Nursing goals at assessment interview, 235
Nutrition groups in inpatient program, 260
Nutritional counseling, 261
Nystagmus, 37, 132
Obstructive hydrocephalus, 133
Obstructive pulmonary disease, 94
Occupational history, 32-33
Occupational therapy groups in inpatient program, 260
Octopamine, 96
Ocular motility, 37-38
Ocular palsies, 44, 139
Oculomotor paralysis, 29
Oculomotor-trochlear-abducens system, 38
Off-the-shelf medications, 159, 244, 250
Olfactory nerve testing, 37
Oligemia, 86
Ongoing treatment considerations, 235-242
Onset of headache, 27
Ophthalmoplegic migraine, 51, 192-193
Opiate withdrawal model of migraine, 10, 12
Opiate-containing fibers, moderating trigeminovascular system, 2
Oppenheim reflex, 41
Optic nerve testing, 37
Oral contraceptives, 30, 31, 95, 212
Orange peel thick skin, 29
Orbital bruits, 201
Orbital swelling, 115
Organic disease and headache, 27
Orgasmic cephalgia, 44-45
Orientation groups in inpatient program, 259
Orphenadrine citrate, 108
Osteoarthritis, 49-50

Osteomyelitis of skull, 50
Osteoporosis, 50
Over-scheduling, 221
Over-the-counter analgesics, 159, 244, 250
Oxazepam, 107
Oxprenolol, 73
Oxygen inhalation, 119, 125
Oxygen therapy, 251
Paget's disease, 49
Pain lifestyle, 261
Pain mechanism, 13-14
Pain pathways, 163
Pain sensation testing, 40
Pain sensitive structures, 1, 129-130
Pain signal transmission, 71-72
Pallor, 29, 84, 115, 134
Palpitations, 29
Pamelor, 104, 180, 245
Para-chlorophenylalanine, 71
Paraflex, 108
Parafon Forte, 108
Paralysis, 85
Paranasal sinus disease, 141-142
Paraphasia, 37
Parathyroid adenoma, 144
Parathyroid endocrinopathy, 134
Parenchymal hemorrhage, 136
Parenchymal lesion, 45
Parenchymal tumor, 47
Parenteral medication, 93, 247
Paresis, 85
Paresthesia, 29
Pargyline HCl, 107
Parlodel, 10, 11, 145
Parnate, 107, 150
Paroxysmal headache, 27, 188
Participation of patient in treatment, 218, 257
Passive relaxation, 220
Pathogenesis of cluster headache, 119-121
Pathophysiology and pharmacology of headache and medications, 63-78
Patient evaluations in inpatient unit, 260-261
Patient goals, realistic, 241
Patient program, inpatient unit, 259-260
Pattern-shift VEP, 54-55
Pentazocine, 12
Peptidergic system, 13
Periactin, 21, 71, 161, 162, 203, 248
Periodontal disease, 140
Peripheral neuropathy, 40
Peripheral pain impulses, 163
Peripheral vascular disease, 123, 167
Peripheral vs. central effects, 162
Perphenazine, 105
Personality factors, 116
Pertofrane, 104
Pharmacy groups in inpatient program, 260
Pharyngitis, 154
Phenelzine sulfate, 106, 107, 180, 245, 248
Phenergan, 158, 164, 246

Phenothiazine therapy, 181
Phenothiazines, 105, 203
Phentolamine, 149
Phenylethylamine, 95-96, 190
Phenylpropanolamine, 149-150
Phenytoin, 105, 203, 248, 255
Pheochromocytoma, 54, 134
Philosophy of inpatient treatment, 257-259
Phobias, 29, 44, 115, 200
Phosphorylation potential, 87
Photic stimulation, 52
Photoperiodicity, 112
Photoplethysmographic measures of vascular lability, 216
Phrenilin, 108
Physical aspects of inpatient unit, 258-259
Physical examination, 201
Physical exertion, 30, 191
Physical therapy, 108, 203, 261
  inpatient program groups, 259-260
Physiological profile, 216
Pia mater, 1
Pickled food, 149
Pillow, cervical orthopedic, 108
Pindolol, 73
Pineal tumor, 47
Piribedil, 10, 11
Pituitary adenoma, 140
Pituitary apoplexy, 140
Pituitary lesions, 48
Pituitary tumor, 47
Pizotifen, 21, 71, 72, 78, 195, 212
Plasma cyclic adenosine monophosphate, 90
Plasma dopamine-hydroxylase activity, 10
Plasma estradiol level, 95
Plasma phenylsulphatransferase, 10
Plasma progesterone, 95
Plateau waves, 134
Platelet 5-HT release, 211-212
Platelet activity, 12, 136
Platelet monoaminoxidase b (MAOb), 10, 12
Platelet serotonin content, 70
Pleasure, need for, 221
Pleocytosis, 53
Pleuropulmonary fibrosis, 94
Poliomyelitis, 187
Polyuria, 29
Pondimin, 212
Porphyrin metabolites, 54
Portable EMG units, 220
Post attack phase of migraine, 14
Post-head-trauma syndrome, 255
Post-herpetic neuralgia, 119
Post-spinal headache, 52, 53
Post-traumatic cephalalgia, 197-204
  mechanisms of, 198-199
  treatment, 201-204
Post-traumatic headache, 255
Posterior fossa tumors, 131
Potassium moderating trigeminovascular system, 2

Potential, evoked, 11, 54-55, 216
Potential biochemical modulators of trigeminovascular system, 2
PQRST model for intake interview, 235
Prazepam, 107
Prazosin HCl, 210
Precipitating factors, 30, 189
Predisposition to type of headache, 209
Prednisone, 123
Pregnancy, 30, 95, 123
Premenstrual migraine, 30
Premonitory symptoms, 191
Pressor amines, 148
Pressure changes, intracranial, 133-134
Preventive treatment, 93-94, 179-181, 195, 247-249, 251-252
Procardia, 21, 94, 180, 248, 252
Prochlorperazine, 194, 246
Prodromal symptoms, 29
Prodrome (aura), 12
Progesterone, 2, 31, 95, 212
Proglycem, 210
Progressive relaxation, 220
Prolactin, 53, 121
Prolactinoma, 145, 211
Promethazine HCl, 164, 246, 247
Pronation-supination test, 39
Prophylactic medication, 122-125, 195
Propoxyphene, 108
Propranolol, 72-73, 91, 94, 107, 180, 195, 203, 209, 210, 248
Proserotoninergic agent, 75
Prosody, assessment of, 37
Prostacyclin production, 21
Prostaglandin, 147
Prostatic hypertrophy, 94
Protein extracts, 149
Protriptyline, 103, 104, 202
Prozac, 245
Pseudotumor cerebri (PTC), 133, 147
Psychasthenia, 56
Psychiatric disorders, 31, 32, 230-231
Psychic distress, 102
Psychobiology, 224
Psychological considerations, 29, 56-57, 165, 223-232
  primary headache disorders and, 224, 225-229
Psychomotor agitation or retardation, 32
Psychophysiological factors, 216-217, 224, 229-230
Psychosocial stress, 95
Psychotherapy, 108, 179, 196, 261
PTC (pseudotumor cerebri), 133, 147
Ptosis, 5, 29, 115, 116, 117
Pupils, 5, 11, 37
Purulent meningitis, 134-135
Pyloric sphincter, 92
Pyridoxine, 161, 162, 164
Radiofrequency lesions of trigeminal ganglion, 125
Radionuclide cisternography, 50-51
Radionuclide scans, 50

Raeder's paratrigeminal neuralgia, 117
Ranitidine, 212
Rapid eye movement (REM) sleep, 28-29, 115, 116, 119, 122
Raskin protocol, 171
Reactive hypoglycemia, 144
Rebound phenomena, 31, 92, 144, 178-179
Receptor pharmacology, 67-68
Recreational drug usage, 32
Rectal administration of medication, 92
Recurrent headache, 187-188
Red wine, 30, 149
Reflex examination, 41
Refractoriness, 178-179
Regitine, 149
Reglan, 92, 93, 158, 164, 194, 246
Relative hypoglycemia, 144
Relaxation therapy, 165, 204, 220, 244, 259
REM (rapid eye movement) sleep, 28-29, 115, 116, 119, 122
Reserpine, 31, 210, 212
Respiratory problems, 31
Retroperitoneal fibrosis, 94, 248, 253
Reye's syndrome, 194
Rheumatoid disease, 50
Rhinocerebral mucormycosis, 143
Rhinorrhea, 5, 29, 115, 116
Rinne test, 38
Ritalin, 203
Robaxin, 203
Rotational vertigo, 44
Rush, 148
Safety of cerebral angiography, 51-52
SAH (aneurysmal subarachnoid hemorrhage), 45
Salami, 96, 148
Salicylates, 163, 243
Sansert, 21, 69, 93-94, 123, 181, 195, 203, 212, 248, 253
Sarcoid meningitis, 52
Sarcoidosis, 134
Scalp and facial relaxation, 220
Scalp hyperalgesia, 115
Scalp lacerations, 198
Scalp tenderness, 200
Scintillating scotoma, 29, 76, 84, 86
Secondary gain assessment, 226, 227, 230
Sectral, 73
Sedative-hypnotics, 158
Sedimentation rate, 53
Seizure disorder, 31
Seizure equivalent headache, 255
Selection of diagnostic tests, 44-46
Self-diagnosis of headache pain, 235
Self-regulation, 218, 220-221
Sensitivity to light and noise, 83
Sensory systems, 11, 40
Sentinel headache, 135
Serax, 107
Serotonin, 2, 11-12, 70-71, 90, 106
 agonists, 69-70, 181

receptor function, 19-22, 170
 uptake, 75
Serotoninergic system, 103, 162-163
Sertraline HCl, 245
Serum IgE levels, 190
Serum protein electrophoresis, 53
Sexual activity, 30, 102
Shark liver, 148
Sherry, 149
Short history, 46
Shoulder and neck relaxation, 220
Sibelium, 94
Sinequan, 103-104, 180, 245
Sinus headache, 141-143
Sinus problems, 31, 46, 49, 130
Sinus vein thrombosis, 211
Skin, furrowed, 29
Skipping meals, 96
Skull anomalies, 49
Skull fractures, 197
SLE (systemic lupus erythematosus), 49
Sleep
 apnea, 119
 assessment of, 32
 cluster attacks in, 115
 disturbance, 30, 102, 103, 152, 154, 159
 headache attack during, 28-29
 in headache treatment, 219-220
Smoked food, 149
Smoking, 32, 116, 150, 179
Smooth muscle cells, 75
Snout reflex, 41
Social work groups in inpatient program, 259
Socially acceptable diagnosis, 103
Sodium chromoglycate, 190
Soft touch deficit, 40
Soma, 108
Somatoform disorders, 230
Somatosensory disturbance, 84-85, 86
Somatosensory evoked potentials (SSEP), 55
Sorbitrate, 149
Sound, sensitivity to, 29, 200
Spastic tonus, 39
Sphenoid mucocoele, 142-143
Sphenoid sinus pain, 142
Sphenopalatine block, 254
Spinal accessory nerve testing, 38
Spinal cord, 103
Spinal tap, 45, 52-53, 210
Splenectomy, 12
Spondylosis, 108
Spousal headache, 150-151
Spreading depression, 71, 76, 85-87
SSEP (somatosensory evoked potential), 55
Station and gait evaluation, 40
Status migrainosus, 92-93
Stereognosis, 40
Steroid therapy, 253
Steroids, 123, 151, 158, 247, 251-252
Stransky reflex, 41

Stress, 30, 33, 95, 189-190
Stress management, 221, 179
Stretch, severe, moderating trigeminovascular system, 2
Stroke, 136-137
Subacute meningitis, 135
Subarachnoid hemorrhage, 52, 132, 199, 210
Subchronic cluster headache, 111, 124-125
Subdural hematoma, 48, 50, 132, 199
Subgaleal hematomas, 198
Subperiosteal hematomas, 198
Substance abuse, 177
Substance P, 5-6, 7, 13, 88, 136, 246
Substance Y, 13
Sudden onset, 44-46
Suicide ideation, 32, 102, 114, 230
Sulpiride, 211
Sumatriptan, 7, 13, 20, 69-70, 125, 246, 251
Sumatriptan succinate, 93
Sunlight, 96
Superficial temporal artery, 87-88
Supportive psychotherapy, 232
Surgery for cluster headache, 124-125
Surmontil, 103
Symmetry, sensory, testing of, 40
Sympathetic nervous system, 90
Sympathetics moderating trigeminovascular system, 2
Sympathomimetics, 31, 106, 149
Symptomatic agents, detoxification from overuse of, 179
Symptomatic treatment, 125
Symptomatology, 224
Symptoms, change in, 27
Syndromes recently described, 154-155
Syphilis, central nervous system, 53
Systemic lupus erythematosus (SLE), 49
Tachycardia, 105, 144
Tachykinin substance P, 5-6
Tagamet, 212
Talwin, 12
Tamoxifen citrate, 249
TCAs (tricyclic antidepressants), 31, 73-75, 141, 163, 180, 202, 244, 248, 250
Tegretol, 119, 203, 248
Teichopsia, 84
Temperature sensation assessment, 40
Temporal arteritis, 53, 54, 119
Temporal artery biopsy, 54
Temporal artery pulsation amplitude, 93
Temporal artery swelling, 115
Temporomandibular (TM) disorders, 140-141
Temporomandibular joint (TMJ) disorders, 31, 50, 140-141, 201
Tenderness, 36
Tenormin, 73, 94, 248
TENS (transcutaneous electrical stimulation), 108, 203
Tension-type headache (TH), 28, 29, 63
  acute, 102, 243-244
  in children, 193
  chronic, 73-75, 101-109
  comprehensive treatment approach, 243-245
  defined by Ad Hoc Committee, 176
  vs. migraine, 11, 175
  psychological considerations, 227-228
Tentorium, 129
Testosterone, 121
Tetracycline, 134, 187
TH, See Tension-type headache
Thalamic nuclei, 163
Thermal rings, 220
Thermography, 57-58
Thirst, 134
Thoughts of death, 32, 102, 114, 230
Thrombocytopenia, 12
Thyroid endocrinopathy, 134
TIAs (transient ischemic attacks), 85, 136
Tic douloureux, 28, 29
Tigan, 246
Time management, 221
Time of headache onset, 28-29
Time zone-change headache, 151-152
Timing of attacks, 115
Timing of diagnostic tests, 44-46
Timolol maleate, 73, 94
Tissue oxygenation, inadequate, 74
TMAs (transient migrainous accompaniments), 77, 85
TM (temporomandibular) disorders, 140-141
TMJ (temporomandibular joint) disorders, 31, 50, 140-141, 201
Tofranil, 74, 103, 104, 180
Tolfenamic acid, 147
Tomograms, 46, 50
Tongue wiggle test, 40
Tonsillar herniation, 131, 133
Tonsils, cerebellar, 48
Topography (EEG brain mapping), 52
Torcula herophili, 130
Tranquilizers, minor, 107-108
Transcranial Doppler, 55-56
Transcutaneous electrical stimulation (TENS), 108, 203
Transderm Nitro, 150-151
Transdermal nitroglycerin, 150-151
Transformation concept, 176-177
Transient ischemic attacks (TIAs), 85, 136
Transient migrainous accompaniments (TMAs), 77, 85
Tranylcypromine sulfate, 107, 150
Trauma, 27, 31, 187
Travel, 115, 189
Trazodone HCl, 104, 245
Treatment, 91, 121-125, 175-182, 193-196, 218-219
Tremor, 40
Triavil, 105
Tricyclic antidepressants (TCAs), 31, 73-75, 141, 163, 180, 244, 248, 250
  toxicities and side effects, 202

Tricyclics, 103-105, 107
Trigeminal nerve, 1, 2, 38, 129
Trigeminal neuralgia, 114, 119
Trigeminothalamic tract, 71
Trigeminovascular system, 2-3
　diagram, 3
　intracranial blood vessel innervation, 11
　neuropeptides and, 5-6
　substance P release in, 246
Trigger identification, 238
Trigger point injections, 204
Trimethobenzamide HCl, 246
Trimipramine maleate, 103
Trochlear nerve, 37-48
Tryptophan, 162-163
Tuberculosis, 135
Tuberculous meningitis, 187
Tumor, 4, 46, 47, 124, 188
　brain, 50, 130-133, 135
　pseudotumor cerebri (PTC), 133, 147
Type A behavior, 57, 221, 228
Types of headache, 26-27
Tyramine, 11, 30, 96, 148-149, 190
Tyramine-containing foods, 106, 149
Tyramine-restricted diet, 238
Tyrosine, 150
Ulcer disease, 31
Ultrasound, 203
Unidentified bright objects (UBOs), 48-49
Unusual headache types, 139-155
Urecholine, 105
Urinary incontinence, 133
Urinary retention, 105
Urine tests, 54
Vacuum headache, 143
Vagus nerve testing, 38
Valium, 74, 107
Valsalva maneuver, 135, 255
Valsalva phenomenon, 131
Vanillylmandelic acid (VMA), 54, 90
Vascular headaches, 57
　animal studies and human headache, 6
　antimigraine drugs in, 7-8
　clinical anatomical correlations, 4-5
　pathophysiology of, 1-7
　comprehensive treatment approach, 245-250
Vascular lability, 216
Vascular smooth muscle cells, 75
Vasculitis, 132
Vasoactive intestinal polypeptide (VIP), 136
Vasoactive medications, 30, 158
Vasoconstriction-induced cerebral hypoxia, 85-86
Vasoconstrictor effects, 68, 70-71
Vasoconstrictors, 31, 64, 92
Vasodilation, 76, 115, 149
Vasodilator headache, 207-209
Veins sensitive to pain, 130
VEP (visual evoked potential), 54-55
Verapamil, 21, 76, 94, 124, 180, 203, 247, 252, 253
Vertebro-basilar migraine, 192

Vertigo, 29, 44, 132, 192
Vibratory sensation testing, 40
VIP (vasoactive intestinal polypeptide), 136
Viral meningitis, 44
Vision, impaired, 44, 85, 105, 188, 192, 211
Visken, 73
Vistaril, 246
Visual evoked potential (VEP), 54-55
Vital signs, 36
Vitamin A, 54, 188, 147
Vitamin B_6, 161, 162, 164
Vivactil, 103, 104, 202
VMA (vanillylmandelic acid), 54, 90
Vomiting, 29, 31, 46, 83, 84, 132, 134, 150
　in children, 191-192
　post traumatic, 200
　projectile, 133
Von Frey hairs, 40
Vulnerability and symptomatology, 224
Warning headache, 45
Wartenburg wheel, 40
Weather changes, 30, 36
Wechsler Adult Intelligence Scale (WAIS), 201-202
Wechsler Memory Scale, 202
Weekend headaches, 146
Weight change, 32, 94, 102, 106, 187, 230
White matter, 48-49
Wigraine, 158, 251
Wine, 30, 122, 149
Withdrawal, 31, 32, 158
World Federation of Neurology, 188
Worthless feelings, 32, 230
Wrong-sided headache, 4
Xanax, 164
Xanthines, 31
Xanthochromia, 45, 135
Xenon-clearance technique, 71
Yawning, 29
Yeast, 149
Ytterbium, 50
Zantac, 212
Zimelidine, 212
Zoloft, 245
Zostrix, 253
Zung Depression Scale, 57, 216, 229